AREND BOUHUYS, M.D.

THE PHYSIOLOGY OF BREATHING

A Textbook for Medical Students

Grune & Stratton
A Subsidiary of Harcourt Brace Jovanovich, Publishers
New York · San Francisco · London

Library of Congress Cataloging in Publication Data

Bouhuys, Arend, 1925-
The physiology of breathing.

Consists of chapters, rev. and updated, from the author's Breathing.
Bibliography: p.
Includes index.
1. Lungs—Diseases. 2. Respiration. 3. Environmentally induced diseases. I. Title.
[DNLM: 1. Respiration. WF102 B759p]
RC732.B653 612'.2 76-46724
ISBN 0-8089-0984-3

Grune & Stratton, Inc.
111 Fifth Avenue
New York, New York 10003

Distributed in the United Kingdom by
Academic Press, Inc. (London) Ltd.
24/28 Oval Road, London NW1

Library of Congress Catalog Number 76-46724
International Standard Book Number 0-8089-0984-3
Printed in the United States of America

To the Memory of Gunnar Lundin
(May 26, 1910 - June 8, 1967)

Anaximenes, son of Eurystratus of Miletus, declared that air is the principle of existing things; for from it all things come-to-be and into it they are again dissolved.

Aetius

Contents

Preface

This book contains the chapters on physiology of breathing, previously published in a book of broader scope.* It appears in response to several suggestions that these chapters might serve as a textbook for medical students. For this edition, all chapters have been updated and revised where necessary. Several illustrations have been replaced or improved. A section on carbon dioxide transport has been added to Chapter 6. Chapter 10 has largely been rewritten to include results of recent work on the control of breathing. Chapter 12 has been written to introduce students to applications of respiratory physiology in studies of environmental lung disease.

The book is intended to provide students of medicine with a comprehensive framework of knowledge concerning respiratory physiology, emphasizing areas which are important in physiopathology. The text is extensively referenced, so that the reader can find his way to the original articles and reviews which I have used in preparing the text. Hence, the critical reader can decide whether or not he agrees with my interpretations and summarizing statements. I welcome comments, particularly from those who disagree, as well as suggestions for additional material that might be covered in a text of this scope.

Arend Bouhuys, M.D., Dr. med. Sci.

Professor of Medicine and Epidemiology,
Director, Yale University Lung Research Center,
Fellow of the John B. Pierce Foundation,
Yale University School of Medicine,
New Haven, Connecticut

* *Breathing—Physiology, Environment and Lung Disease,* by A. Bouhuys, Grune & Stratton, 1974, 511 pp.

Acknowledgments

I am indebted to my colleagues and the staff of the Yale University Lung Research Center, who have contributed their work, thoughts, and criticism to this book.

I am also grateful to many sponsoring agencies and institutions which have supported my research and that of the Lung Research Center, including the National Heart and Lung Institute, the National Institute for Occupational Safety and Health, the National Air Pollution Control Agency, the Connecticut Lung Association, the John B. Pierce Foundation, and the estate of the late Beulah S. Hinds.

The manuscript was prepared during my tenure of a Josiah Macy, Jr., Faculty Scholarship at the Université de Paris-Sud, during the academic year 1975–1976. I am indebted to Professor E. E. Baulieu for his interest and help during my sabbatical leave. Several colleagues were again kind enough to send me comments and criticisms on the manuscript. I thank Drs. J. Hildebrandt, R. E. Hyatt, M. J. Jaeger, E. K. Motoyama, A. B. Otis, S. A. Rooney, D. Stanescu, S. Weismann, J. B. West, and especially Drs. R. H. Kellogg and R. A. Mitchell for detailed reviews of Chapter 10. Again, any remaining errors and omissions are my own.

Jeanne E. Remington, M. A., and Juanita Havill, M. A. provided invaluable editorial assistance. My wife, Fenna G. Bouhuys, revised many illustrations and prepared the new ones. Marion M. Bruch, Juanita Havill, and my wife helped with proofreading, reference checking, and indexing.

I am also indebted to the following authors, publishers and journals who gave their permission to use illustrations and tabular material for inclusion in the book.

Authors: R. Benesch, E. J. Caldwell, R. M. Cherniack, F. J. Clark, S. W. Clarke, C. D. Cook, H. W. Davenport, P. Dejours, J. Emery, L. E. Farhi, M. J. Fisher, R. E. Forster, D. L. Fry, J. Georg, J. B. Glazier, W. W. L. Glenn, R. E. Hyatt, R. Lefrançois, J. Mead, C. C. Michel, J. Milic-Emili, E. K. Motoyama, E. Nattie, L. Nardone, J. T. Parer, H. Parker, J. B. Paton, J. Piiper, D. F. Proctor, H. Rahn, P. E. Bauwerda, P. W. Scherer, R. C. Schroter, H. Spencer, N. C. Staub, S. M. Tenney, E. R. Weibel, J. B. West, H. Yamabayashi. Also, B. Møller, J. A. Pierce, and W. B. Schwartz.

Publishers and Journals: Academic Press (*Computers and Biomedical Research*); *Acta Physiologica Scandinavica;* American Association for the Advancement of Science (*Science*); New York Academy of Sciences (*Annals* and *Transactions*); American Physiological Society (*Journal of Applied Physiology; American Journal of Physiology; Handbook of Physiology*); Butterworth's; *Clinical Science;* Elsevier/North-Holland (*Respiration Physiology*); Federation of American Societies for Experimental Biology (*Federation Proceedings*); Wm. Heinemann Medical Books, Ltd.; *Journal of Clinical Investigation; The Journal of Pharmacology and Experimental Therapeutics;* S. Karger; Lippincott (*Annals of Surgery*); McGraw-Hill; Macmillan Journals (*Nature*); Medical-Technical Publ. Co.; Pergamon Press; *Pflügers Archiv;* The Physiological Society (*Journal of Physiology*); Springer-Verlag (*Pneumonologie*); University of Chicago Press; Vigot Frēres (*Le Poumon et Le Coeur*). Also, Charles C. Thomas; British Medical Association (*Thorax*); Amercan Academy of Pediatrics (*Pediatrics*).

The staff members of Grune & Stratton, Inc., have been most helpful in seeing the manuscript through the production stage.

To all these persons, and many others, my sincere thanks.

Introduction

Unless we understand the function of an organ system, we cannot fully understand the diseases that affect it. The physiology of today remains the medicine of tomorrow—and in the years since E. H. Starling first wrote these words, the scope of both physiology and of medicine have greatly expanded and become more diversified. Today, most respiratory physiologists are specialists in one or a few of the areas covered by chapters in this book. They have partitioned the simple act of breathing, which anyone can observe, into its minutest components. They have analyzed the main objective of breathing—transport of oxygen and carbon dioxide—in great detail. They have also discovered how the central nervous system controls the mechanical act of breathing, so that gas transport can be optimal under a variety of conditions.

Unicellular organisms can acquire oxygen and excrete carbon dioxide simply by diffusion between the cell and its medium. Higher organisms, including man and other mammals, need increasingly complex, specialized gas transport systems to supply all tissues with enough oxygen and to remove CO_2. They cannot rely on gas exchange by diffusion alone, because of their size and the relative impermeability of the skin to gases. In addition, the diversity of their tissues and their varying demands for oxygen supply and carbon dioxide excretion impose the need for a gas transport system that is regulated to adapt itself to metabolic demands. The development of gas transport systems in the animal kingdom is a main topic of comparative respiratory physiology.[2] This book, on the other hand, concerns itself mainly with the objectives of the student of human health and medicine: to understand how the human gas transport system works, what can go wrong with it, and how one can assess its function in health and disease.

A resting human needs an oxygen supply of about 0.3 liters per minute. During heavy exercise, the need for oxygen may increase to 4 liters per minute or even more. The lungs are a gas-exchanger of a degree of efficiency not yet matched by any "artificial lung" designed by man. In a volume less than 10 liters, they contain a surface area of about 80 m^2 where air and blood can exchange O_2 and CO_2. At rest, only part of this surface area is used; during heavy exercise, increased blood flow through the lung capillaries is a principal device which allows increased gas exchange.

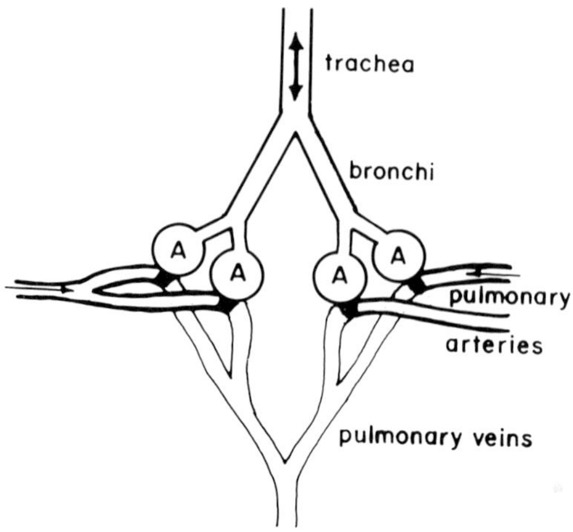

Fig. 1. Design of the gas-exchange system in the lungs. A = alveoli, where gas exchange occurs between alveolar gas and blood in capillaries (dark areas in blood vessels).

The large surface area of the air-blood barrier is created by the design shown schematically in Fig. **1**. Atmospheric air is brought to the gas-exchanging surfaces by a system of branched tubes, the bronchial tree, which end in thin-walled sacs, the alveoli. In the alveoli, an extremely thin alveolocapillary membrane (Fig. 6-1, p. 100) separates alveolar air from venous blood, carried to capillary blood vessels in the alveolar walls by a second system of branched tubes, the pulmonary artery and its branches. During the passage of blood through the alveoli, O_2 is taken up and CO_2 is excreted; i.e., blood becomes arterialized. A third system of branched tubes, the pulmonary veins, collects the arterialized capillary blood and carries it to the left atrium and ventricle. From there, it is distributed to all body tissues through the aorta and its branches, the systemic arteries.

The continuous exchange of gases between alveolar air and pulmonary capillary blood can only be maintained if the partial pressure of oxygen in alveolar air is higher, and that of carbon dioxide lower, than the corresponding partial pressures in venous blood arriving in the lung capillaries. This is accomplished by discontinuous, rhythmic dilution of alveolar air with atmospheric air, which contains almost no CO_2 and has a P_{O_2} higher than that of alveolar air. Periodic entry of atmospheric air into the alveoli is assured by cyclical increases of lung volume (inspiration), followed by equal decreases of lung volume (expiration) which remove a portion of alveolar air from the lungs. These rhythmic volume changes—ventilation—of the lungs (at a rate of about 15 per minute and a volume, the tidal volume, of about 500 ml at rest; see Fig. 7-1, p. 150) are brought about by rhythmic volume changes (at the same rate and volume) of the chest cage, the bony and muscular structure which contains the lungs (see Fig. 7-2, p. 157). The chest cage is able to increase and decrease its volume actively, by contraction of inspiratory or expiratory respiratory muscles which are attached to the chest cage.

Hence, ventilation of the lungs is brought about by a pump—the chest cage; the lungs follow the volume changes of the chest cage passively. The rate of ventilation can be altered by changing the rate of the breathing movements or the tidal volume, or both. The ventilation of the lungs is regulated by the central nervous system, which sends nerve impulses to the respiratory muscles (see, e.g., Fig. 10-4, p. 240). Changes in these nerve impulses can have their origin in our will, e.g., when we voluntarily hold the breath, or when we consciously breathe faster or deeper. But under many other conditions, changes in the signals sent by the central nervous system to the muscles of breathing are initiated unconsciously, automatically. This involuntary control system includes sensors which detect changes in the partial pressures of oxygen and carbon dioxide in blood, other sensors which detect changes in lung volume, and yet others which assess the degree of contraction of respiratory muscles. In this way, the central nervous system receives information on the mechanical process of breathing and on its consequences in terms of changes in blood gas tensions. In response to this information, groups of nerve cells in the brain stem adjust their rate of firing in accordance with changes in requirements for ventilation of the lungs. The impulses generated by the brain stem "centers" (the ventilatory drive) reach other groups of nerve cells, most of them in the spinal cord, which coordinate the signals sent to the respiratory muscles in accordance with the ventilatory drive.

Thus, the main aspects of the human and mammalian breathing apparatus which need to be discussed in detail are:

(1) Gas transport;
(2) Mechanics of breathing;
(3) Control of breathing.

This book begins with two additional topics: the development of the breathing apparatus (Chap. 1) and the morphology and function of the conducting airways, i.e., the upper airways and the part of the bronchial tree which does not participate in gas exchange (Chap. 2). These airways are more than passive conduits for inspired and expired gas: they participate in heat and water exchange and help in protecting the lungs against entry and accumulation of foreign matter.

Gas transport between atmospheric air and the tissues is discussed in Chaps. 3–6. First, Chapter 3 deals with gas transport mechanisms in the conducting airways, and with the volume of these airways, the anatomical dead space. Next in the chain of events is the distribution of inspired gas to different regions of the lungs and its mixing with alveolar gas (Chap. 4). Chapter 5 deals with the "dialogue" between air and blood in the alveoli, where O_2 and CO_2 exchange is chiefly determined by the ratio of alveolar ventilation and lung capillary blood flow. Chapter 6 traces oxygen transport from alveolar gas to the cells' mitochondria by diffusion through alveolocapillary and red cell membranes, binding to hemoglobin, and diffusion from capillary blood into the cells. The second part of Chapter 6 describes the transport of carbon dioxide in the opposite direction, from the cells to the alveoli, through solution and chemical binding of CO_2 in blood; it includes discussion of the relations between CO_2 transport and the acid-base balance.

The section on *mechanics of breathing* (Chaps. 7–10) focuses, in part, on a simple pumping function: as the lungs and chest suck in atmospheric air and expel air containing less oxygen and more carbon dioxide, alveolar air is renewed. Although, for many purposes, such a simple model is sufficient, lung mechanics is more than the study of an ingenious pump system ventilating through a complex system of pipes. It also involves the basic physical properties of lung tissue and the details of lung structure which determine transmission of forces; lung mechanics can lead to study of airways and lungs as biological systems. Measurement of mechanical parameters, although an imperfect reflection of the physical system, helps assess changes in lungs and airways which result from disease, drugs, and other agents. In an attempt to treat lung mechanics in this broader sense, Chapter 7 describes the properties of the lungs and chest cage during volume displacements. The relationships between driving pressures and airflow through airways are discussed in Chapter 8. Chapter 9 describes flow-volume curves and their applications.

The *control of breathing* is discussed in two different contexts. Chapter 10 describes breathing mainly as an involuntary motor act, controlled by a neuronal network in the brain stem which initiates rhythmic breathing and modifies its pattern guided by information concerning lung inflation, respiratory muscle tension, and arterial blood gas composition received from different types of sensors. Chapter 11 focuses on breathing as a voluntary motor act in the service of interhuman communication via speech, singing, and wind-instrument playing. This function of the breathing apparatus emphasizes the integration of the control of breathing with the control of other motor acts.

Clinical applications of respiratory physiology are discussed in each chapter. In addition, Chapter 12 contains a more comprehensive discussion of applied respiratory physiology in the study of environmental lung diseases caused by smoking, occupational exposures, and air pollution. It is now clear that morbidity and mortality due to chronic lung diseases and lung cancer could be greatly reduced if everyone at all times inspired air free from smoke, dusts, fumes, and noxious gases. There are many examples of controlled studies in man and in animals, using methods of respiratory physiology, which have shown relations between environmental exposures and lung diseases. Tests which can detect minor changes in lung function, due to inhalation of noxious agents in our environment, can further refine our knowledge of environmental lung diseases.

The subject matter of this book is sometimes called "classical" respiratory physiology, perhaps because it concerns topics in which physiologists have had a long-standing interest. It is therefore possible to present a systematic discussion of concepts, experimental data, and areas of ignorance. More recently, biochemists, pharmacologists, and cell biologists have in increasing numbers turned to the study of the lungs. All lung diseases involve responses of cells to exogenous or endogenous factors. As a tissue, the lungs are a heterogeneous mixture of many different types of cells, involved in a wide variety of activities. Biochemists prefer to study basic principles in simpler systems. Yet, to understand lung diseases one needs to study lung tissue and lung cells. Some biochemical processes (e.g., formation of surfactant, p. 8) are specialized functions of the lungs and cannot be studied in other tissues. Other events, like the ciliary beat (p. 37) are similar in human bronchi, oysters, and unicellular organisms. Yet other processes (e.g., smooth muscle contraction, mucous gland secretion, fibroblast proliferation) are not unique to lung tissue, but their occurrence in lung tissue has special significance for the development of lung diseases. Hence, biochemical studies of these events usually take their cue from questions raised by physicians and physiologists who detect abnormalities in the structure and function of the lungs and wonder how these came about.

Because tissue and cellular responses in the lungs are diverse, it is not surprising that people with a wide variety of expertise are needed to unravel the problems posed by lung diseases. Immunologists and pharmacologists study asthma and other hypersensitivity lung diseases. Protein chemists study the formation of collagen. Lipid chemists investigate the pathways of surfactant formation. Tissue and cell culture specialists try to tease lung tissue apart and to obtain homogeneous cultures of viable cells. Thus, the cell biology of the lungs is highly diverse in its approaches, depending largely on which disease or tissue response one wants to study.

Some of the types of lung cells which the reader will encounter in various chapters of this book are:

Type I alveolar cells, which are destroyed by high concentrations of oxygen, ozone, and other toxic gases (p. 101, 301);

Type II alveolar cells, which are destroyed in repair of the alveolar epithelium when Type I cells have been destroyed, and which normally produce surfactant (see Chap. 1);

Alveolar macrophage cells, which phagocytose bacteria and dust particles (p. 294);

Mast cells, which release histamine and other chemical mediators in allergic reactions (p. 35);

Fibroblasts, which form collagen and may proliferate to form dense fibrous tissue in the lungs (p. 301);

Airway smooth muscle cells, which affect airway caliber in asthma and other diseases with airway obstruction (p. 296);

Mucous glands and goblet cells, which secrete airway mucus (Chap. 2).

Much recent work on lung metabolism and on lung cells is discussed in two recent books.[1,3] There is little question that basic research on lung cell biology holds many promises for the future. I believe that these promises stand the best chance of coming true if, at the same time, the methods and concepts of "classical" respiratory physiology continue to be improved and refined. The combination of the two approaches is a powerful one if one wants to relate responses of cells and tissues to events that can be observed in vivo in animals and in man. In this respect, we are fortunate in having chosen the lungs for our studies: so few other systems in the body yield as much information on their function, with simple methods, as the lungs do. This means that the physiologist can study not just patients, but also large groups of healthy subjects, including those who may have incipient or unrecognized lung disease. The detection and description of these early stages of lung diseases, together with the study of the development of cellular and humoral responses in lung cells and tissue, is just one example of an area where cell biologists and biochemists, on the one hand, and respiratory physiologists, physicians, and epidemiologists, on the other hand, can work together towards prevention and better treatment of lung diseases.

References

1. Bouhuys A (ed): Lung Cells in Disease. Proceedings of a Brook Lodge Conference. Amsterdam, Elsevier/North-Holland Biomedical Press, 1976
2. Dejours P: Principles of Comparative Respiratory Physiology. Amsterdam, North-Holland/American Elsevier, 1975
3. Junod AF, de Haller R (eds): Lung Metabolism: Proteolysis and Antiproteolysis, Biochemical Pharmacology, Handling of Bioactive Substances. New York, Academic Press, 1975

THE PHYSIOLOGY OF BREATHING

Chapter 1

Development of the Breathing Apparatus

Growth and differentiation of tissues and organs are regulated by information contained in the genetic code. How this information is transcribed during the development of a fertilized egg into a full-grown organism remains a mystery. Gross morphological development is well understood in a descriptive sense, but we do not know the mechanisms that bring about the rapid and profound changes in a developing organism. How the biochemical machinery of the body and its capacity to respond to exogenous agents, such as drugs, develop is virtually unknown. The surfactant system of the lungs is a prime example of the difficulties remaining in this field. In this chapter, we will consider chiefly the lungs' morphological development, the maturation of the surfactant system, and the maturation of the neuromuscular system that controls chest motion and affects airway caliber. We will also review aspects of lung and chest growth that can be measured in vivo. Several other developmental aspects of breathing, such as fetal gas exchange and the initiation of breathing in newborn infants, have been discussed in recent monographs and reviews[4, 25, 29] (see also Chap. 10, p. 254).

MORPHOLOGICAL DEVELOPMENT

When the human fetus is about 3 mm long, the lungs begin to form. A groove develops from the foregut, forming two pouches, with a tissue mass around them: the *primary lung bud.* Next, the proximal foregut divides into esophagus and trachea, with the latter connecting to the primary lung bud. The bronchial tree develops by division of the primary lung bud. During the first four months of fetal life—the *pseudoglandular period*—the whole tissue mass grows rapidly. The primitive airways that are formed are open from the beginning: at no stage of lung development is the tissue solid.[29] The *canalicular period* follows, and the newly formed bronchi divide further and the amount of connective tissue between them decreases. Increased numbers of blood vessels now enter the lungs. Although the epithelium flattens out, there is still enough tissue between epithelium and blood vessels to prevent effective gas exchange. At about the 25th week of gestation the *terminal sac period* [39] begins (Fig. 1-1). At this stage, in a human fetus of about 30 weeks' gestation, flattened epithelium was found in the terminal bronchioles and saccules, but no alveoli had as yet formed.[14] The airways terminated in relatively wide saccules from which, presumably, alveoli develop later on. Although there was a considerable amount of interstitial tissue between epithelium and blood vessels, the lung had some gas exchange capability; the infant survived 19 hours. Several generations of saccules are formed, and each generation lengthens during the last weeks of gestation. At birth the saccules have shallow, primitive alveoli in their walls.[15] At this stage, each saccule probably has its own capillary network, so that there are two capillary networks, separated by fibroblasts, in each intersaccular septum.[19, 73]

After birth the saccules are converted into alveolar ducts, and the primitive alveoli assume the shape of true alveoli. At the same time, the two capillary networks in the septa merge to one.[19] Most alveoli are formed after birth. At first, up to age 3 in man, they increase only in number; thereafter also in size. From age 8 on, alveolar surface area and volume increase further, mainly because the alveoli continue to grow in size.[39]

The development of an elastic tissue network may be an essential factor in the formation of new alveoli.[29] At birth there are only a few elastic fibers around terminal airways; during postnatal growth collagen fibers are converted into elastic fibers, making this network more extensive and dense.

The elastic fibers curve around existing alveoli and indent their walls (Fig. 1-2). This is the first method of alveoli formation—*peripheral alveolar segmentation.* Similarly, the septa between the alveoli are indented; this is called *alveolar*

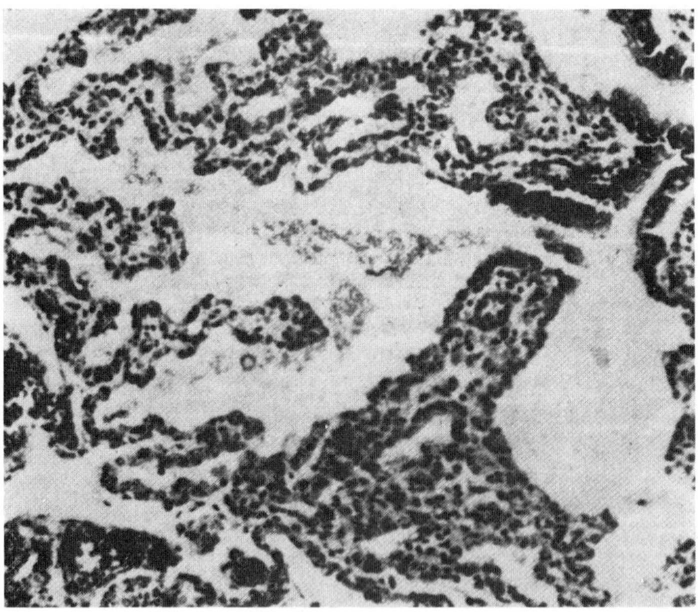

Fig. 1-1. Photograph (×140) from the lung of a stillborn human fetus of 30 weeks' gestation. The lumen is distended with liquor amnii. The bronchial tree terminates in saccules. Distinct connective tissue is obvious between the cavities. From Emery.[29]

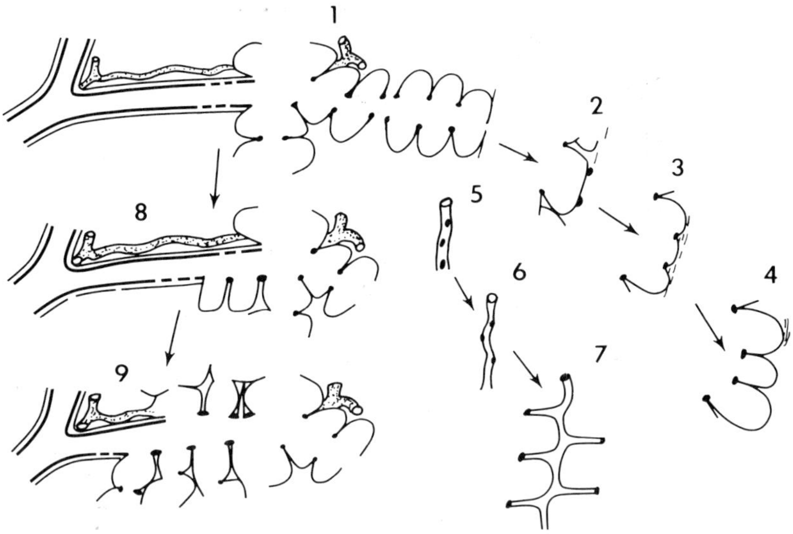

Fig. 1-2. Diagram showing methods of proliferation of alveoli as suggested by changes in the elastic tissue: (*1*) at birth; (*2*, *3*, and *4*) peripheral alveolar segmentation; (*5*, *6*, and *7*) alveolar wall compoundment; (*8* and *9*) fragmentation of terminal respiratory passage. From Emery.[29]

wall compoundment. Finally, there is a thick layer of elastic fibers in bronchiolar walls. Gaps develop in this network, and alveoli form by protrusion through holes in the elastic structure. Eventually, little of the bronchiolar wall remains but the ends of the septa (Fig. 1-3). This formation of alveoli by "eating away at the bronchioles" is called *fragmentation of terminal respiratory passages.*

In man, the total number of epithelialized airways increases slightly from birth up to age 1; from that age on the number declines. At the same time, the total number of alveoli increases rapidly. This is indirect evidence for conversion of conducting airways into alveolar ducts and alveoli. Boyden and Tompsett[15] observed in dog lung lobes that some airways disappeared in the process of alveolar formation. During the first 10 days after birth, conducting airways were rapidly altered into gas-exchanging units. Shortly before birth, airways lined with cuboid epithelium could be found at a distance less than 0.5 mm from the pleura. Ten days after birth, in another specimen, this distance was more than 3 mm. Boyden and Tompsett propose that the terminal nonrespiratory passages become "drawn out" during the rapid process of lung expansion after birth and that new alveoli develop from these as shown in Figure 1-2 (*8* and *9*). As many as six generations of airways, counting from the lobar stem bronchus, are transformed to respiratory units in this process. From these descriptions it appears that alveolar development is slower in man than in the dog. Schwieler and Skoglund[65] found considerable variability in the number of branches on the main stem bronchi of two lobes in 6- to 11-week-old cats. The anatomist is at a technical disadvantage when making the number of observations that satisfies statisticians!

From this theory of lung development one would expect that early damage to terminal conducting airways could permanently arrest alveolar formation.[29] Alveolar hypoplasia may, in fact, occur peripheral to obstructed airways,[56] but it

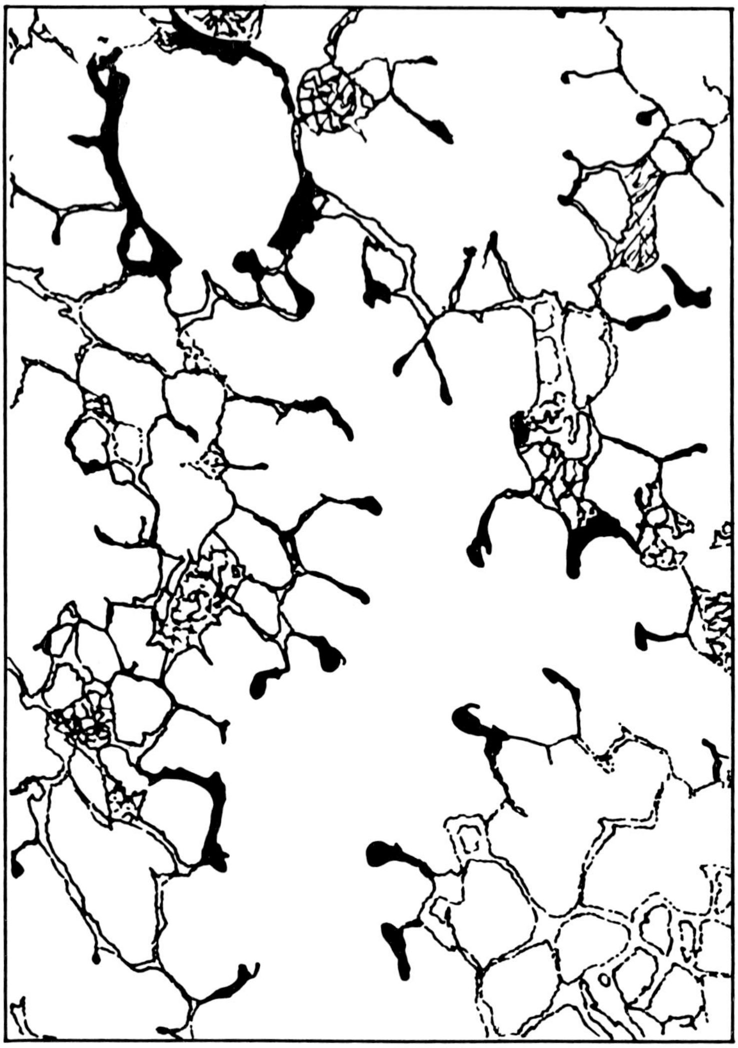

Fig. 1-3. Alveolar duct and alveoli, drawn after a preparation made by Staub.[70] The rings of smooth muscle surrounding the entrance to the alveoli are seen as thickened endings of interalveolar septa.

is not certain whether, for instance, children who survive severe attacks of bronchiolitis sustain permanent damage to lung growth. Although controlled studies to answer this question are difficult to perform, it might help to know whether the total lung capacity remains small in children who have had severe bronchiolitis.

New alveoli are formed until at least age 7.[27] Data on a large number of lung samples have suggested that new alveoli might continue to form until early adulthood.[30] In any case, the increase in the number of alveoli during the teens is small. Large numbers of new alveoli are formed during the first decade of life, and at this age developmental arrest resulting from lung disease or even effects of pollutants on small airways might conceivably lead to permanent lung damage.

Cigarette smoke is perhaps the pollutant most worthy of concern in this context (Chap. 12).

Several aspects of morphological development have been traced in groups of small animals raised under controlled conditions. Rats treated with growth hormone become abnormally large, and their lung weight, lung volume, and alveolar surface area all grow in proportion to body weight.[9] This is due to formation of new alveoli rather than to expansion of existing ones. If expansion were the main factor, alveolar surface would increase in proportion to the two-thirds power of lung volume; in fact, it increases more than that.

In newborn small animals, such as mice and rats, few alveoli are present at birth and these are similar in size to those of newborn infants and calves (diameter, 90–140 μm).[10] Adult animals of these species have quite different alveolar diameters (about 20 μm in mice; 280 in men). Bartlett[10] has pointed out that if newborn mice had more alveoli, their diameter would be very small and they would be highly susceptible to collapse.

Comparatively little is known about the development of specific tissue components of the lungs. A variety of *mucosal cells* occurs in small bronchioles of premature infants.[61] In the rabbit, functional airway *smooth muscle* is present in the trachea at birth.[64] In smooth muscle cells (vas deferens of mice[77]), the Golgi apparatus and ribosomes appear at an early stage, while thin and thick myofilaments follow much later. There are apparently large differences between the development times of various kinds of smooth muscle. Bundles of *nerve fibers* are present around the trachea of a 35-mm long human fetus and begin to penetrate its wall to form an intrachondral plexus in the 100-mm fetus.[71] Nerve fibers to tracheal smooth muscle can be identified in the 100-mm fetus, and to mucous glands in the 140-mm long fetus. In the same study, nerve fibers to pulmonary arteries and veins were found in the 65-mm long fetus. The continued postnatal development of the *pulmonary arterial system* has been studied in human lung specimens.[24]

DEVELOPMENT OF THE ALVEOLAR LINING

Respiratory physiologists often picture the lungs as consisting of bubbles (alveoli) at the end of tubes (airways). Morphologists may scoff at such a naive idea, but this has been a productive model of the lungs. It led Von Neergaard[49] to realize that surface force could play an essential role in the lungs' recoil force. By comparing the recoil of air-filled lungs with that of liquid-filled lungs, he found that two-thirds to three-quarters of the total lung recoil force is caused by surface tension at the alveolar air-liquid interface. Recent measurements of stress relaxation[40] have suggested that surface tension accounts for ⅞ of the total viscoelastic force, and tissue proper for only ⅛, not far from Von Neergaard's estimate. Von Neergaard also realized that the newborn animal must overcome surface forces in the alveoli when inflating the lungs for the first time, and that this requires a large inspiratory force. But this force might be less if "the surface tension of the alveoli is decreased, in comparison with other physiological solutions, through enrichment by surface-active substances, according to Gibbs-

Thomson's law." This suggestion of Von Neergaard has been amply confirmed, although it took nearly 30 years.

The more recent history of lung surfactant is well known and has been ably reviewed.[34, 53, 72] Studies of fetal lambs have shown that surfactant material begins to develop at a well-defined moment during gestation (after about 128 days of a 147-day gestation).[51] After about 135 days' gestation, enough surfactant has been formed to allow safe transition to air breathing after birth. When delivered before 135 days' gestation, newborn lambs do not breathe well and their condition resembles the respiratory distress syndrome of human newborns.[57] This happens even when asphyxia is prevented, so that prematurity, and not asphyxia, appears to be the crucial event. In these studies the appearance of lung surfactant was usually deduced from measurements of the surface tension of lung extracts. More recently the anatomical substrate for surfactant formation has been clarified by electron microscope studies of the two main types of cells in the alveolar wall. Kikkawa et al.[43] compared the morphological appearance of alveolar type II epithelial cells (i.e., large cells with inclusion bodies; Fig. 1-4) with the absence or presence of surface activity in lung extracts, at various stages of development in fetal and newborn lambs. Surface activity was first detected a few days after osmiophilic inclusion bodies appeared in type II cells. These bodies first appear at about 121 days' gestation, and they increase in number and size as the lungs mature. In human and monkey lungs, the osmiophilic inclusions form concentric layers; in other mammals the inclusions consist of transverse lamellae.[54] Large osmiophilic bodies are often found near the cell surface, where it is likely that they deposit their contents. Several investigators have now shown a lining layer of similar osmiophilic material on the surface of the alveolar epithelium. Although

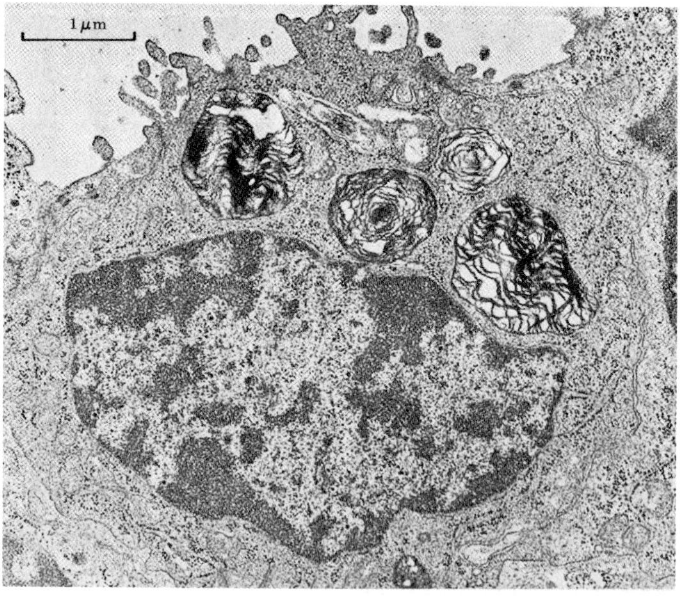

Fig. 1-4. Type II cell in lung of a rabbit fetus (27th day of gestation). There are four lamellar bodies in the cytoplasm. Electron micrograph courtesy of Dr. Linda Nardone.

the layer's origin in the osmiophilic bodies of the type II cells is not fully established, it appears likely. The presence of the layer correlates with surface activity in lung extracts, and the layer is absent in immature animals whose lungs collapse after birth. The surface lining layer remains particularly well conserved when tissue is fixed by perfusing the pulmonary vessels rather than by filling the air spaces with liquid.[33]

The chemical nature of the surfactant material in vivo is not certain. Most likely it is a phospholipid compound. In particular, disaturated lecithin is probably an important component of surfactant; its presence correlates with alveolar surface area in 11 different vertebrate species, including man, and surfactant shows a similar correlation.[21] Phosphatidylglycerol is an additional surface-active component of surfactant.[59] In vivo, the lipid component of surfactant may be bound to protein. Although tissue extractions may yield a protein-free lipid, this may result from lipoprotein breakdown during the preparative procedures.[62] King and Clements[44] have extracted four highly surface-active fractions, at least 40 times enriched, from dog lung. All consisted of lipid and protein, and all decreased surface tension and formed films on air-liquid interfaces. All four contained large amounts of lecithin.

Lung tissue can synthesize phospholipids from acetate in vitro; most of the acetate is incorporated in lecithin.[47] It is not certain which cells perform the synthesis, but type I cells are unlikely candidates since they possess few intracellular organelles. Type II cells, in contrast, appear to be highly active metabolically and thus more suitable for this role. *De novo* synthesis of fatty acids occurs in the soluble fraction of rabbit fetal lung; synthesis by elongation of smaller chain fatty acids in mitochondria and microsomes is of lesser importance.[36] Recent work by Page-Roberts[52] shows that a purified lamellar body fraction from rat lung was surface-active and had a much higher phospholipid content than that of mitochondrial and microsomal fractions. Further studies[60] show that the phospholipid content of the lamellar body fraction is similar to that of lung wash (which represents surfactant), and that its saturated fatty acid content is much higher than that in other fractions. These findings support the importance of the lamellar body in storing surfactant.

In humans, prematurity and its accompanying lack of surfactant production are associated with a severe and often fatal condition known as the idiopathic respiratory distress syndrome (IRDS) of the newborn. As a result of insufficient surfactant, the lungs have a greatly increased recoil force and tend to collapse during each expiration, often resulting in atelectasis. Recently, clinical improvement has been obtained when such infants were ventilated with continuous positive airway pressure, to counteract the lung's increased recoil.[35] Another feature of the respiratory distress syndrome is the formation of curious hyaline membranes in the air spaces of the lungs. The membranes are probably formed from fibrin and fibrinogen, derived from transudation of plasma into the air spaces.[43] In the healthy fetal lamb, the alveolar epithelium is an effective barrier against passage of such large molecules as proteins, and thus normal alveolar fluid contains very little protein.[50] When immature lambs are ventilated, this barrier breaks and the alveolar epithelium then becomes permeable to proteins. Therefore, leakage of the alveolar epithelium appears to promote hyaline membrane formation in the lungs of infants with respiratory distress.

The respiratory distress syndrome is self-limiting—if the infant survives long enough, the lungs mature and sufficient surfactant will be formed. Clinically, most surviving infants appear to have no permanent pulmonary damage, although lung fibrosis occurs in some.[67] Thus, such symptomatic treatment as continuous positive pressure may be essential for survival. In addition, it may be possible to speed up surfactant formation with drugs. There is evidence that treating the unborn rabbit with corticosteroids may accelerate surfactant formation and increase survival chances after transition to air breathing.[45, 46] Proteins with the specific property of binding glucocorticoids (hormone receptors) have been demonstrated in the soluble fraction (cytosol) as well as in the nuclear fraction of fetal lung tissue.[3, 5] Direct injection of cortisol or thyroxine into the rabbit fetus (2–3 days before premature delivery) caused an earlier appearance of surfactant and maturation of type II cells. Also, the lungs were better aerated after delivery than those of control litter mates.[46, 76] Experiments with drugs that affect microsomal or mitochondrial metabolism or specific steps in the synthesis of lung lipids could help unravel the events in lung maturation and at the same time yield important therapeutic results. Along these lines, Kikkawa and Motoyama[42] have recently treated rabbits with an inhibitor of cholesterol synthesis (AY-9944) and found that this delayed lung tissue maturation while at the same time abnormally large numbers of type II cells appeared. Morphological development and surfactant maturation did not proceed at the same pace. It seems obvious that there are specific biochemical pathways for surfactant formation, and these appear to be, in part, independent of tissue growth and alveolar formation.

NEUROMUSCULAR MATURATION

Coordination of breathing requires a mature neuromuscular apparatus to move the chest bellows. To do this, all components of the system must function adequately—coordinating centers as well as peripheral nerve fibers, neuromuscular junctions, and muscle fibers. The newborn infant lacks coordinated control over many motor acts; there is also evidence that central as well as peripheral nerve fibers need to mature considerably after birth in many animals. But the steps that limit motor control development are not clear. Is it the learning process, or is it immaturity of one or other anatomical components of the system? With more insight into this basic question, we might eventually be able to correlate physiological events at the cellular level with behavioral aspects of development in infants and children. In respiration, this may improve understanding not only of the development of control over breathing itself (Chap. 10), but also of other motor acts, such as speech, that use the respiratory bellows (Chap. 11).

Here we describe some aspects of development of peripheral neuromuscular elements. Peripheral myelinated nerve fibers mature considerably after birth, increasing in both number and diameter.[69] When mature, the fibers are better able to transmit impulses continually and at high frequencies.[63] In part, their relative functional incompetence in the immature stage may be a consequence of their small size. In addition, metabolic factors may be important.[64] Autonomic nerve fibers, too, increase in number and size during postnatal development[78] For instance, the hearts of 1–2-day-old rabbits contain few adrenergic fibers; they also contain little epinephrine.[31]

Physiological experiments also suggest that post-natal maturation occurs in peripheral nerve fibers. In our laboratory, Schwieler developed a technique that provides information on the functional competence of vagal and sympathetic nerve fibers to the trachea and the heart in rabbits.[64] Supramaximal stimulation at different rates was used in tracheotomized animals varying in age from less than 1 day to more than 6 months. The effects on the trachea were measured by recording the pressure inside a thin-walled balloon placed in a segment of the trachea above the tracheostomy. The response to vagal stimulation is shown in Figure 1-5. In older animals, contractions are well maintained at stimulation frequencies up to 200 impulses per second. In younger animals, however, they decrease before the end of the stimulation period at 30 and 50 impulses per second, and at 100 impulses per second the initial amplitude is also reduced. This decreasing response was not due to smooth muscle exhaustion, because less than 1 minute later a sustained maximum response could again be obtained by simply reducing the stimulation rate to 20 or 30 impulses per second. It also seemed unlikely that the neuromuscular junction limited the response to high-frequency stimulation. Other experiments showed that physostigmine can prevent the decrease of vagal responses at high stimulation frequencies. This made it clear that the end organ can follow repetitive stimuli at high frequencies, if only enough transmitter substance is available. Thus, these experiments suggested that the ability of immature vagal efferent fibers to conduct impulses at high rates is limited. In addition, these immature fibers are highly sensitive to effects of general anesthesia. For instance, in the results shown in Figure 1-6, sodium pentobarbital decreases the heart's response to vagal stimulation. The effect is seen in an adult as well as in an immature animal, but in the latter much less of the drug is required.

The response to stimulation of efferent sympathetic fibers often depends on the initial state of the tracheal muscle. For instance, in the experiment outlined in Figure 1-7, vagal stimulation contracted the tracheal muscle, while sympathetic stimulation alone had no effect. Only when the muscle tone was first increased by stimulating the vagus did sympathetic stimulation result in tracheal muscle

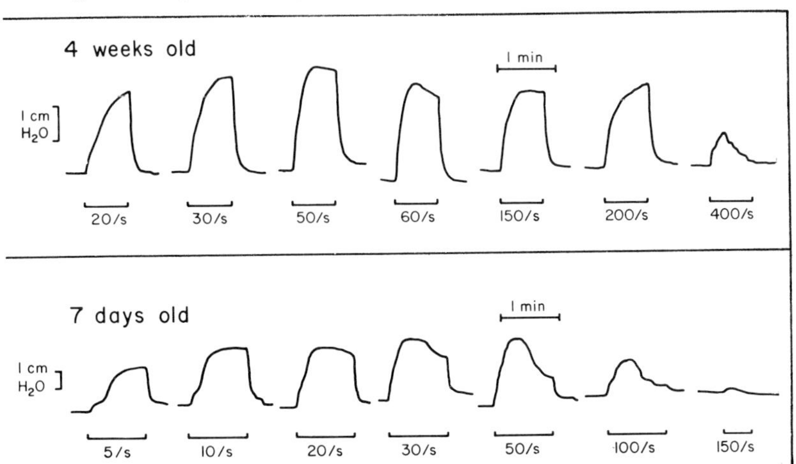

Fig. 1-5. Intratracheal pressure changes in response to supramaximal vagal stimulation in a 4-week-old and a 7-day-old rabbit. From Schwieler et al.[48]

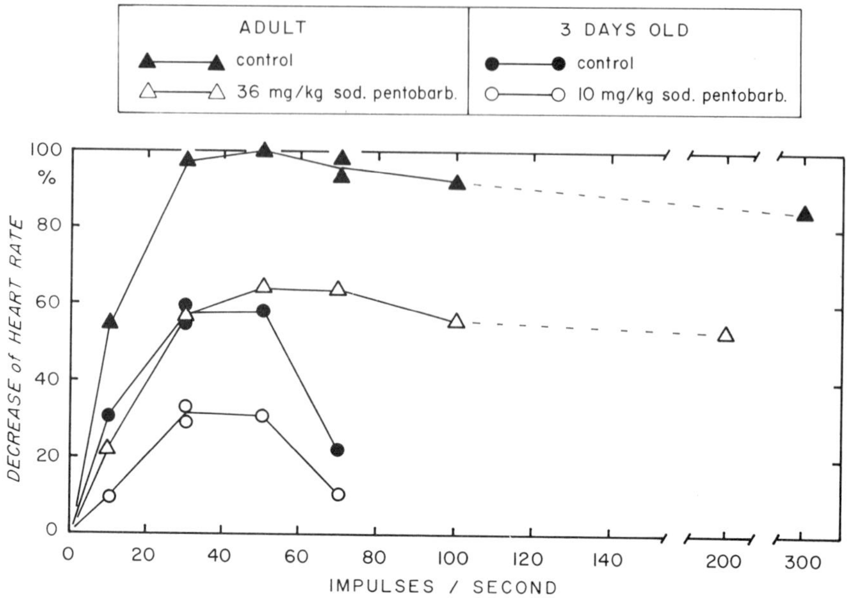

Fig. 1-6. Effect of sodium pentobarbital on heart rate response to supramaximal vagal stimulation in an adult and a 3-day-old rabbit. Control responses were obtained 1–2 hours after administering 1.5 gm/kg urethan and 20 mg/kg sodium pentobarbital to adult animal and 1 g/kg urethan and 10 mg/kg sodium pentobarbital to 3-day-old animal. Each dot represents decrease in mean heart rate (as a percentage of control value) produced by vagal stimulation for 20 sec. About 4 times more sodium pentobarbital is required in adult animal to produce a response decrease similar to that in 3-day-old animal. From Schwieler et al.[64]

relaxation. Like the vagal responses, sustained sympathetic responses in newborn animals occurred only at low stimulation frequencies.

From these results, as well as from other studies,[2, 26] it seems clear that the rabbit's trachea and heart have a functional efferent autonomic innervation at birth or very soon thereafter. But, apparently, important functional changes occur during the first 4–6 postnatal weeks, and these enable the nerve fibers to better conduct impulses at high stimulation rates for prolonged periods of time. Yet, the immature nerve fibers appear to participate effectively in reflex events. For instance, Downing[26] observed baroreceptor reflex activity on the heart in

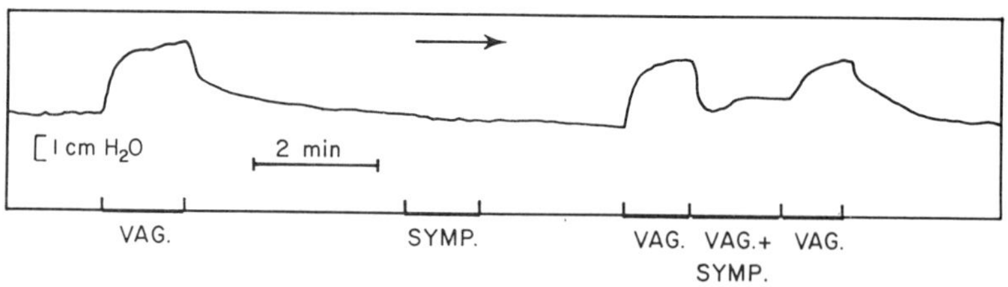

Fig. 1-7. Intratracheal pressure changes in response to supramaximal stimulation of right cervical vagal and sympathetic trunks at a stimulation frequency of 30 impulses per second in a 5-week-old rabbit. Tracheal smooth muscle relaxes in response to sympathetic stimulation only during simultaneous vagal stimulation. Upward deflection = pressure increase. From Schwieler et al.[64]

newborn rabbits. It seems likely, however, that the immature fibers can handle only short-lasting responses. During some of these evoked responses, vagal and sympathetic fibers fire at rates up to about 60 per second,[75] and immature fibers can transmit such impulse traffic only for short periods of time. In contrast with its competence during electrical stimulation and baroreceptor reflexes, the heart in newborn rabbits and other immature animals apparently does not respond to tonic vagal influences.[1, 2, 74] Vagotomy or atropine administration do not increase heart rate until a few weeks after birth. Perhaps even low-frequency stimuli (involved in maintaining vagal tone) are poorly conducted over long periods of time in immature autonomic fibers.

Impulse transmission decreases at high stimulation frequencies in immature pyramidal neurons in kittens,[41] as well as in preganglionic and postganglionic autonomic fibers. Since similar results have been obtained with somatic sensory nerve fibers,[28, 68] this may be a property of immature nerve fibers in general. It is hard to assess the physiological significance of nerve fiber immaturity in the development of such integrated responses as breathing and speech. If central[41] and peripheral[28, 64, 68, 69] neurons have common immature features, it is difficult to determine which component limits development of integrated motor acts and responses. Perhaps responses that require only low-frequency impulse traffic can develop earlier than those that require high rates of nerve-impulse conduction.

LUNG VOLUMES AND MECHANICS IN GROWING CHILDREN

Morphological data on lung development are difficult to obtain in sufficient quantity. On the other hand, measurements of lung volumes and other aspects of lung function are easily made, at least in older children, and these can clarify several aspects of growth. As children grow, their chest cages, lungs, and airways increase in size. This results in bigger lung volumes, larger maximum flow rates, and reduced resistance to airflow through airways. These changes correlate with height and age of the growing individual. Measurements of volumes and flow rates are useful to determine whether the lungs of a pediatric patient conform to normal limits,[55] but they can also increase understanding of lung growth in healthy children. The rationale and technical aspects of several of the tests are discussed in other chapters; here I discuss aspects that bear on lung and chest growth in older children, in whom accurate data can be obtained relatively simply.

Lung Volumes

Measurements of lung volumes are basic to most other lung function tests. The use of the body plethysmograph allows repeated and accurate studies of lung volumes, even in small children. Other methods, using gas dilution, require several minutes of quiet breathing through a mouthpiece, and errors due to leakage around the mouthpiece are a constant worry. With the plethysmograph, each volume measurement takes only a few seconds. Most children learn the maneuvers easily, and they like the space-age environment of the body box. The methods are also well suited for studying children with lung diseases.[80, 81]

Figure 1-8 shows data for total lung capacity (TLC), vital capacity (VC), and forced expiratory volume in 1 second ($FEV_{1.0}$) in boys and girls. (For defini-

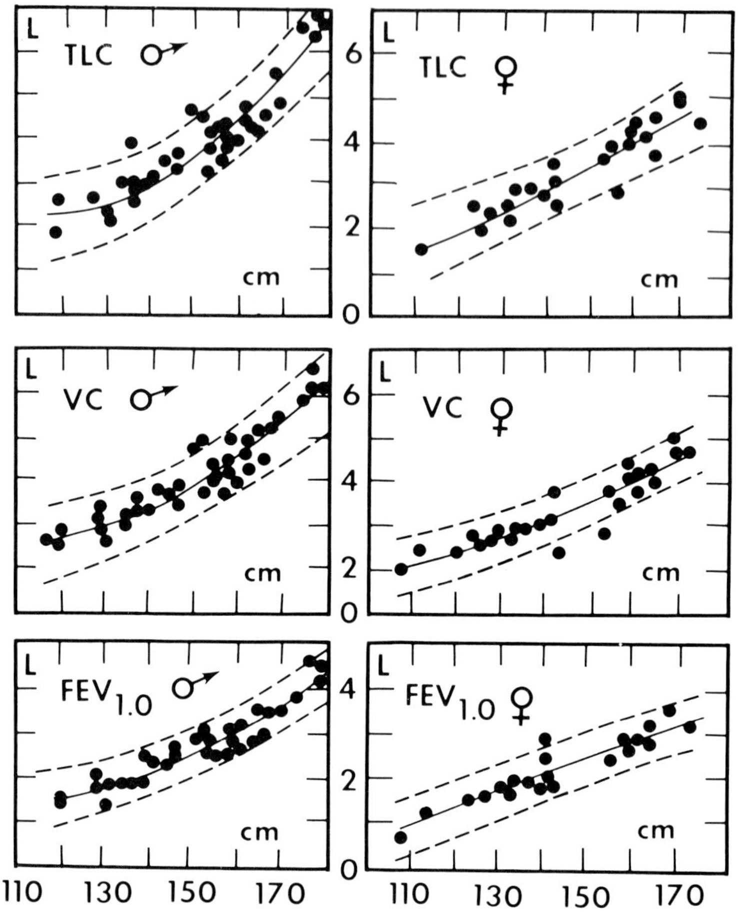

Fig. 1-8. TLC, VC, and $FEV_{1.0}$ versus body height (standing) in boys and girls. The drawn lines are regression equations; 95% confidence limits indicated by dashed lines. Age range 6–18 yrs. From Zapletal et al.[82]

tion of these variables, see p. 217.) In teen-agers, both TLC and VC increase with height much more in boys than in girls. Table 1-1 contains additional data on lung volume in the same group of children and adolescents. The relations between lung volume and body height clearly depend on the degree of lung inflation. At minimum volume (RV), lung volume is linearly related to height in both sexes (Table 1-1). At maximum inflation (TLC), lung volume increases progressively more (per unit height increase) as growth proceeds, particularly in boys. A recent study of 8–16-year-old British children[22] gave results similar to those of Zapletal et al. in U.S. white children (Table 1-1).[82] But these data cannot be extrapolated to older adolescents, since lung growth, as measured with function tests, does not proceed at an equal rate from childhood to adulthood.[66] TLC and VC values for adolescents may differ from those of adults of the same height and sex.[11] Observations in the age group 16–24 years are limited, and hence the prediction of "normal" TLC and VC data in this age range is relatively uncertain.

Table 1-1
Statistical Analysis of Lung Volumes (L) Versus Body Height (cm)

y	Sex	N	a *	b	c	130 cm	150 cm	170 cm
TLC	♂	37	+15.1397	−0.22713	+0.001002	2.55 ±0.51	3.62 ±0.46	5.49 ±0.47
	♀	24	+1.7592	−0.03394	+0.000300	2.41 ±0.40	3.41 ±0.40	4.66 ±0.42
VC	♂	39	+7.9942	−0.12509	+0.000605	1.96 ±0.40	2.85 ±0.35	4.21 ±0.43
	♀	26	+0.1694	−0.01217	+0.000189	1.78 ±0.27	2.60 ±0.25	3.56 ±0.27
FRC	♂	37	+9.3716	−0.14152	−0.000602	1.15 ±0.36	1.70 ±0.34	2.71 ±0.36
	♀	24	−2.1776	+0.02556	0	1.11 ±0.27	1.66 ±0.25	2.17 ±0.28
RV	♂	37	−1.0519	+0.01270	0	0.60 ±0.27	0.85 ±0.26	1.11 ±0.29
	♀	24	−0.8046	+0.01092	0	0.61 ±0.23	0.83 ±0.22	1.05 ±0.24
$FEV_{1.0}$	♂	33	+6.6314	−0.10261	+0.000499	1.73 ±0.31	2.47 ±0.29	3.61 ±0.32
	♀	21	−3.0378	+0.03640	0	1.69 ±0.30	2.42 ±0.29	3.15 ±0.30

* a, b, c=Coefficients in regression equations of the type $y=a+bx+cx^2$, where y is the measurement and x is height in cm. N=number of observations. Data for height 130, 150, and 170 cm are predicted values ± standard error for future individual measurements according to the regression analysis. Age range 6–18 years. Data from reference 82.

Pleural Pressure

A recent study of Zapletal et al.[79] suggests that lung elastic recoil increases with height in children who are less than 150 cm tall. For instance, in a 120-cm-tall child, the average Pst(l) at 90 percent of TLC was 13.8 cm H_2O, compared with 19.2 cm H_2O in a child 160 cm tall, and 20.4 cm H_2O in a 180-cm tall person. Several factors may account for the increase of static lung recoil in small children. The increased density of the lung's elastic fiber network[29] may be important, as was confirmed by Hartung in the discussion of Zapletal's paper.[79] Another contributing factor may be unbalanced growth of the chest and lungs, with the chest growing slightly faster, leading to some added stretch of lung tissue. It is sometimes thought that much of lung growth after about age 8 is merely inflation of preexisting tissue. Chest cage growth may well be the primary factor, but without an increase in lung tissue mass, lung inflation would lead to much larger increases of lung recoil force than are actually found. In young children, increased lung elastic recoil, as well as more rapid chest cage growth, lead to increased static recoil pressures. In older children (over 150 cm tall), further growth of the chest and lungs appears to proceed in a balanced fashion, with increased lung tissue mass keeping pace with the increased chest volume. Thus, several quantitatively ill-described factors (chest cage recoil, muscle force), each of which is a function of development and growth, must affect lung size and TLC. In spite of this, TLC appears to be a useful guide to lung size in growing children and adolescents.

Maximum Expiratory Flow-Volume (MEFV) Curves

These curves[82] provide an impressive picture of lung growth (Fig. 1-9). They are obtained by recording flow rates during a maximally forced expiration, starting at TLC (i.e., after maximum inspiration), as a function of lung volume (see Chap. 9). Both vital capacity (on the abscissa) and maximum expiratory flow rates (on the ordinate) increase, and hence MEFV curves become much larger as children grow. Quantitative information on flow can be obtained by reading instantaneous maximum flow rates (MEF) at different volume points, e.g., 25 or 50 percent of VC, or 50 percent of TLC.

Such flow rates on MEFV curves correlate positively with body height (Fig. 1-10), but their relationship to lung volume is even more interesting. To compare flow rates among four subjects with widely differing lung volumes, lung volume is expressed as a percentage of TLC on the abscissa in Figure 1-9*B*. Concurrently, flow rates (in liters per second) of each individual are divided by his TLC and expressed as TLC per second.[12] This sizing adjustment is required because a maximum flow of, say, 2 liters/sec, is large for small lungs, but small for large lungs. The growth of the MEFV curve is almost solely related to TLC and not to sex; growth produces a geometrically similar enlargement of the MEFV curve. This is also shown in Figure 1-10*B*; maximum flow rates, at a fixed lung-

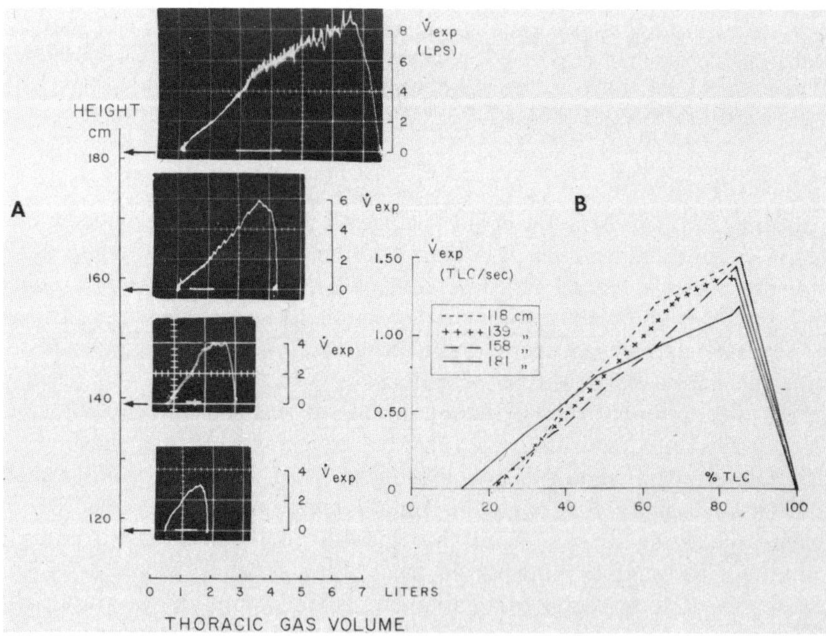

Fig. 1-9. *A*. MEFV curves of 4 boys; standing height indicated on scale at left. All curves have been lined up to fit the TGV scale at the bottom. TLC at right-hand side, RV at left-hand side on each curve. *B*. MEFV curves of *A* replotted with lung volume in percentage of TLC on abscissa and maximum flow rates in TLC per second on ordinate. From Zapletal et al.[82]

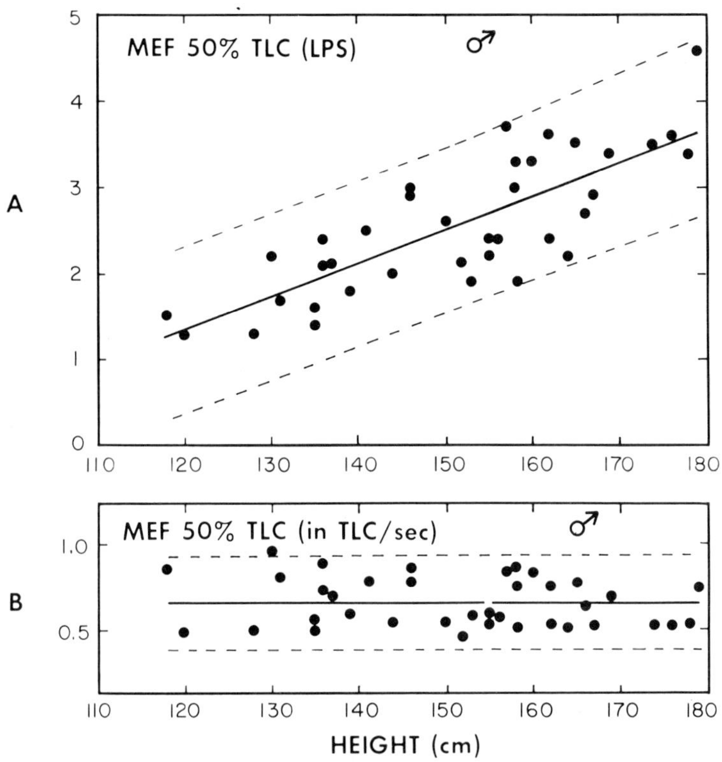

Fig. 1-10. *A*. Maximum expiratory flow rate at 50% TLC versus standing height in boys. Drawn line, regression equation; dashed lines, 95% confidence limits. *B*. Same data with flow rates in TLC per second. Drawn and dashed lines—average and 95% confidence limits, respectively. Age range 6–18 yrs. Data from reference 82.

volume level, become independent of height when expressed in units of TLC per second. This is, of course, just another way of stating that maximum flow is proportional to TLC in a group of subjects of widely varying body and lung sizes. The rule holds true at all volumes within the vital capacity range at which flow rates were measured; Tables 1-2 and 1-3 summarize these data.

Airway Conductance

Similar relations hold for airway conductance (Chap. 8). Measurements of conductance (Gaw) during panting need to be combined with determinations of lung volume (thoracic gas volume, TGV) measured with the body plethysmograph. Values for conductance at functional residual capacity (FRC) are shown in Figure 1-11. As with the maximum flow rates, division of Gaw by each individual's TLC yields a ratio that does not correlate with body height. Average values for these ratios at different lung volumes are given in Table 1-3.

Models of Lung Growth

As lung size increases, maximum expiratory flow rates and airway conductance increase in proportion to TLC. The simplest model that can explain this finding

Table 1-2
Statistical Analysis of MEF Versus Body Height

y	Sex	N	a *	b	r	130 cm	150 cm	170 cm
MEF 25% VC	♂	39	−2.3069	+0.02817	+0.76	1.36 ±0.41	1.92 ±0.40	2.48 ±0.43
	♀	26	−1.8576	+0.02483	+0.76	1.35 ±0.42	1.87 ±0.40	2.36 ±0.43
MEF 50% VC	♂	39	−4.5848	+0.05430	+0.87	2.48 ±0.50	3.35 ±0.47	4.65 ±0.53
	♀	26	−3.3655	+0.04477	+0.86	2.45 ±0.50	3.35 ±0.49	4.25 ±0.53
MEF 75% VC	♂	39	−6.8220	+0.07811	+0.86	3.32 ±0.75	4.89 ±0.73	6.46 ±0.80
	♀	26	−5.1934	+0.06367	+0.82	3.08 ±0.87	4.36 ±0.85	5.63 ±0.92
MEF 50% TLC	♂	37	−3.4163	+0.03946	+0.80	1.73 ±0.50	2.50 ±0.46	3.29 ±0.50
	♀	24	−2.3030	+0.03162	+0.80	1.81 ±0.42	2.44 ±0.41	3.07 ±0.44
MEF 60% TLC	♂	37	−5.1176	+0.05660	+0.87	2.24 ±0.53	3.37 ±0.52	4.50 ±0.55
	♀	24	−3.3956	+0.04413	+0.85	2.34 ±0.47	3.22 ±0.47	4.11 ±0.52
PEF	♂	39	−6.9865	+0.08060	+0.85	3.49 ±0.84	5.10 ±0.82	6.72 ±0.90
	♀	26	−5.3794	+0.06594	+0.82	3.19 ±0.87	4.51 ±0.84	5.83 ±0.92

* a, b=Coefficients in regression equations of the type $y=a+bx$, where y is the measurement and x is height in cm. N=number of observations. r=correlation coefficient of measured variable vs. height; all values are significant at $P < 0.001$. Data for height 130, 150, and 170 cm are predicted values ± standard error for future individual measurements according to the regression analysis. MEF is given in liters per second. Data from reference 82. Definition of MEF measurements: see Table 9-1, p. 217.

is a lung-airway system which grows isotropically, i.e., with equal relative increases of linear dimensions.[82] In such a model, airway volume grows in proportion to lung volume, and linear dimensions of alveoli and airways increase in proportion to the cube root of volume. If we represent airways by a single cylindrical tube in which airflow is laminar, Gaw will be proportional to TLC. The proportionality of maximum expiratory flow rates and TLC fits the same model. Other functional data, as well as anatomical measurements, support the hypothesis of isotropic growth. For instance, Hart et al.[37] have shown that anatomical dead space increases approximately in proportion to TLC (Table 1-4). For alveoli, Dunnill[27] concluded that between about 7 and 18 years of age alveolar diameter increases with the cube root of the change in lung volume. The same is true for frontal and sagittal bronchial diameters.[13, 82] Hislop et al.[38] recently measured airway diameters in human lung specimens from the main bronchi to the terminal bronchioles and concluded that "the infant bronchial tree may be regarded as a miniature

Table 1-3
MEF in TLC per Second and Gaw in TLC per Second per cm H_2O at Different Lung Volumes

	MEF, TLC per Second		Gaw, TLC per Second per cm H_2O	
Volume Level	Boys (N=37) *	Girls (N=24)	N	Boys and Girls
25% VC	0.50 ± 0.12	0.55 ± 0.12	21	0.071 ± 0.017
50% VC	0.93 ± 0.14	0.98 ± 0.16	21	0.105 ± 0.025
75% VC	1.27 ± 0.18	1.27 ± 0.24	21	0.141 ± 0.038
50% TLC	0.66 ± 0.14	0.72 ± 0.14	22	0.090 ± 0.020
60% TLC	0.88 ± 0.13	0.94 ± 0.15	21	0.106 ± 0.026
FRC			25	0.085 ± 0.015
PEF	1.33 ± 0.21	1.31 ± 0.24		

* N = number of observations. Values are means ± SD. Age range 6–18 yrs. Data from reference 82.

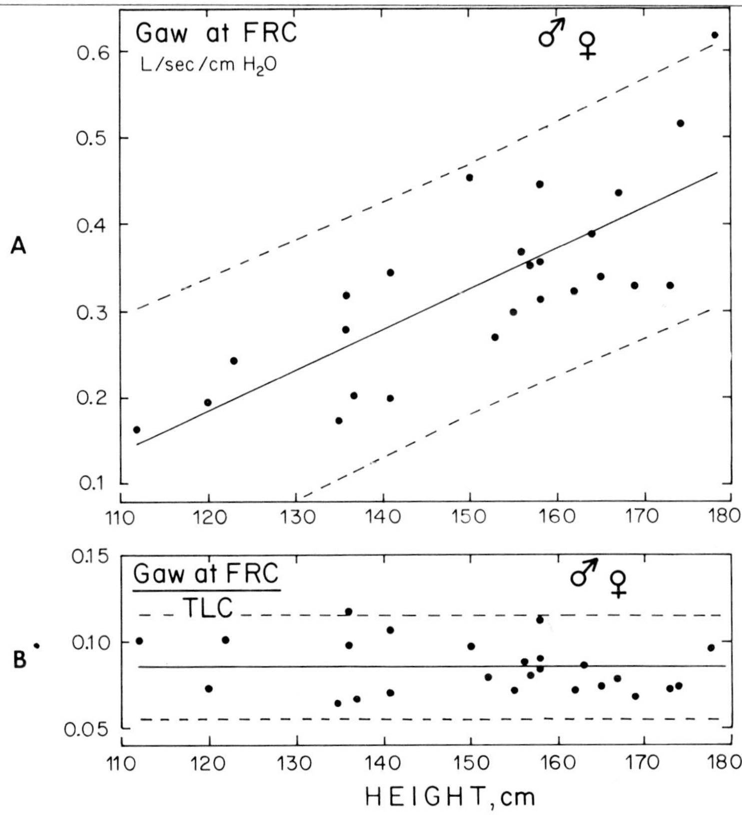

Fig. 1-11. *A*. Airway conductance at FRC versus standing height. *B*. Same data with conductance in TLC per second per cm H_2O. Regression lines and 95% confidence limits as in Fig. 1–10; Gaw at FRC = −0.3819 + 0.00472×height (cm). Age range 6–18 yrs. Data from reference 82.

Table 1-4
Anatomical Dead Space in Children

Body Height (cm)	V_D * (liters)	TLC (liters) † M	TLC (liters) † F	$\frac{V_D}{TLC} \times 100$ M	$\frac{V_D}{TLC} \times 100$ F
125	0.068	2.4	2.2	2.83	3.09
150	0.105	3.6	3.4	2.92	3.09
175	0.150	6.0	5.0	2.50	3.00

* Average data of Hart et al.;[37] data for both sexes were pooled since they did not differ significantly.

† Average data of Zapletal et al.[82] for males and females.

version of the adult pattern and . . . this . . . persists during postnatal growth." Thus, isotropic growth appears to be the rule throughout the bronchial tree.

Applications

The data in the preceding paragraphs simplify the interpretation of mechanical tests of lung function in children in the age range suitable for this type of measurement. Since airway conductance and maximum expiratory flow rates are proportional to TLC, one can distinguish between the effects of growth and of disease on lung mechanics. This should be especially helpful in longitudinal studies of children throughout their growth periods. TLC is an easily measured value related to overall growth of the lungs and chest cage. Therefore, it seems a better standard for comparison than body height, since the latter does not directly reflect chest and lung growth. These concepts have been applied in clinical studies of lung function in children with asthma and cystic fibrosis.[80]

Even a simple visual inspection of MEFV curves yields valuable information. The curves in Figure 1-9 are typical of those found in children and adolescents. In children with lung disease or in those who regularly smoke cigarettes, MEFV curves are shaped differently (Chap. 9). In healthy children, the MEFV curve can be used to predict certain performance limits during exercise and other activities. For instance, maximum flow rates required for playing wind instruments (Chap. 11) can be up to 2 liters/sec. A small boy (Fig. 1-9*A*, lowest curve) can achieve such a flow rate only over a volume range of about 0.8 liters. That is, he can maintain a tone on a horn that requires a flow of 2 liters/sec for only 0.4 seconds at the most. With such a physiological handicap, it is amazing that so many small children do well in compositions written for people with lungs like those that, in Figure 1-9, provided the top MEFV curve!

EXOGENOUS FACTORS IN LUNG DEVELOPMENT

Several recent studies suggest that environmental factors can influence lung growth. We already discussed the effect of corticosteroid hormone on surfactant development (p. 10). Bartlett[7] found that lung development was impaired in young rats kept in a hyperoxic environment (46.8 percent oxygen) for 2 weeks. This was probably due to a local effect of oxygen. In experiments with young rats kept for about 3 weeks at simulated high altitude (inspired O_2 tension 95 mm Hg), morphometric data obtained independently by two groups of investigators [8, 20] showed a significant increase in alveolar surface area. Mean alveolar diameter remained unchanged,[8] and calculated diffusion capacity increased.[20] This apparently useful adaptation of lung growth to a hypoxic environment is not a result of hyperventilation; rats kept for 3 weeks in 5 percent CO_2 in air were unaffected.[8]

Exercise (for 20 days at sea level) did not influence lung growth of rats significantly,[6] and treatment with thiouracil or thyroxin to decrease or increase, respectively, metabolic rates also had no effect.[6]

Even adult rats are capable of increasing lung weight and alveolar surface area when subjected to hypoxia.[23] Their alveoli and alveolar ducts increase in size but not in number; in hypoxic immature rats both number and size of alveoli and alveolar ducts increase.[23] There is some evidence that lung growth may be enhanced in humans at high altitude. High-altitude natives as well as persons who moved to high altitude (3400–3840 m) at an early age have significantly larger (approx. 10%) vital capacities (adjusted for age, height, and weight) than sea-level residents and persons acclimatized to altitude later in life.[32]

When one lung is surgically removed, because of disease in man or experimentally in animals, the remaining lung undergoes compensatory growth. This process is more effective in immature rats than in adult ones. In the young animal, proliferation of alveoli may occur near the pleural surface,[48] and the alveoli increase considerably in size.[18] In the adult rat, only a moderate increase in alveolar size occurs and hence alveolar surface area increases less during compensatory growth than it does in the immature rat.

How compensatory lung growth after removal of one lung is stimulated is unknown. Hypoxemia after surgery is at best a minor contributing factor;[48] increased mechanical stress upon the remaining lung may be more important. But humoral factors other than hypoxemia may be crucial. For instance, when the left lung is removed in pregnant rats, the weight of the lungs of their fetuses increases 20–40%, and these fetal lungs then contain 3–4 times as many mitoses as control fetal lungs.[58] This response of the fetal lung occurs within five days after pneumonectomy in the mother, a time course similar to that of the compensatory growth response in immature and adult rats.[18] Growth hormone increases the post-pneumonectomy growth response in adult rats, while excision of the hypophysis prior to lung excision inhibits compensatory growth.[16] In man, acromegaly is associated with increased lung size.[17] Besides growth hormone, tissue-specific inhibitors of mitosis (chalones) may be involved in regulating compensatory lung growth.[48]

SUMMARY

During intrauterine development, the lungs go through a pseudoglandular, a canalicular, and finally a terminal sac period. Most alveoli are formed after birth, partly by segmentation of existing alveolar units, partly by fragmentation of terminal bronchioles. New alveoli continue to form at least until the age of about 8 years, and some alveolar formation may continue in the teens.

The newborn infant's lungs may collapse and he may develop the respiratory distress syndrome if birth occurs prematurely, before sufficient surfactant material is formed. Surfactant, which is mainly composed of surface-active phospholipids, may be synthesized by alveolar type II epithelial cells and is secreted to form an alveolar surface lining that decreases surface tension at the air-liquid interface. Surfactant begins to form during the last weeks of prenatal development, and recent work indicates that corticosteroids and other drugs can accelerate this process.

Airway smooth muscle is well developed at birth and is supplied with functional vagal and sympathetic nerve fibers (in animals). During postnatal development, these fibers increase in size and become better able to conduct high-frequency impulses. Somatic nerve fibers undergo a similar postnatal development. Maturation of somatic fibers may be a prerequisite for the development of motor control of breathing; the functional importance of autonomic nerve fiber maturation is less clear.

As children grow, their chest cages and lungs become larger. Total lung capacity, vital capacity, and maximum expiratory flow rates increase, while airflow resistance in the bronchi decreases. During growth maximum flow rates and airway conductance increase in proportion to the total lung capacity, so that the ratios MEF/TLC and Gaw/TLC are constant at any relative lung volume (in percentage TLC). This facilitates the interpretation of lung-function tests in growing children. Static lung recoil pressure increases in young children. Lung-function data support the hypothesis that the lungs and airways as a whole grow isotropically, and morphological studies have confirmed this view. The lungs of rats kept at high altitudes grow faster and have a larger gas exchange surface area than those of rats kept at sea level, and this adaptive mechanism may also operate in children born and raised at high altitudes. Compensatory lung growth, probably under control of humoral factors, occurs at any age within one week after surgical removal of one lung in rats.

REFERENCES

1. Adolph EF: Ranges of heart rates and their regulations at various ages (rat). Am J Physiol 212:595–602, 1967
2. Anrep B von: Ueber die entwicklung hemmenden Funktionen bei Neugeborenen. Arch Ges Physiol 21:78–80, 1880
3. Avery ME: Pharmacological approaches to the acceleration of fetal lung maturation. Brit Med Bull 31:13–17, 1975
4. Avery ME, Wang NS, Taeusch HW Jr: The lung of the newborn infant. Sci Am 228: 74–85, 1973
5. Ballard PL, Ballard RA: Cytoplasmic receptor for glucocorticoids in lung of the human fetus and neonate. J Clin Invest 53:477–486, 1974
6. Bartlett D Jr: Postnatal growth of the mammalian lung: influence of exercise and thyroid activity. Respir Physiol 9: 50–57, 1970
7. Bartlett D Jr: Postnatal growth of the mammalian lung: influence of low and high oxygen tensions. Respir Physiol 9: 58–64, 1970
8. Bartlett D Jr, Remmers JE: Effects of high altitude exposure on the lungs of young rats. Respir Physiol 13:116–125, 1971
9. Bartlett D Jr: Postnatal growth of the

mammalian lung: influence of excess growth hormone. Respir Physiol 12:297–304, 1971

10. Bartlett D Jr: Postnatal development of the mammalian lung, in Goss RJ (ed): Regulation of Organ and Tissue Growth. New York, Academic Press, 1972, pp 197–209
11. Boren HG, Kory RC, Syner JC: The Veterans-Administration-Army cooperative study of pulmonary function. II. The lung volume and its subdivisions in normal men. Am J Med 41:96–114, 1966
12. Bouhuys A, Jonson B: Alveolar pressure, airflow rate, and lung inflation in man. J Appl Physiol 22:1086–1100, 1967
13. Boyd E: Outline of physical growth and development. Minneapolis, Burgess, 1942
14. Boyden EA: The pattern of the terminal air spaces in a premature infant of 30–32 weeks that lived nineteen and a quarter hours. Am J Anat 126:31–40, 1969
15. Boyden EA, Tompsett DH: The postnatal growth of the lung in the dog. Acta Anat (Basel) 47:185–215, 1961
16. Brody JS, Buhain WJ: Hormonal influence on post-pneumonectomy lung growth in the rat. Respir Physiol 19: 344–355, 1973
17. Brody JS, Fisher AB, Gocmen A, DuBois AB: Acromegalic pneumonomegaly: lung growth in the adult. J Clin Invest 49:1051–1060, 1970
18. Buhain WJ, Brody JS: Compensatory growth of the lung following pneumonectomy. J Appl Physiol 35:898–902, 1973
19. Burri PH: The postnatal growth of the rat lung. III. Morphology. Anat Rec 180:77–98, 1974
20. Burri PH, Weibel ER: Estimation de paramètres fonctionnels du poumon par morphométrie: Adaptation du poumon en croissance au taux d'oxygène dans l'air ambiant. Bull Physiopathol Respir (Nancy) 6:495–499, 1970
21. Clements JA: Comparative lipid chemistry of lungs. Arch Intern Med 127: 387–390, 1971
22. Cotes JE, Dabbs JM, Hall AM, Axford AT, Laurence KM: Lung volumes, ventilatory capacity, and transfer factor in healthy British boy and girl twins. Thorax 28:709–715, 1973
23. Cunningham EL, Brody JS, Jain BP: Lung growth induced by hypoxia. J Appl Physiol 37:362–366, 1974
24. Davies G, Reid L: Growth of the alveoli and pulmonary arteries in childhood. Thorax 25:669–681, 1970
25. De Reuck AVS, Porter R (eds): Development of the Lung, Ciba Foundation Symposium. Boston, Little, Brown & Co, 1967
26. Downing SE: Baroreceptor reflexes in newborn rabbits. J Physiol (Lond) 150: 201–213, 1960
27. Dunnill MS: Postnatal growth of the lung. Thorax 17:329–333, 1962
28. Ekholm J: Postnatal changes in cutaneous reflexes and in the discharge pattern of cutaneous and articular sense organs. A morphological and physiological study in the cat. Acta Physiol Scand (Suppl) 297:1–130, 1967
29. Emery J (ed): The Anatomy of the Developing Lung. London, William Heineman Medical Books, 1969
30. Emery JL, Wilcock PF: The post-natal development of the lung. Acta Anat (Basel) 65:10–29, 1966
31. Friedman WF, Pool PE, Jacobowitz D, Seagrens C, Braunwald E: Sympathetic innervation of the developing rabbit heart. Biochemical and histochemical comparisons of fetal, neonatal, and adult myocardium. Circ Res 23:25–32, 1968
32. Frisancho AR, Velásquez T, Sanchez J: Influence of developmental adaptation on lung function at high altitude. Human Biol 45:583–594, 1973
33. Gil J: Ultrastructure of lung fixed under physiologically defined conditions. Arch Intern Med 127:896–902, 1971
34. Goerke J: Lung surfactant. Biochim Biophys Acta 344:241–261, 1974
35. Gregory GA, Kitterman JA, Phibbs RH, Tooley WH, Hamilton WK: Treatment of the idiopathic respiratory-distress syndrome with continuous positive airway pressure. N Engl J Med 284:1333–1340, 1971
36. Gross I, Warshaw JB: Enzyme activities related to fatty acid synthesis in developing mammalian lung. Pediatr Res 8:193–199, 1974
37. Hart MC, Orzalesi MM, Cook CD: Relation between anatomic respiratory dead space and body size and lung volume. J Appl Physiol 18:519–522, 1963
38. Hislop A, Muir DCF, Jacobsen M, Simon G, Reid L: Postnatal growth and function of the pre-acinar airways.

Thorax 27:265–274, 1972
39. Hislop A, Reid L: Development of the acinus in the human lung. Thorax 29: 90–94, 1974
40. Horie T, Hildebrandt J: Dynamic compliance, limit cycles, and static equilibria of excised cat lung. J Appl Physiol 31: 423–430, 1971
41. Huttenlocher PR: Functional properties of pyramidal neurons during development of cerebral cortex in the kitten. Fed Proc 28:825, 1969
42. Kikkawa Y, Motoyama EK: Effect of AY-9944, a cholesterol biosynthesis inhibitor, on fetal lung development and on the development of Type II alveolar epithelial cells. Lab Invest 28:48–54, 1973
43. Kikkawa Y, Motoyama EK, Cook CD: The ultrastructure of the lungs of lambs. Am J Pathol 47:877–903, 1965
44. King RJ, Clements JA: Surface active materials from dog lung. I. Method of isolation; II. Composition and physiological correlations; III. Thermal analysis. Am J Physiol 223:707–733, 1972
45. Kotas RV, Avery ME: Accelerated appearance of pulmonary surfactant in the fetal rabbit. J Appl Physiol 30:358–361, 1971
46. Motoyama EK, Orzalesi MM, Kikkawa Y, Kaibara M, Wu B, Zigas CJ, Cook CD: Effect of cortisol on the maturation of fetal rabbit lungs. Pediatrics 48:547–555, 1971
47. Nasr K, Heinemann HO: Lipid synthesis by rabbit lung tissue in vitro. Am J Physiol 208:118–121, 1965
48. Nattie EE, Wiley CW, Bartlett D Jr: Adaptive growth of the lung following pneumonectomy in rats. J Appl Physiol 37:491–495, 1974
49. Neergaard K von: Neue Auffassungen ueber einen Grundbegriff der Atemmechanik. Z Ges Exper Med 66:373–394, 1929
50. Normand ICS, Reynolds EOR, Strang LB: Passage of macromolecules between alveolar and interstitial spaces in foetal and newly ventilated lungs of the lamb. J Physiol (Lond) 210:151–164, 1970
51. Orzalesi MM, Motoyama EK, Jacobson HN, Kikkawa Y, Reynolds EOR, Cook CD: The development of the lungs of lambs. Pediatrics 35:373–381, 1965
52. Page-Roberts BA: Preparation and partial characterization of a lamellar body fraction from rat lung. Biochim Biophys Acta 260:334–338, 1972
53. Pattle RE: Surface lining of lung alveoli. Physiol Rev 45:48–79, 1965
54. Pattle RE, Gandy G, Schock C, Creasey JM: Lung inclusion bodies: different ultrastructure in simian and non-simian mammals. Experientia 30:797–798, 1974
55. Polgar G, Promadhat V: Pulmonary Function Testing in Children: Techniques and Standards. Philadelphia, WB Saunders Co Inc, 1971
56. Reid L, Simon G: The role of alveolar hypoplasia in some types of emphysema. Br J Dis Chest 58:158–168, 1964
57. Reynolds EOR, Jacobson HN, Motoyama EK, Kikkawa Y, Craig JM, Orzalesi MM, Cook CD: The effect of immaturity and prenatal asphyxia on the lungs and pulmonary function of newborn lambs: the experimental production of respiratory distress. Pediatrics 35:382–392, 1965
58. Romanova LK, Zhikhareva IA: On the humoral regulation of restorative growth in the lungs, kidneys and liver [in Russian, English summary]. Biull Eksp Biol Med 73(1):84–87, 1972
59. Rooney SA, Canavan PM, Motoyama EK: The identification of phosphatidylglycerol in the rat, rabbit, monkey and human lung. Biochim Biophys Acta 360:56–67, 1974
60. Rooney SA, Page-Roberts BA, Motoyama EK: Role of lamellar inclusions in surfactant production: studies on phospholipid composition and biosynthesis in rat and rabbit lung subcellular fractions. J Lipid Res 16:418–425, 1975
61. Rosan RC, Lauweryns JM: Mucosal cells of the small bronchioles of prematurely born human infants (600–1700 g). Beitr Pathol 147:145–174, 1972
62. Scarpelli EM, Colacicco G, Chang SJ: Significance of methods for isolation and characterization of pulmonary surfactants. Respir Physiol 12:179–198, 1971
63. Schwieler GH: Respiratory regulation during postnatal development in cats and rabbits, and some of its morphological substrate. Acta Physiol Scand (Suppl) 304:1–120, 1968
64. Schwieler GH, Douglas JS, Bouhuys A: Postnatal development of autonomic efferent innervation in the rabbit. Am J

Physiol 219:391–397, 1970
65. Schwieler GH, Skoglund S: Individual variations in the bronchial tree in cats of different ages with special reference to the post-natal development. Acta Anat (Basel) 56:70–78, 1964
66. Seely JB, Guzman CA, Becklake MR: Heart and lung function at rest and during exercise in adolescence. J Appl Physiol 36:34–40, 1974
67. Shepard FM, Johnston RB Jr, Klatte EC, Burko H, Stahlman M: Residual pulmonary findings in clinical hyaline-membrane disease. N Engl J Med 279: 1063–1071, 1968
68. Skoglund S: The activity of muscle receptors in the kitten. Acta Physiol Scand 50:203–221, 1960
69. Skoglund S, Romero C: Postnatal growth of spinal nerves and roots. A morphological study in the cat with physiological correlations. Acta Physiol Scand 66 (Suppl) 260:1–50, 1965
70. Staub NC: The interdependence of pulmonary structure and function. Anesthesiology 24:831–854, 1963
71. Taylor IM, Smith RB: Intrinsic innervation of the human foetal lung between the 35 and 140 mm crown-rump length stages. Biol Neonate 18:193–202, 1971
72. Tierney DF: Lung metabolism and biochemistry. Annu Rev Physiol 36:209–231, 1974
73. Weibel ER: Morphological basis of alveolar-capillary gas exchange. Physiol Rev 53:419–495, 1973
74. Wekstein DR: Heart rate of the preweanling rat and its autonomic control. Am J Physiol 208:1259–1262, 1965
75. Widdicombe JG: Action potentials in parasympathetic and sympathetic efferent fibres to the trachea and lungs of dogs and cats. J Physiol (Lond) 186:56–88, 1966
76. Wu B, Kikkawa Y, Orzalesi MM, Motoyama EK, Kaibara M, Zigas CJ, Cook CD: The effect of thyroxine on the maturation of fetal rabbit lungs. Biol Neonate 22:161–168, 1973
77. Yamauchi A, Burnstock G: Development of smooth muscle. J Anat 104:1–15, 1969
78. Yamauchi A, Burnstock G: Post-natal development of the innervation of the mouse vas deferens. A fine structural study. J Anat 104:17–32, 1969
79. Zapletal A, Misur M, Samanek M: Static recoil pressure of the lungs in children. Bull Physiopathol Respir (Nancy) 7:139–143, 1971
80. Zapletal A, Motoyama EK, Gibson LE, Bouhuys A: Pulmonary mechanics in asthma and cystic fibrosis. Pediatrics 48:64–72, 1971
81. Zapletal A, Motoyama EK, van de Woestijne KP, Gibson LE, Bouhuys A: Use of the body plethysmography in children. Prog Respir Res 4:228–235, 1969
82. Zapletal A, Motoyama EK, van de Woestijne KP, Hunt VR, Bouhuys A: Maximum expiratory flow-volume curves and airway conductance in children and adolescents. J Appl Physiol 26:308–316, 1969

Chapter 2

Conducting Airways

The main purpose of the airways that lead from the atmosphere to the alveoli is to conduct inspired air to the gas-exchanging surfaces and to eliminate expired air. In addition, they have other important functions—warming and humidifying air, removing aerosol particles and soluble gases from inspired air, producing voice sounds, and chemically monitoring inspired air. The latter depends on special receptors for the sense of smell, while the air-conditioning functions depend on the mucosal surface area, the nature of airflow over it, and the properties of its mucus. The voice function makes more subtle demands on upper airway function to generate and to articulate speech sounds. This task, the essence of human communication, is associated with important changes in the shape and structure of the upper airways during man's evolution (Chap. 11).

UPPER AIRWAYS

Nose

During quiet breathing, a healthy person breathes through the nose. Although its volume is only about 20 ml, folds make the mucosal surface area large—about 160 cm^2 (Fig. 2-1)—rendering the nose an effective air-conditioning device. Unless it is first passed through the nose, dry air damages the mucosa of airways; for patients who must breathe through a tracheostomy tube, special air-conditioning devices prevent drying and crust formation in the trachea ("artificial nose").[27, 60] The effectiveness of air conditioning in the upper airways is apparent, for instance, in experiments with dogs exposed to inspired air at −40°C and at +40°C during normal breathing.[2] Just below the larynx, inspired air was fully saturated with water vapor and had reached body temperature (37°C), regardless of the inspired air temperature.

A man who inspires dry air at 0°C must evaporate about 420 gm water per 24 hours to saturate all inspired air with water vapor. Since this requires about

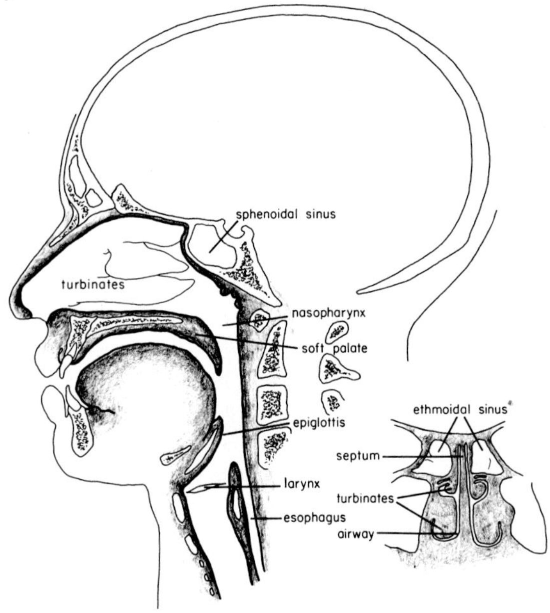

Fig. 2-1. Sagittal section through the human head to show anatomical relations in the upper airways. *Inset.* A transverse section through the nose shows how mucosal folds (turbinates) narrow the airway passage and provide a large surface area for heat and water exchange. From reference 42.

2200 calories/24 hr, he would use nearly all of his metabolic heat production merely to warm and humidify the air he inspired. Clearly, protective mechanisms prevent this—much of the added heat and water are recovered on expiration. Cold inspired air cools the nasal mucosa, and the expired air meets a cool mucosa on its return. Hence, expired air cools when it reaches the front portion of the nose, and water condenses on the mucosa. This water is available for evaporation during the next inspiration of cold air. Any excess water on the mucosal surface causes the "runny nose" when one is out in the cold. With this type of countercurrent heat exchange mechanism,[54] the nose recovers water and calories from the expired air before they are lost to the atmosphere. In contrast, when the inspired air is warm, the mucosa remains warm during inspiration, and the expired air leaves the nose at a temperature of 37°C, saturated with water vapor. Thus, the upper airways contribute to heat loss when we are in a warm environment.

To facilitate air conditioning, then, it makes sense to breathe through the nose. But the anatomy that enables the nose to be effective for this purpose—narrow passages between well-vascularized mucosal folds—creates a high resistance to airflow. Just as in our houses, effective air conditioning requires energy. The nose's resistance to airflow is about twice that of the mouth (Chap. 8), and during quiet breathing, the nasal passages contribute nearly half the total flow resistance. We normally prefer to accept the extra work that breathing through the nose requires, only switching to mouth breathing during talking, sighing, and exercise. The control mechanisms that determine the choice of mouth or nose breathing are not clear. Opening the mouth is a part of the act of talking or sighing. I doubt whether it can be explained in terms of flow rate increases or some other local mechanical event, since it does not seem to follow but rather to anticipate these events. We may have learned mouth breathing during exercise simply because we discovered it was easier during hard work. Subjectively, the decreased effort during mouth breathing is obvious whenever we breathe at increased frequency and at high flow rates. Very little air passes through the nose when we breathe through the mouth, because of the nose's high resistance in contrast to the low resistance of the oral cavity. In newborn infants, the morphology of the nasal and oral passages suggests that the reverse is true; the obligate nose breathing of infants may be due to a lower nasal flow resistance.[36]

Linear air velocities in the nose are not uniform and may reach high values in certain areas even when total flow rates are moderate.[43] The highest velocities occur in the anterior part of the middle meatus. High velocities during inspiration lead to partial collapse of the alae nasi and may, along with accompanying sensations, trigger the switch to mouth breathing.

Pharynx

Well-known accidents can occur at this crossroad, with food, liquid, or air taking inappropriate directions (Fig. 2-1). Fenn[13] wondered about the possible advantages of this curious design. Why should we have a crossing of food and air passages at all? One answer may be structural economy—the tongue helps to process food, to speak, and to condition air somewhat during mouth breathing. In primates and other mammals, the pharynx is much less developed than in man,[29] and the epiglottis and larynx are much closer to the nasopharynx. Thus, the dangers of food and liquid running into the airway are much less in animals than they are in man. The pharynx is essential for articulated speech (Chap. 11), and perhaps the disadvantages of the human design are simply accidental to its advantages for communication.

The crossing of food and air allows interaction between the senses of taste and smell. Of the two, smell is more sensitive, and although some of its survival function has been lost during man's evolution, it retains great psychological importance. It leaves long-term memory imprints, as those immortalized by Proust's description of the smell of madeleines dipped in tea.[44] Proctor[43] has observed that the nasal sensors are placed outside the mainstream of the inspired air, so that they are not really in a good position to sample the air. This may be another design disadvantage that man incurred when his upper airways adapted to speech.

Swallowing

Bosma[4] has reviewed the pharyngeal stages of deglutition. Triggered by the arrival of a food bolus at the back of the mouth, a fixed sequence of movements, lasting 0.3–0.5 seconds, passes the bolus from the mouth to the esophagus. The tongue brings the bolus into the middle part of the pharynx (oropharynx), while the palate prevents it from entering the nasopharynx. While the bolus passes over the epiglottis, swallowing begins with a headward movement of the pharynx, accompanied by upward motion of the hyoid bone and its attachments, including the larynx. During this time, the epiglottis curves down over the airway, and breathing is momentarily interrupted. As the pharyngeal sphincter muscle propels the food bolus downward, the hypopharyngeal sphincter muscle at the entrance of the esophagus relaxes. This allows food to enter the esophagus; at all other times, the hypopharyngeal sphincter is tightly closed, preventing air from entering the esophagus, where—as elsewhere in the chest cage—pressure is normally less than atmospheric.

The nervous control of swallowing is closely linked with that of breathing. During a swallow, breathing is interrupted, and every swallow is followed by an expiration. In newborn infants, swallowing, suckling, and breathing follow in a fixed sequence.[4] Swallowing is a good example of a motor act in which an obligatory series of motor events can be triggered voluntarily or by reflex. It fits the concept of a programmed motor act (Chap. 11). Bosma[4] stresses its all-or-nothing character, independent of afferent modification. Much training, not always successful, is required to teach laryngectomized patients to use their hypopharyngeal sphincter in a quite different way, namely, as a substitute larynx (esophageal speech[11]).

Larynx

The larynx acts as a valve that prevents food or liquid from entering the trachea. It is also a major obstacle for the respiratory physiologist: since the larynx is a major site of flow resistance during breathing, it complicates the measurement of lower airway resistance. The use of the larynx during phonation and speech is discussed elsewhere (Chap. 11). One component of the larynx, the cricoid cartilage, located at the upper end of the trachea, has special importance during breathing. The only complete cartilaginous ring around the trachea, the cricoid cartilage alone can keep the trachea open during forced inspirations, when the pressures inside the trachea are less than atmospheric. Without the tethering function of the cricoid cartilage, the trachea would be much more subject to dynamic compression during forced inspirations.

The glottal opening is larger in men than in women, and, as a consequence, unilateral paralysis of a vocal fold causes more respiratory embarrassment in women than in men. Schiratzki[53] documented this with measurements of subglottic pressure and upper airway resistance. In patients with vocal fold paralysis, lung volume and forced expiratory volumes ($FEV_{1.0}$; Chap. 9) are often normal, while maximum voluntary ventilation (MVV) may be low.[53] This is one of the rather rare instances where the MVV test, which requires the subject to breathe in and out as deep as possible and at a high rate of breathing, detects an abnormal condition that may not be revealed by the $FEV_{1.0}$ and other tests based on single expirations. There appear to be no reports on visual observations of paralyzed vocal folds during maximum voluntary ventilation maneuvers. One suspects that the passive to-and-fro movements of the paralyzed fold, "in the wind" as it were, create much extra energy loss and increase laryngeal resistance.

THE BRONCHIAL TREE

Morphology of Branches

Table 2-1 gives names, numbers, and dimensions of the trachea and its branches. Figure 2-2 illustrates the main features of large conducting airways (*A*) and of the transition between conducting and gas-exchanging airways in terminal lung units (*B*). Illustrations of airway morphology are available elsewhere.[20, 56] To correlate form and function, quantitative morphological data are a prerequisite; this "morphometric" approach to the study of lung structure was introduced by Weibel and Gomez.[63] The quantitative data thus obtained can be used to develop concepts or models of lung morphology that clarify lung and airway physiology. The first of these is Weibel's model (Fig. 2-3).[62]

The first generations of the bronchi are named after easily recognized parts of the lungs with surface landmarks—lobes and segments. Subsequent generations decrease in size and gradually lose the cartilaginous support in their walls as they branch further. The last generation of "small bronchi" contains little cartilage. The next several generations are given a distinct name, bronchioles; they are distinguished from bronchi by the absence of cartilage. Yet further along, alveoli appear in the walls; because of their participation in gas exchange, these airways are called respiratory bronchioles. The walls of the airways become more and more studded with alveoli, until nothing remains of their walls but the septa between alveoli (Fig. 1-3); the bronchioles have then become alveolar ducts. These branch through a few more generations of decreasing length and terminate in the alveoli. The average total pathway length from the cricoid cartilage to the alveoli is about 24 cm, half of which is the length of the trachea; individual pathway lengths vary considerably. Ross documented this for the dog lung.[51]

In Weibel's model, each airway that branches is assumed to divide into two equivalent branches (*regular dichotomy.*) Weibel also described another model,[62] based on the assumption of *irregular dichotomy,* but this has not been as widely used. Parker et al.[40] found dichotomous branching in small but not in larger airways. The problem of defining the type of branching is illustrated in the diagrams of Figure 2-4, which express the same bronchial tree two different ways. One model (*B*) considers all branching points as Y junctions leading into two equivalent branches. The other (*A*) considers them as T junctions: the smaller branch is a minor sidebranch, the other continues as the main stem of the T. As models, these two concepts differ importantly. Which one is more realistic depends on precise measurements of branching angles at the junctions and of all branch diameters. Since lung volume affects airway diameters and branching angles, one's choice of model might differ depending on lung inflation.

Several quantitative observations confirm the general validity of the regular dichotomy model introduced by Weibel.[62] Parker et al.[40] counted alveoli and alveolar ducts in one lobule, about 0.34 ml of inflated human lung tissue, and found an average of 13 alveoli per alveolar duct or sac. Weibel estimated the total number of alveoli at 300×10^6; with the data of Parker et al., this gives a total of $300/13 = 23 \times 10^6$ alveolar sacs and ducts (16×10^6 in generations 19–23 of Weibel's model). Horsfield and Cumming[22] found 224×10^3 most distal respira-

Table 2–1
The Bronchial Tree

Generation	Name	Diameter † (cm)	Length † (cm)	Total Cross Section † (cm^2)	Number per Generation †	Small Airway Counts
0	Trachea	1.8	12.0	2.54	1	
1	Main bronchi	1.22	4.76	2.33	2	
2	Lobar bronchi	0.83	1.90	2.13	4	
3	Segmental bronchi	0.56	0.76	2.00	8	
4	Subsegmental bronchi	0.45	1.27	2.48	16	
5		0.35	1.07	3.11	32	
thru	Small bronchi					
10		0.13	0.46	13.4	1.02×10^3	
11		0.109	0.39	19.6	2.05×10^3	
thru	Bronchioles					
13		0.082	0.27	44.5	8.19×10^3	7.6×10^3 §
14		0.074	0.23	69.4	16.38×10^3	13.4×10^3 §
&	Terminal bronchioles					
15		0.066	0.20	113.0	32.77×10^3	24.8×10^3 §
16		0.060	0.165	180.0	65.54×10^3	51.6×10^3 §
thru	Respiratory bronchioles					
18		0.050	0.117	534.0	262.14×10^3	224×10^3 §
19		0.047	0.099	944.0	524.29×10^3	} 23×10^6 § (19 thru 23)
thru	Alveolar ducts					
23 *		0.041	0.050	11800.0	8.39×10^6	
24	Alveoli	244 μm ††	238 μm ††	43–80 m^2 ‖		300×10^6 ††

Nomenclature according to Staub.[56]
* 23rd generation also named alveolar sacs.
† Data from Weibel;[62] regular dichotomy model based on lungs inflated to 4.8 liters = 75% of TLC.
†† Average data from 5 normal lungs. (see pp. 61, 66 in ref. 62).
§ Data of Parker et al.[40] for alveolar ducts and generation 18; others derived from their counts of small airways in human lung lobule.
‖ Total alveolar surface area. (see p. 67 in ref. 62).

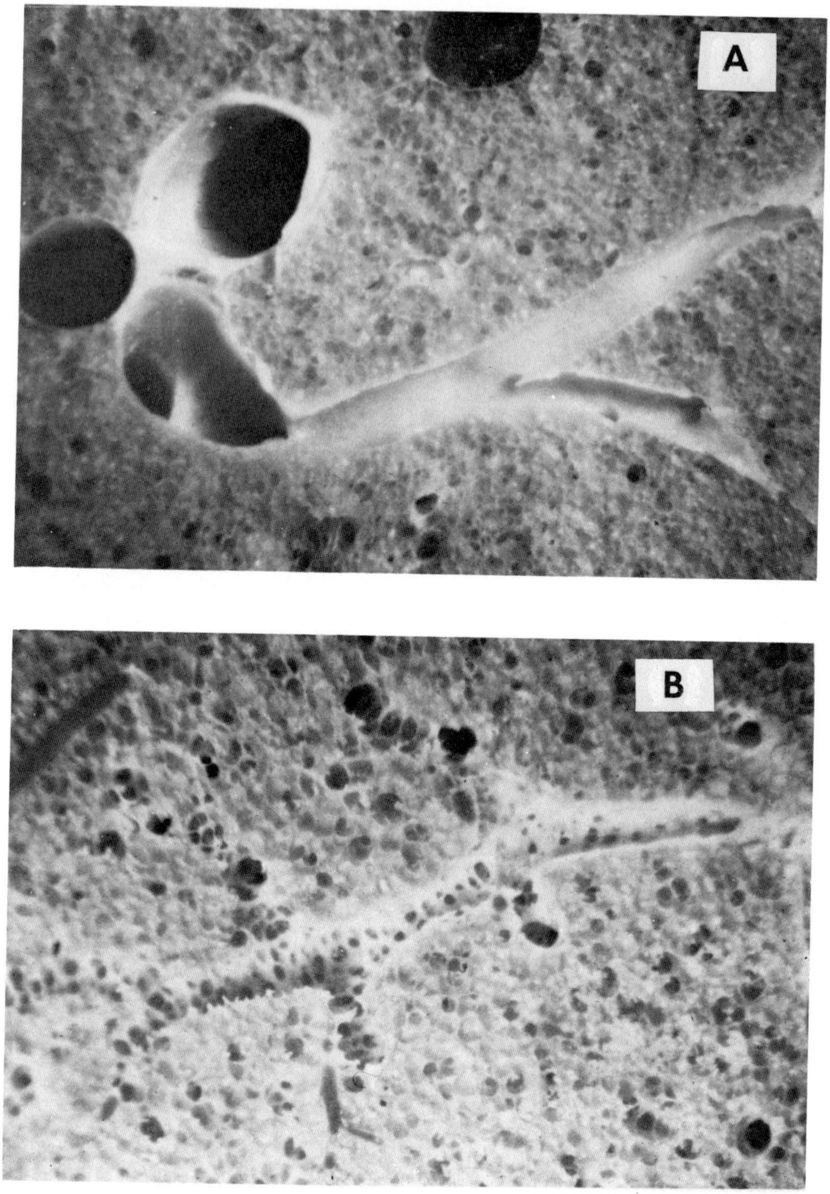

Fig. 2-2. Microscopic sections of rapidly frozen cat lungs, prepared by Staub. *A*. Segmental bronchus and branches. A small bronchus emerges from the lower branch and its longitudinal section shows another branching. The pulmonary artery is close to the airway (*left*); the pulmonary vein is at a distance from the airway (*top*). The airway branches are embedded in peripheral lung tissue. *B*. Transition of a terminal bronchiole with scattered alveoli in its wall (*upper right*) into more alveolated respiratory bronchioles and alveolar ducts, toward the left. The transition between conducting and gas-exchanging airways cannot be defined precisely. Reproduced with permission from teaching slides of Dr. Norman Staub (see also reference 56).

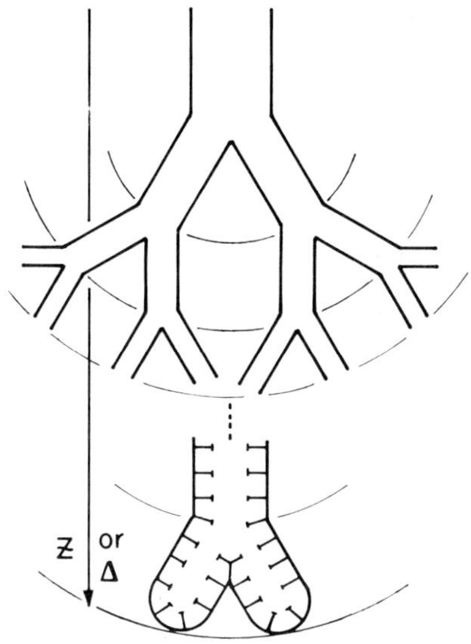

Fig. 2-3. Airway generations in the regular dichotomy model; z indicates length of pathway from entrance to trachea. Modified from Weibel.[62]

tory bronchioles (262 × 10^3 in Weibel's model). Estimates for the larger bronchioles (Table 2-1; last column) also reasonably agree with the regular dichotomy model.

Weibel's model has been criticized as "being based more on a mathematical concept than on direct observation."[40] Such criticism ignores the basic requirements of a good model—it must be based on facts, and it must summarize and

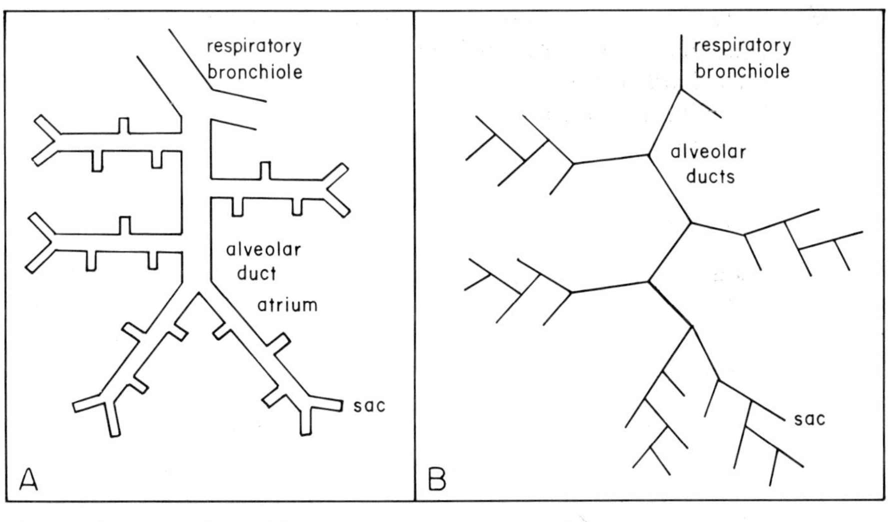

Fig. 2-4. The same branching pattern of the bronchial tree can be schematized in different diagrammatic models. Discussion in text. From Parker et al.[40]

simplify them in a mathematical concept. Since Weibel's model fits this definition, it is a useful representation of airway dimensions. Few physiologists, for instance, were aware of the tremendous increase in total cross-sectional area of the airway as one approaches the alveoli until Weibel's data brought this fact home. Although more data have become available since Weibel's book was published in 1962, these have as yet not led to an equally elegant and useful concept of bronchial tree structure. Other models, such as those of Figure 2-4, are more complex than Weibel's and seem to be about equally far removed from anatomic reality. They will supersede Weibel's model only if it can be shown that they better predict or describe important features of lung mechanics or gas exchange.

Physiological events are often described as occurring in "small" or "large" airways. This distinction is arbitrary, considering the wide range of airway sizes; the definition depends on one's purposes. Small bronchi are small in relation to other bronchi (generations 1-4; Table 2-1), but large in relation to bronchioles. Hence, cartilage may be a more useful factor than size in distinguishing large from small airways. Airways without cartilage (approximately 11th generation and smaller) would then be small airways, while all cartilaginous airways would be considered large. Among small airways, the bronchiolar walls have well-developed smooth muscle layers and no protection from cartilage. This definition of small airways may be useful in discussions of smooth muscle function. (see Chap. 8, p. 184) Other ways of dividing the bronchial tree into small and large airways are: (1) location downstream (large) or upstream (small) from an equal-pressure point in the airways;[34] (2) blood supply via bronchial (large) or pulmonary (small) blood vessels;[37] (3) dynamic compression during forced expiration occurs only in large and not in small airways;[5] and (4) small airways are those smaller than the airway in which a pressure-measuring catheter is lodged.[31] Each definition is useful in the context for which it was proposed—confusion results when definitions are used inappropriately. Accurate anatomical information on the site of events in airways during life may clarify some of these problems. It is unrealistic, however, to expect that more elaborate morphological studies will necessarily lead to better understanding of function. Morphological data are easily visualized but difficult to quantitate, while functional data are by nature quantitative and conceptual, but often hard to translate into concrete structural form. Thus, one encounters basic difficulties in correlating structural and morphological detail with physiological measurements and concepts.

The Walls of the Airways

Airway walls consist of epithelium, smooth muscle, cartilage, and glands in a framework of connective tissue.[18, 20, 55] The epithelium of the airways is composed of ciliated and goblet cells, together with columnar epithelial and basal cells (Fig. 2-5). In the bronchioles this pseudostratified epithelium is replaced by a simpler cuboidal cell epithelium with fewer goblet cells. Situated between the basal membrane of the epithelium and the cartilage of larger airways are seromucinous glands, ducts of which open onto the epithelial surface; these glands are absent in bronchioles. The smooth muscle network, arranged to allow changes of width as well as of length, discovered by Reisseisen, 1808,[39, 50] consists of transverse and longitudinal fibers. Only transverse fibers are found in deflated lungs, but this

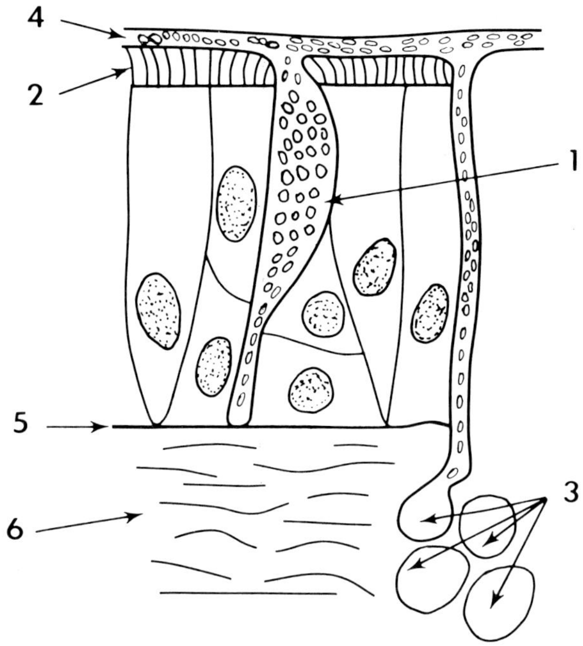

Fig. 2-5. The epithelial layer of the airways with a goblet cell (*1*), cilia (*2*), and a submucous gland (*3*). The cilia beat in the watery layer (sol phase) of the mucus; the mucous layer (gel phase) lies on top of the cilia (*4*). The epithelial layer is separated from the submucosal connective tissue (*6*) by the basement membrane (*5*). Schematic drawing, not to scale.

is an artifact.[32] In small bronchi the amount of smooth muscle increases, occupying the largest fraction of the wall thickness in the terminal bronchioles, where it becomes a conspicuous structure.[32] Nerve fibers, ganglia, and possible sensory elements in airway walls have been described.[28, 32] A dense network of adrenergic nerve fibers, identified by fluorescence labeling of catecholamine stores, is present in respiratory bronchioles of the cat.[7] Mast cells are found around airways and in the pleura of the human lung.[21] Secretory cells without cilia (Clara cells) occur in bronchioles, increasing in number towards the terminal bronchioles.[66] Their structure differs from that of goblet cells. The nature of their secretions is not certain; some believe they contribute toward the production of surfactant (see Chap. 1).

Glands and Goblet Cells

Both glands and goblet cells produce mucus, which coats the epithelial surface of the airways. The number of these structures along the bronchial tree varies greatly among different species and in the same animal. The rabbit, guinea pig, mouse, and hamster are poorly endowed, while the cat has more than man.[24, 48] The rat, which has more glands and goblet cells than most other small animals, responds to irritant exposure with hypertrophy of the glands as well as with development of goblet cells in bronchioles where normally there are none; its mucus-secreting system may be fairly similar to that of man.[48] In the epithelium of trachea and large bronchi, there is about one goblet cell for every five ciliated cells. The number of goblet cells decreases in smaller airways; bronchioles normally contain few or none at all. Although glands and goblet cells are absent, a thin fluid layer can be identified on the mucosal surface in terminal bronchioles if the lungs are fixed by perfusion through the blood vessels.[16] The origin of this fluid is not known.

The seromucinous glands contain some cells that mainly produce serous liquid and others that produce mucus. The nasal mucosa contains similar glands, and the serous cell type appears to be more predominant than it is in lower airways.[6] Mucous glands are commonly hypertrophied in asthma [23] and in chronic bronchitis.[6, 47, 59] As an index of gland hypertrophy, Reid [47] proposed measuring the gland's thickness as a proportion of the total thickness of the bronchial wall in the same airway section. However, this "Reid index" can be determined accurately only in large airways.[59] A Reid index of more than about 0.50 is commonly associated with chronic bronchitis, in which the gland hypertrophy is limited to the bronchial tree and does not involve the nasal mucous glands.[6] Mucous gland hypertrophy correlates well with smoking habits and is more pronounced in airways of people who have smoked much.[35] Smoking does not seem to affect the nasal mucosal glands.[6]

High concentrations (300–400 parts per million) of sulfur dioxide in air induced hypersecretion of mucus and, after several weeks' exposure, extensive glandular hypertrophy as well as development of goblet cells in bronchioles.[48] These changes occurred without evidence of infection. Other authors [35] have concluded that, in man, smoking is more important than infection in the development of mucous gland hypertrophy. Thus, airway infections in chronic bronchitis may often be secondary to such factors as smoking, which not only cause mucous gland hypertrophy but probably also damage the lungs' cleansing mechanisms. The effects of cigarette smoking on human mucous gland hypertrophy may be largely reversible, as evidenced by the disappearance of sputum production in many young people who stop smoking. In Reid's SO_2-exposed rats,[48] however, the effects of 4–6 weeks' exposure did not disappear in a subsequent period of three months without exposure.

Mucus production by glands and goblet cells, and the physical and chemical composition of their secretions, pose interesting problems that have received far less attention than they deserve. Since it is difficult to collect human bronchial secretions without eliciting increased mucus production in the airway, most studies with human material use sputum—a pathological product, an inconstant and heterogeneous mix of abnormal lower airway secretions, saliva, and other extraneous material from the nose and mouth. In recent years, however, histochemical studies together with biochemical measurements of components of mucus have provided some basic information.[65]

Goblet cells have a prominent Golgi apparatus where vacuoles are formed. In the upper part of the cell, vacuoles are transformed into mucous granules and are then discharged on the epithelial surface. A similar process occurs in the seromucinous glands, although they produce a mixture of serous and mucous liquid which is perhaps less viscous than the product of goblet cells. Mucus has so-called viscoelastic properties because it contains long-chain mucoproteins (molecular weight $>200,000$), partly in a fibrillar structure. The peptide skeleton of these chains is combined with mucopolysaccharides containing sulfate and sialic acid radicles. With histochemical methods, these radicles can be marked, and at least six different types of intracellular mucus—occurring in different proportions in goblet and gland cells [49]—can be distinguished. Radioactive-labeled sulfate is incorporated in serous gland cells as well as in goblet cells.[19] According to Reid, proximal goblet cells form more sulfated mucopolysaccharides, while sialic acid appears to be the predominant radicle in smaller airways.[48] Serum albumin and γA-immunoglobulins are the main plasma proteins present in bronchitic sputum as well as in fluid aspirated from lower airways in man.[33] It is not clear whether these proteins are secreted by glandular elements, but at least one other protein, lactoferrin, is.[33] In addition, nonpurulent human airway secretions contain lysozyme.[33]

A baffling question is how the total production of secretion is regulated, using different production sites, so that just enough material is available to coat the airways with a layer of mucus sufficient for protection and for mucociliary transport. The amount of mucus a healthy man produces is not known. Toremalm [61] estimated mucus production to be about 15–20 ml/24 hr in laryngectomized patients with a tracheostomy. The number of secretory cells per unit airway wall surface area is perhaps roughly constant throughout the bronchial tree, so that the amount of mucus produced would be proportional to the surface area to be covered if all cells produced mucus at a constant rate. But it seems unlikely that production is indeed constant. Vagal stimulation in the cat increases mucus flow considerably, while atropine inhibits this effect.[14] Increased secretion could also be elicited by reflex and, more directly, by irritants, the latter unaffected by vagotomy or by atropine.[14] Injected intravenously, pilocarpine increased secretion in the cat.[14] In a different type of experiment, Formijne et al.[15] found that isoproterenol inhibits the incorporation of labeled glucosamine into mucin formed in rat tracheal tissue in vitro. Such data suggest that the secretion of mucous liquid, as well as the formation of one important ingredient of mucus, can be influenced by autonomic mediating substances. Thus, there are potential mechanisms for changes in the amount and composition of mucus produced in the airways, as a function of physiological conditions.

The physical properties of mucus are essential for its protective function as a relatively impermeable cover of the epithelium, for its ability to trap foreign materials, and for its mode of transport by the cilia. This topic is discussed together with other aspects of mucociliary transport later in this chapter.

Cilia

The ciliated epithelium of the airways is the motor organ for transport of mucus and the cells and particles imbedded in it to the pharynx, where it is swallowed. Ciliated epithelium covers the airway mucosa from the larynx down to the terminal bronchioles. There are about 200 cilia on each ciliated cell, with a length of 5–7 μm.[52] Cilia move to and fro with a rapid stroke in the direction of the airway opening and a slow return beat in the opposite direction. In airways with mucus-secretory elements, the cilia move in thin fluid and are covered with a mucous layer. This two-phase liquid system (Fig. 2-5) is essential for mucociliary transport.

Iravani [25] developed an ingenious method to observe ciliary motion in intact small airways in rat lungs in vivo. The ciliary beat is arrhythmic, stroboscopic images are never steady, and some coordination of the beat exists between several adjacent cells. The rate increases from the periphery to the main bronchus, as well as near branches, where the wall surface area is reduced by the opening of the branch.[25] In a 0.2-mm diameter rat airway, beat frequency was 13/sec at 35° C, and 2/sec at 20° C;[25] in the rabbit trachea, 20/sec at 37° C, and 7/sec at 20° C.[17] Species, site, and temperature are the important variables. In addition, the amount of material to be transported probably regulates beat frequency.[25]

The Mucociliary Ladder

The concept that most of the conducting airways are covered with a continuous and coherent sheet of mucus, which normally moves constantly toward the pharynx, has led to use of the term mucociliary ladder for this protective transport mechanism. Cell debris, inhaled particles, and any other matter that gets trapped in the mucus sheet will eventually be removed from the lungs. The rate of this transport is subject to a large number of ill-understood variables. The rate of displacement of a particle or droplet placed on the mucosa provides information only on overall transport. Such data need interpretation in terms of the biological mechanisms that affect the ciliary beat or the amount and the quality of mucus.

Scanning electron micrographs have recently shown that, in the rat, respiratory mucus is present as distinct droplets and plaques rather than as a continuous layer.[67] This finding may explain, in part, why mucociliary transport rates show great variability (see below). If, in fact, large portions of the bronchial mucosa are normally not covered by mucus, the mucociliary ladder concept, as a physiological mechanism, may need rather fundamental revision.

The mucociliary ladder eliminates material once it is subject to the impact of ciliary motion. But in the last 50 μm of the terminal bronchioles of the rat, no ciliary motion occurs.[25] Other protective mechanisms, including phagocytosis (Chap. 12), take over at this level. Presumably, live phagocytes can reach the first rung of the mucociliary ladder by their own motion.

The amount and the physical qualities of bronchial mucus are crucial for mucociliary transport. Several physical scientists have studied the rheological properties, or flow characteristics, of mucus, and the results do not provide easy answers.[9, 10, 30, 45, 57] Everybody who has ever had a cold knows that the secretions of the nasal mucosa vary with the stage of that disease, from thin serous liquid to a sticky and tenacious mucus. A similar difference exists between the sol and gel phases of the mucous layer in the lower airways (Fig. 2-5). Mucus viscosity is a complex concept, since mucus does not follow simple linear stress-shear relations, as do such homogeneous liquids as water and oil. Layers of mucus do not follow a regular laminar flow pattern. In conformance with a property of plastic materials, a certain minimum stress must be exerted before mucus moves at all. Because of its long-chain mucoproteins, mucus can store some of the energy spent on it, so that it can recoil from stretch. Thus, mucus has plastic and elastic, as well as viscous, properties. The same long molecules make mucus into a coherent layer, continuous with the filaments that emerge from the glandular ducts. In physiological conditions, the ciliary beat exerts enough force on the mucus blanket, on top of the cilia, to keep the material moving and to break the filaments that connect the sheet to the glands. Since the ciliary beat is so rapid, the mucus layer has no time to recoil between beats. Therefore it keeps moving as a relatively rigid sheet of material.

It might be useful to express the physical properties of mucus in numbers. Unfortunately, owing to the heterogeneity of the material and its complex properties, no physically meaningful numbers can be measured. Many attempts have been made to measure sputum viscosity. Puchelle and Benis[45] compiled data for human sputum viscosity varying from 0.017 poises to 61×10^5 poises, a difference of some eight orders of magnitude. These numbers include effects of viscosity as well as contributions of plasticity, elasticity, and heterogeneity. Sputum viscosity measurements have not yet been of great help to the clinician. In theory, a very watery mucus would require little energy for transport, but gravity might make it accumulate in the alveoli. Tenacious mucus, on the other hand, is difficult to set in motion but once started it is likely to keep moving because of its elasticity and coherence. On arriving in large airways, this kind of mucus often bypasses mucociliary transport altogether; it acts as a foreign body and elicits cough. During lavage of the lungs, large amounts of mucus can be removed,[58] probably by eliminating air-mucus interfaces rather than by altering the physical properties of mucus per se. Between the extremes of watery mucus and tenacious sputum may be some optimal set of physical properties that best serves the purposes of mucociliary transport. The tolerance for variations around such optimal properties may be rather large; this would decrease the requirements for controlling the quality and quantity of the secretion products.

The rate of particle transport by the mucociliary ladder has been measured in different species. Kilburn has reported transport rates in the lung of the bullfrog,[26] and Baetjer[3] developed a quantitative method for measuring transport rates in the conveniently long necks of chicks in vivo under nearly physiological conditions. She deposited 1 μl of a ^{131}I-labeled solution on the mucosa through a small hole at the lower end of the trachea and followed its progress with two detectors placed 3.2 cm apart over the upper part of the trachea. Transport rates so measured varied from 7.4 to 17.9 mm/min. In man, a labeled inert particle can be placed on the nasal mucosa and its rate of displacement followed with external detectors.[1, 46] These methods produced variable results, even in the same subject during constant, controlled climatic conditions, with average rates from less than 0.10 to 23.6 mm/min in 58 subjects.[1] Often clearance was not continuous throughout the period of measurement, and, in localized areas on the mucosa, virtually no clearance was seen. Foreign materials might preferentially accumulate at such spots.

Mucociliary transport in the human bronchial tree can be studied only with indirect methods. The clearance of particles deposited on the mucosa by aerosol inhalation can be measured with external monitoring methods (Chap. 12). Qualitative observations have been made from serial x-ray films after coating the airways with a contrast medium such as tantalum powder.[38] Parks et al.[41] concluded that exposure to mists, often used to treat patients with lung disease (water aerosolized by heated jet nebulizer or by ultrasonic nebulizer), caused no change in tantalum clearance rate in dogs. So far, there is no objective evidence that this treatment improves the removal of secretions from lower airways. It is sometimes believed that mist droplets, when inhaled into the airways, render mucus less viscous.

However, adding water droplets to air already saturated with water vapor does not result in deposition of significant amounts of water.[64] Also, water and mucus do not mix to form a homogeneous liquid, and addition of water, therefore, does not liquify mucus. After auto- or allotransplantation of a lung in dogs,[12] tantalum clearance was delayed up to 120 days. Decreased glandular mucus secretion, as a consequence of denervation, may be one factor in this delay,[12] but it is difficult to exclude subtle local impediments at the suture site.

Transport measurements reflect an average value of rates that may vary considerably in time and place during the observations. With a method that detects arrival of a marker at some distance, the result depends on the first arrivals, i.e., the faster rates. Short-term changes in transport rates can be detected if they are large enough. Other methods (e.g., tantalum clearance) assess the amount of material that stays behind. This is a function of the slowest transport rates and is the relevant information if one wants to know how much of a toxic material remains in the lungs after a given period of time.

SUMMARY

The conducting airways have an important function in protecting the lungs' gas-exchanging parts from exposure to cold, dry, or contaminated air. The nose's functions of heat and water exchange and the prevention of food and liquid from entering the airways during swallowing are both essential protective mechanisms. The branching pattern of the bronchial tree can be described in different ways; Weibel's regular dichotomy model is adequate for many purposes. Small and large airways need to be defined in some context, and several criteria can be used for this purpose. The bronchial wall's structures—consisting of epithelium, glands, smooth muscle, connective tissue, and cartilage—vary with airway size. Glands, goblet cells, and ciliated epithelium are essential parts of the mucociliary clearance mechanism that helps eliminate foreign matter from the lungs.

REFERENCES

1. Andersen I, Lundquist GR, Proctor DF: Human nasal mucosal function in a controlled climate. Arch Environ Health 23:408–420, 1971
2. Armstrong HG, Burton AC, Hall GE: The physiological effects of breathing cold atmospheric air. J Aviat Med 29: 593–597, 1958
3. Baetjer AM: Effect of ambient temperature and vapor pressure on cilia-mucus clearance rate. J Appl Physiol 23:498–504, 1967
4. Bosma JF: Deglutition: Pharyngeal stage. Physiol Rev 37:275–300, 1957
5. Bouhuys A: Airway dynamics and bronchoactive agents in man, in Bouhuys A (ed): Airway Dynamics; Physiology and Pharmacology. Springfield, Charles C Thomas, 1970, pp 263–282
6. Burton PA, Dixon MF: A comparison of changes in the mucous glands and goblet cells of nasal, sinus, and bronchial mucosa. Thorax 24:180–185, 1969
7. Dahlström A, Fuxe K, Hökfelt T, Norberg KA: Adrenergic innervation of the bronchial muscle of the cat. Acta Physiol Scand 66:507–508, 1966
8. Dalhamn T: Mucous flow and ciliary activity in the trachea of healthy rats exposed to respiratory irritant gases (SO_2, H_3N, HCHO). Acta Physiol Scand 36 (suppl 123):1–161, 1956

9. Davis SS, Dippy JE: The rheological properties of sputum. Biorheology 6: 11–21, 1969
10. Denton R, Forsman W, Hwang SH, Litt M, Miller CE: Viscoelasticity of mucus. Its role in ciliary transport of pulmonary secretions. Am Rev Respir Dis 98:380–391, 1968
11. Diedrich WM: The mechanism of esophageal speech, in: Sound Production in Man. Ann NY Acad Sci 155, Article 1, 1968, pp 303–317
12. Edmunds LH Jr, Stallone RJ, Graf PD, Sagel SS, Greenspan RH: Mucus transport in transplanted lungs of dogs. Surgery 66:15–21, 1969
13. Fenn WO: Perspectives in phonation. In: Sound Production in Man. Ann NY Acad Sci 155, Article 1, 1968, pp 4–8
14. Florey H, Carleton HM, Wells AQ: Mucus secretion in the trachea. Br J Exp Pathol 13:269–284, 1932
15. Formijne P, van der Schoot JB, de Nie I: On the formation of mucin in tracheal mucosa of the rat. Biochim Biophys Acta 83:239–241, 1964
16. Gil J: Ultrastructure of lung fixed under physiologically defined conditions. Arch Intern Med 127:896–902, 1971
17. Hakansson CH, Toremalm NG: Studies on the physiology of the trachea. I. Ciliary activity indirectly recorded by a new "light beam reflex" method. Ann Otol Rhinol Laryngol 74:954–969, 1965
18. Hale FC, Olsen CR, Mickey MR Jr: The measurement of bronchial wall components. Am Rev Respir Dis 98:978–987, 1968
19. Havez R, Deminatti M, Roussel P, Degand P, Randoux A, Biserte G: Étude des glycoprotéines carboxyliques et sulfatées de la sécrétion bronchique humaine. Clin Chim Acta 17:463–477, 1967
20. Hayek H von: Die menschliche Lunge. Berlin, Springer, 1953. (Translation by Krahl VE: The Human Lung, New York, Hafner, 1960)
21. Holczabek W: Die Mastzellen der Lunge des Menschen. Deutsche Z gerichtl Med 54:175–177, 1963
22. Horsfield K, Cumming G: Morphology of the bronchial tree in man. J Appl Physiol 24:373–383,1968
23. Huber HL, Koessler KK: The pathology of bronchial asthma. Arch Intern Med 30:689–760, 1922
24. Hughes T: Microcirculation of the tracheobronchial tree. Nature 206:425–426, 1965
25. Iravani J: Flimmerbewegung in den intrapulmonalen Luftwegen der Ratte. Pfluegers Arch 297:221–237, 1967
26. Kilburn KH: Mucociliary clearance from bullfrog (Rana cantesbiana) lung. J Appl Physiol 23:804–810, 1967
27. Koch Hj, Allander C, Ingelstedt S, Toremalm NG: A method for humidifying inspired air in posttracheotomy care. Ann Otol Rhinol Laryngol 67:991–1004, 1958
28. Larsell O, Dow RS: The innervation of the human lung. Am J Anat 52, 125–146, 1933
29. Lieberman P, Crelin ES: On the speech of Neanderthal man. Linguistic Inquiry 2:203–222, 1971
30. Litt M: Mucus rheology. Relevance to mucociliary clearance. Arch Intern Med 126:417–423, 1970
31. Macklem PT, Mead J: Resistance of central and peripheral airways measured by a retrograde catheter. J Appl Physiol 22:395–401, 1967
32. Macklin CC: The musculature of the bronchi and lungs. Physiol Rev 9:1–60, 1929
33. Masson PL, Heremans JF, Prignot J: Studies on the proteins of human bronchial secretions. Biochim Biophys Acta 111:466–478, 1965
34. Mead J, Turner JM, Macklem PT, Little JB: Significance of the relationship between static recoil and maximum expiratory flow. J Appl Physiol 22:95–108, 1967
35. Megahed GE, Senna GA, Eissa MH, Saleh SZ, Eissa HA: Smoking versus infection as the aetiology of mucous gland hypertrophy in chronic bronchitis. Thorax 22:271–278, 1967
36. Moss ML: Veloepiglottic sphincter and obligate nose breathing in the neonate. J Pediatr 67:330–331, 1965
37. Nadel JA, Corn M, Zwi S, Flesch J, Graf P: Location and mechanism of airway constriction after inhalation of histamine aerosol and inorganic sulfate aerosol, in Davies CN (ed): Inhaled Particles and Vapours II. London, Pergamon, 1966, pp 55–67
38. Nadel JA: New technique for studying structural changes of airways in vivo using powdered tantalum, in Bouhuys A

(ed): Airway Dynamics; Physiology and Pharmacology. Springfield, Charles C Thomas, 1970, pp 73–83

39. Oreckin-Duchemin H: Documents sur la vie et l'oeuvre de F.D. Reisseisen (1773–1828). Université de Strasbourg, Faculté de Médecine, 1971
40. Parker H, Horsfield K, Cumming G: Morphology of distal airways in the human lung. J Appl Physiol 31:386–391, 1971
41. Parks CR, Woodrum DE, Graham CB, Cheney FW, Hodson WA: Effect of water nebulization on normal canine pulmonary mucociliary clearance. Am Rev Respir Dis 104:99–106, 1971
42. Proctor DF: Physiology of the upper airway, in Fenn WO, Rahn H (eds): Handbook of Physiology, Section 3: Respiration, vol 1. Washington, D.C., American Physiological Society, 1964, pp 309–345
43. Proctor DF: Airborne disease and the upper respiratory tract. Bacteriol Rev 30:498–513, 1966
44. Proust, Marcel: A la recherche du temps perdu, I. Du Côté de chez Swann. Paris, Bibliothèque de la Pléiade, Edition Gallimard, pp 44–48, 1954
45. Puchelle E, Benis AM: Propriétés d'écoulement des secrétions bronchiques. Bull Physiopathol Respir (Nancy) 7:673–712, 1971
46. Quinlan MF, Salman SD, Swift DL, Wagner HN, Jr, Proctor DF: Measurement of mucociliary function in man. Am Rev Respir Dis 99:13–23, 1969
47. Reid L: Measurement of the bronchial mucous gland layer: A diagnostic yardstick in chronic bronchitis. Thorax 15:132–141, 1960
48. Reid L: An experimental study of hypersecretion of mucus in the bronchial tree. Br J Exp Pathol 44:437–445, 1963
49. Reid L: Histochemical and enzyme studies of bronchial mucus. Med Thorac 22:61–68, 1965
50. Reisseisen FD: Ueber den Bau der Lungen. Berlin, Rücker, 1822 (First published as thesis, Koenigliche Akademie der Wissenschaften, 1808)
51. Ross BB: Influence of bronchial tree structure on ventilation in the dog's lung as inferred from measurements of a plastic cast. J Appl Physiol 10:1–14, 1957
52. Satir P: Cilia. Sci Am 204:108–116, 1961
53. Schiratzki H: Upper airway resistance during mouth breathing in patients with unilateral and bilateral paralysis of the recurrent laryngeal nerve. Acta Otolaryngol (Stockh) 59:475–496, 1965
54. Schmidt-Nielsen K, Hainsworth FR, Murrish DE: Counter-current heat exchange in the respiratory passages: Effect on water and heat balance. Respir Physiol 9:263–276, 1970
55. Sorokin SP: Respiratory system, in: Greep RO (ed): Histology. New York, McGraw-Hill, 1966, p 573
56. Staub NC: The interdependence of pulmonary structure and function. Anesthesiology 24:831–854, 1963
57. Sturgess JM, Palfrey AJ, Reid L: The viscosity of bronchial secretion. Clin Sci 38:145–156, 1970
58. Thompson HT, Pryor WJ, Hill J: Bronchial lavage in the treatment of obstructive lung disease. Thorax 21: 557–559, 1966
59. Thurlbeck WM, Angus GE: The variation of Reid index measurements within the major bronchial tree. Am Rev Respir Dis 95:551–555, 1967
60. Toremalm NG: A heat-and-moisture exchanger for post-tracheotomy care. Acta Otolaryngol (Stockh) 52:461–472, 1960
61. Toremalm NG: The daily amount of tracheo-bronchial secretions in man, a method for continuous tracheal aspiration in laryngectomized and tracheotomized patients. Acta Otolaryngol [Suppl] (Stockh) 158:43–53, 1960
62. Weibel ER: Morphometry of the Human Lung. Berlin, Springer-Verlag, 1963
63. Weibel ER, Gomez DM: Architecture of the human lung. Science 137:577–585, 1962
64. Wolfsdorf J, Swift DL, Avery ME: Mist therapy reconsidered; an evaluation of the respiratory deposition of labelled water aerosols produced by jet and ultrasonic nebulizers. Pediatrics 43:799–808, 1969
65. Yeager H Jr: Tracheobronchial secretions. Am J Med 50:493–509, 1971
66. Smith P, Heath D, Moosavi H: The Clara cell. Thorax 29:147–163, 1974
67. Van As A, Webster I: The morphology of mucus in mammalian pulmonary airways. Environ Res 7:1–12, 1974

Chapter 3

Anatomical Dead Space

In 1894, Loewy measured the volume of a plaster of paris cast of the human bronchi and found a value of 144 ml.[17] Nearly 80 years and many controversies later, the simplest answer to the question, "What is the volume of the conducting airways?" is still: about 150 ml. Because the conducting airways do not participate in gas exchange, this volume is called the anatomical dead space. Its size has important effects on gas exchange, and, if nothing else, it is a source of confusion for medical students and a delight for engineers who enjoy complex plumbing problems. The physiologist must neither oversimplify nor introduce needless complexities. Theoretical analyses that go far beyond what can be measured experimentally are unlikely to increase our understanding of gas exchange or lung disease. The Appendix (p. 56) summarizes several definitions of dead space. In this chapter, I discuss only anatomical dead space; physiological dead space is a concept closely linked with alveolar gas exchange (see Chap. 5).

MORPHOLOGICAL MEASUREMENTS

Loewy's estimate of 144 ml[17] was for the volume of the bronchial tree only. Rohrer[24, 25] did a more complete study, measuring the airway dimensions of a nearly collapsed right lung, down to bronchi of 1 mm in diameter (total volume for both lungs from the carina down—72 ml). He also estimated the volumes of the trachea (45 ml), pharynx (30 ml), and nose (15 ml). Thus, excluding airways less than 1 mm in diameter, he arrived at a value of 162 ml for the total dead space during nose breathing. A more recent estimate[19] is 138 ml for the total dead space, of which 72 ml is in the extrathoracic part of the airways. Thus, about 50 percent of the dead space is in the upper airways, and this volume depends greatly on the position of the jaw.[19]

Weibel's symmetrical model[37] (see also p. 31) is based on measurements made on a single lung specimen inflated to about 75 percent of total lung capacity

(4800 ml volume). This model has an anatomical dead space (from the glottis to the last, 16th generation of unalveolated bronchioles) of 175 ml. Thus, this would yield a total dead space of about 220 ml, assuming 45 ml for the pharynx and nose. In Weibel's model, the volume corresponding to Rohrer's 72 ml (carina to 1 mm bronchi) is less, about 60 ml, in spite of the larger lung volume. The volume of successive generations of airways in the bronchial tree (in Weibel's model) is indicated in Figure 3-4. The trachea and main bronchi contribute about 40 ml, the next 4 generations only 12 ml. Beyond the 10th generation, airway volume rapidly increases, owing to the large increase in total cross-sectional area of the smaller airways (Table 2-1, p. 31).

Loewy and Rohrer both knew that they had underestimated the volume of the small airways in their dead space values. The 17th generation, which carries the first few alveoli, has a volume of about 40 ml (Weibel's model, Fig. 3-4). It is difficult to determine which part of this generation should be assigned to the conducting and which part to gas-exchanging airways, since they gradually merge (Fig. 2-2*B*). Since the aggregate volume of these transition generations is large, morphological determinations of anatomical dead space volume have a large margin of uncertainty.

As a rule of thumb, anatomical dead space in man (in milliliters) is numerically equal to body weight in pounds (i.e., 2.22 ml/kg body wt.).[22] Anatomical data in animals are few: 150 ml in inflated dog lungs,[26] 380 ml in the cow,[23] 1600 ml in the giraffe,[23] and 150 to 300 liters in fin whales.[30]

PHYSIOLOGICAL MEASUREMENTS

Physiological measurements depend on the fact that gas in the dead space retains the composition of inspired air, while gas in the alveoli contains less O_2 and much more CO_2 than inspired air.

Hence, dead space can be measured only for gases which are not absorbed or excreted in the upper airways and the bronchial tree. For instance, the dead space for water vapor is minimal since inspired gas is rapidly saturated with water vapor (Chap. 2, p. 26). Differences between O_2 and CO_2 dead space are discussed in Chap. 5 (p. 94).

During expiration, dead space gas emerges first, and alveolar gas later. Apparently, Wollaston (1766–1828) was the first to notice that the last portion of the expired air extinguishes a candle, and he concluded that this was because of its CO_2 content. In 1845, Vierordt[35] reported the first quantitative measurements: 3.72 percent CO_2 in the first half and 5.44 percent in the second half of the air expired during a deep expiration. Gréhant[13] concluded from an experiment with hydrogen inspiration that 170 ml of inspired gas was expired without change in composition.

In 1891, Christian Bohr[4] formalized these concepts in the following equation

$$V_E \cdot F_E = V_D \cdot F_D + V_A \cdot F_A, \tag{1}$$

where V_E, V_D, and V_A are the volume of expired gas, dead space gas, and alveolar gas, respectively, and F_E, F_D, and F_A are the average fractional concentrations of a reference gas in these volumes. The equation states that the amount of reference gas in the total breath equals the sum of the amounts contained in the first portion expired (the dead space) and the last portion expired (the alveolar gas). Since $V_E = V_D + V_A$, Eq. (1) can be rearranged to solve for V_D

$$V_D/V_E = (F_A - F_E)/(F_A - F_D) \quad (2)$$

Since no gas exchange takes place in the dead space, F_D equals the inspired gas concentration. The equation is usually solved with data for carbon dioxide (during air breathing) and nitrogen (after inspiration of 100% oxygen). In both cases F_D is close to zero and can be ignored, so that Eq. (2) simplifies to

$$\frac{V_D}{V_E} = \frac{F_A - F_E}{F_A} \quad (3)$$

V_E and F_E are measured by collecting the expired gas and determining its CO_2 or N_2 concentration. The remaining unknowns are V_D and F_A. Thus, one may use Eq. (3) to calculate V_D if F_A is known, or F_A if V_D is known or assumed. The controversy surrounding the Bohr equation and dead space has resulted from the difficulty in deciding acceptable values for F_A.

The Bohr equation treats expired air as if it consists of two distinct portions—dead space gas, with inspired gas concentration $F_I = F_D$, and alveolar air, with gas concentration F_A. The equation represents the situation at the end of inspiration as if the conducting airways were filled with inspired air, separated by a sharp gas front (i.e., a distinct boundary without intermixing of gas) from the alveolar gas in the respiratory zone. In this case, if one inspired 100 percent oxygen and analyzed the next expiration for nitrogen with a rapid analyzer, a recording like that of Figure 3-1*A* would be obtained. The first portion of expired air (*OA*) would contain no N_2 at all (pure oxygen from dead space), while the second portion (*AD*) would contain a constant N_2 concentration. The vertical line *AB* is recorded at the moment that the sharp front between dead space gas and alveolar gas passes the sampling site. In this graph, the rectangle *ABCD* represents the amount of N_2 expired (surface area $AD \times AB = V_E \times F_E$).

Actually, no sharp front as implied in Figure 3-1*A* exists. Because of gas mixing (see below), a more gradual concentration change occurs. A test record from a rapid gas analyzer[9, 18] is shown schematically in Figure 3-1*B*. Some of the first recordings, made by Mundt et al.[18] with hydrogen as the test gas, are reproduced in Figure 3-2.

Only the first portion of the expired gas in Figure 3-1*B* contains no N_2 at all. In the next portion, N_2 concentration rises in an S-shaped pattern until a plateau value is reached. At *C*, a new oxygen inspiration begins, and the N_2 concentration seen by the analyzer drops to zero. Fowler[9] indicated a graphical technique to calculate dead space shown in Figure 3-1*A* and *B*. To determine the virtual volume of the anatomical dead space, we must find the virtual sharp front as it occurs in the idealized condition of *A*. Since the surface area under a concentration-volume curve represents an amount of gas, this can be done by finding the rectangle *ABCD* of graph *A* that has the same surface area as the recording of graph *B*. To do this, a line *AB* is placed halfway up the S-shaped portion of *B*, so that the area of the two hatched triangles is equal.

To determine anatomical dead space as in Figure 3-1*B*, a graph of percentage of expired N_2 must be plotted against expired volume. This can be recorded

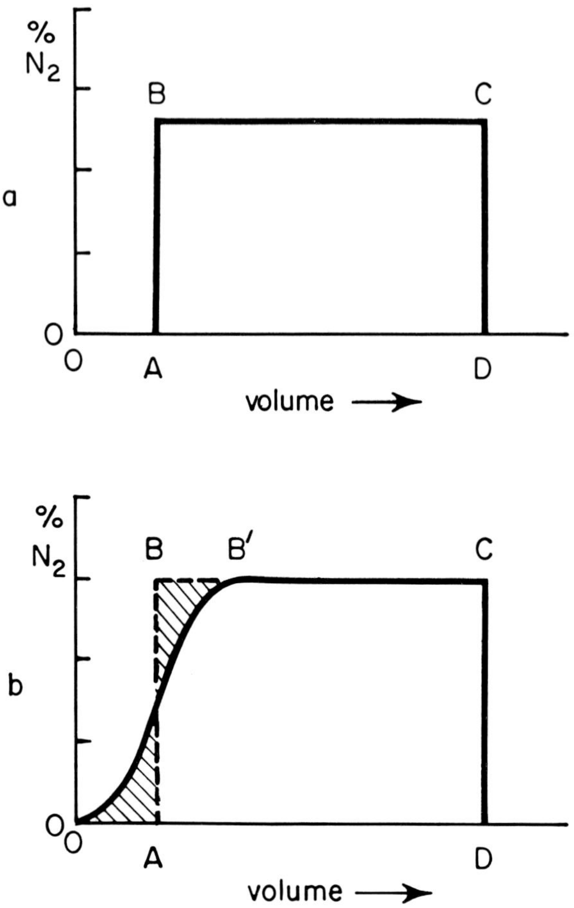

Fig. 3-1. (*A*). Idealized single-breath N_2 curve, assuming a square front of N_2 traveling through the airways. (*B*) Actual shape of single-breath curve (*OB′CD*). Line *AB* represents the vertical N_2 front, placed so that the surface area *OB′CD* equals surface area of *ABCD*. *OA* = anatomical dead space; *OD* = total expired volume.

directly with electronic equipment (Fig. 3-3). The calculation of dead space in Figure 3-1 can be used only if the plateau *B′C* is flat, or nearly so. The line *B′C* represents alveolar N_2 concentrations, and if *B′C* slopes upward (as in many patients with lung disease), this means that alveolar gas is not homogeneous (Chap. 4). Under these conditions, the definition of average F_A becomes arbitrary, and application of Bohr's equation is questionable. Modified dead space measurements are feasible but do not fully solve the problem.[10]

When alveolar gas is not homogeneous, there are different methods for obtaining an average F_A value. One is to make a more or less educated guess from alveolar gas concentration data; e.g., one could select the halfway point on line *B′C*. Another method is to record the rate of mixing of lung gas with gas in a spirometer.[3] The Bohr equation shows why these methods often yield V_D values

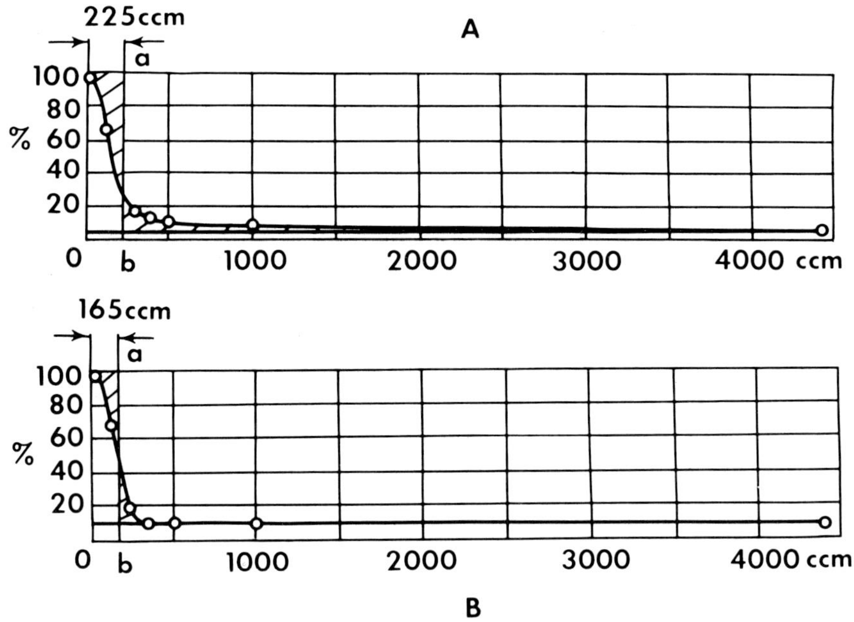

Fig. 3-2. Single-breath records of H_2 concentration in expired air (ordinate) versus expired volume (abscissa) after one inspiration of H_2. In both graphs, the vertical line ab represents the virtual front between dead space and alveolar gas. The hatched areas on either side of line ab have an equal surface area. *A*. If F_A is taken to equal the lowest H_2 concentration recorded in expired air, V_D is calculated by graphical analysis at 225 ml. *B*. If F_A is taken to equal the H_2 concentration at the transition point between the second and the third phase of the record, a V_D value of 165 ml is calculated. This value approximates the anatomical dead space; the larger value calculated from *A* includes an additional volume which reflects the slope of the alveolar plateau. From Mundt et al.[18]

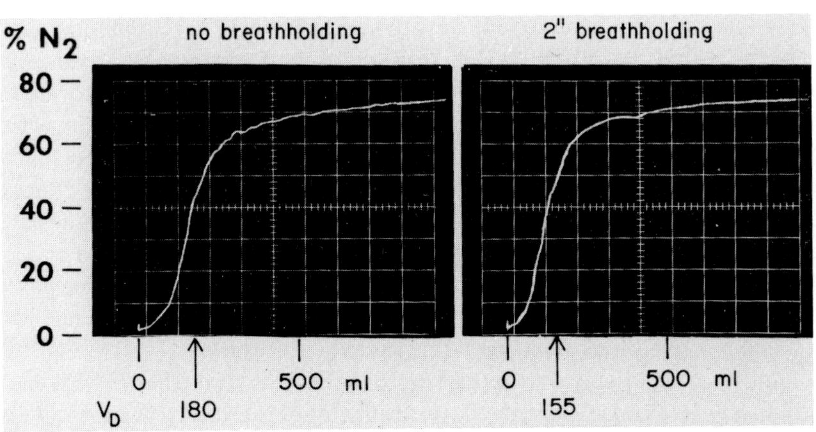

Fig. 3-3. Single-breath N_2 curves in a healthy subject. Two-second breath holding reduces dead space from 180 to 155 ml, end-inspiratory volume and other parameters being equal. Data from Chiang, Snyder, and Bouhuys (unpublished).

that include an increment resulting from nonuniform gas distribution. With 100% O_2 inspiration, Eq. (1) transforms to: $V_E \times F_E = V_A \times F_A$, or, the quantity of N_2 in expired gas equals the amount contributed by alveolar gas. $V_E \times F_E$ is determined experimentally. If one chooses an unduly high F_A value, e.g., at the end of the sloping plateau, V_A becomes too small and thus V_D too large (Fig. 3-2*A*). This effect of nonuniform ventilation was recognized by Mundt et al.[18] and is well illustrated in their curves (Fig. 3-2). Other methods of obtaining an average F_A use the pulmonary circulation as an averaging circuit. This leads to F_A values weighted in favor of lung regions with high perfusion rates. These methods give values for physiological dead space, discussed in Chapter 5.

In healthy subjects, a wide variety of methods [1, 3, 7, 9, 21, 27] gives values close to the anatomical volume of the conducting airways. In patients with nonuniform lung ventilation, no satisfactory method to arrive at such a value has as yet been devised.

THE INSPIRED GAS FRONT AND DIFFUSION DURING INSPIRATION

Yandell Henderson et al.[15] noted in 1915 that some alveolar gas already emerged at the mouth when only 50 ml gas had been expired, an observation confirmed in more recent work.[6] They believed that this resulted from a laminar airflow pattern in the airways, with a peak linear velocity in the middle of the stream twice as large as the mean velocity (parabolic gas front). In this way, some alveolar gas, traveling at peak velocity, would reach the airway opening early during expiration. "The authors of this paper were obviously aware of the complications in mass transport by convection and diffusion during the unsteady flow of a non-uniform gas mixture in a pipe." [39]

A more detailed analysis of gas transport in conducting airways does not support the assumption of a parabolic gas front. Gas moves into the trachea and large airways by bulk transport in the direction of a pressure gradient (convective transport). The exact flow pattern is not clear; turbulent flow very likely prevails in the trachea and may even extend to segmental bronchi.[20] Branching also affects flow patterns,[31] and it is unlikely that fully developed laminar flow occurs at all in the airways. Wilson and Lin [39] estimated that the purely convective forms of transport dominate until the eighth generation. In these large airways, convection is so fast that no appreciable time is available for diffusion. When the tubes narrow and convection velocities slow down, radial diffusion, which smoothes out concentration differences along the radius of the tube, becomes an additional transport mode. This coupling of axial convection and radial diffusion as a combined mode of gas transport is called Taylor diffusion. Beyond the 12th generation, axial gas velocity becomes so slow that no radial concentration differences occur. Hence, transport occurs by convective block flow coupled with axial diffusion.[39]

A model of dead space proposed by Scherer [28, 29] lumps convective transport and radial (Taylor) diffusion since both result in net forward transport. This model illustrates several features of gas transport in the airways. An important feature of the bronchial tree is the increase of total cross-sectional area as a function of airway generation number (Table 2-1), or of distance into the airway (Fig. 3-4). No

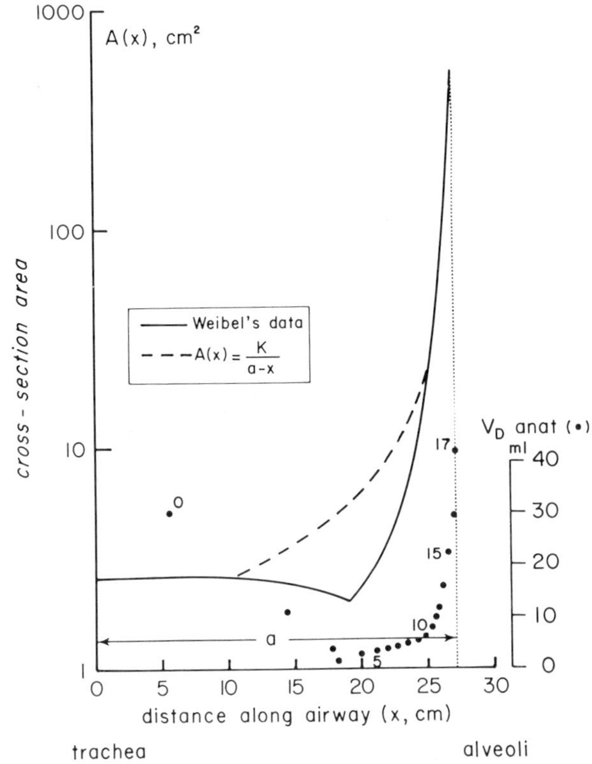

Fig. 3-4. Total cross-sectional area of all airways $[A(x)]$ as a function of distance into the bronchial tree; 0 is at the oral entrance of the trachea. The dashed line is the hyperbola used in Scherer's model (see text). The right-hand ordinate refers to the points which indicate the anatomical dead space volume of airway generations 0-17 (0 = trachea). The point for each generation has been placed at the mid-point of its length. Data from Weibel.[37]

accurate mathematical equation has as yet been fitted to this area function curve. As a rough approximation, a hyperbola is suitable.[28]

How would a front of pure oxygen move into a lung represented by this model? Near the entrance the cross-sectional area is small, hence velocities must be high. As cross-sectional areas increase, velocities decrease, approaching zero in the peripheral airways near the respiratory zone. To quantitate this movement of the front, Scherer assumed a tidal volume of 500 ml and a sine-wave entrance velocity. From the hyperbola, which describes the relationship between airway cross-sectional area and distance along the airway, one can compute the position and velocity of the oxygen front at any moment during the inspiration. Figure 3-5 shows the result. During the first 0.1 second, as the front begins to enter the airways, the velocity of the air entering the trachea is almost equal to the velocity of the front, which is then still in large airways with a cross section nearly equal to that of the trachea. At about 0.3 seconds, front velocity begins to decrease, as the front enters airways with an increasing cross-sectional area. At 1.0 second, velocity

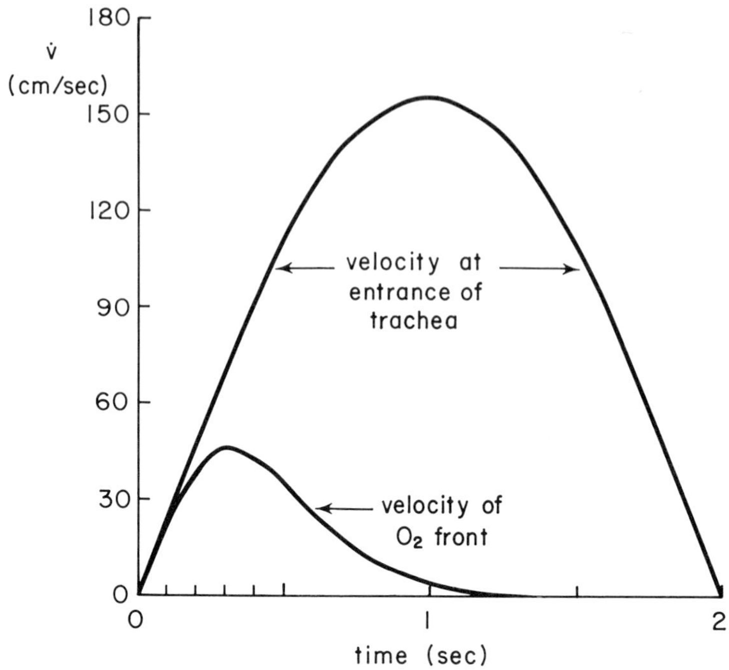

Fig. 3-5. Linear velocity of the gas front ($\dot{v}$) moving into the airways as represented by the hyperbolic function of Figure 3-4. The input velocity (at entrance of trachea) is a sinus function. When $\dot{v}$ at the trachea entrance is at its maximum, the O_2 front is already in small airways and has slowed down considerably. After Scherer.[28]

at the trachea entrance has reached its maximum, and half the tidal volume (250 ml) has entered the airways. The surface area under the area-function curve of Figure 3-4 has the dimensions of volume (abscissa in cm, ordinate in cm^2); when 250 ml air has entered the airways, the front must be situated in very small airways, close to 27 cm from the trachea entrance. Hence, front velocity has decreased to nearly zero.

So far, the front has been treated as if it were a sharp gas concentration boundary throughout inspiration. But inspiration takes a certain time, and diffusion around the front will occur. Scherer [28] separated the effects of bulk flow and diffusion by changing coordinates. An apocryphal analog may illustrate this. Consider a group of people who start a train journey together at the bar of a commuter train out of Grand Central Station bound for Connecticut. Bulk flow begins when the train leaves and picks up speed. While this happens, the commuters pick up their drinks and disperse through the train. To measure their speed of dispersion, an observer must be on the train, not beside the track. To place an observer on the train means establishing the speed of the train as a reference velocity. The dispersion of the commuters is measured with respect to the position of the bar, which itself moves at the reference velocity. Similarly, Scherer used the position of the oxygen front at any time as his zero coordinate. He also assumed that radial diffusion is fast compared with axial diffusion; therefore, only axial diffusion along a single pathway into the lung was considered.

Figure 3-6 illustrates diffusion on both sides of the front. In the trachea, at

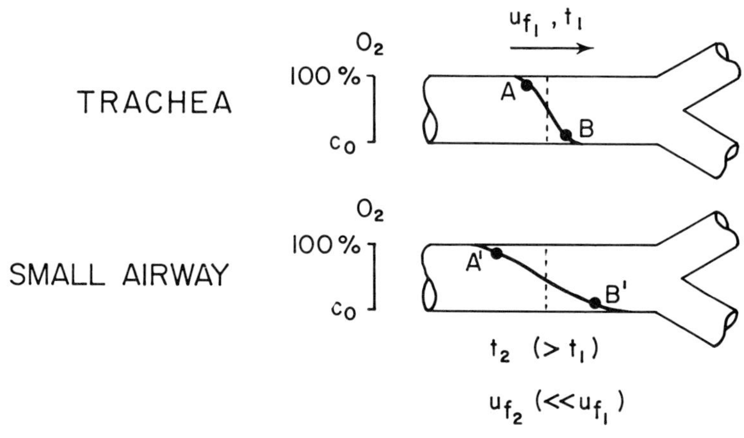

Fig. 3-6. Diffusion around the oxygen front which moves into the airways. In the trachea the diffusion zone is short; in a small airway it has increased in width. $c_0 =$ oxygen concentration in gas in airways before O_2 front moves in. Uf_1 and Uf_2 are the velocities of the front at times t_1 and t_2 respectively.

time t_1, there is a narrow zone around the front in which oxygen concentration changes from 100 percent to c_0. An instant later, at time t_2, the front is in a small airway and its velocity has decreased. In the interval $t_2 - t_1$, diffusion has enlarged the length of airway in which O_2 concentration decreases from 100% to c_0. The speed of individual molecules differs. For instance, a molecule moving from A to A' during t_2-t_1 has covered less distance than a molecule moving from B to B' in the same time interval. However, these differences are small, and for the analysis one may consider all molecules to move with the velocity of the front. In the new coordinate system one may solve the diffusion equation, assuming that there is an infinite oxygen reservoir at the mouth, and that at the alveolar end of the airway there is an infinite reservoir of well-mixed alveolar gas. With these boundary conditions, we ignore the complexities of alveolar mixing and consider only diffusion in pipes. We consider the alveoli as a source of gas with a constant nitrogen concentration. (Gas mixing in the alveolar units themselves is discussed in Chap. 4.) Assume that the lower diagram of Figure 3-6 represents the front and the diffusion zone around it at the end of inspiration. During expiration, the front and diffusion zone move back to the airway opening, now at increasing velocities since the front moves into larger airways, with a decreasing cross-sectional area. As soon as the front has left the small airways, diffusion becomes a minor transport mode because of the increased dimensions and gas velocities. An analyzer sampling gas expired at the mouth will therefore inscribe the S-shaped curve of Figure 3-1B, reflecting the blurring of the gas front caused by diffusion.

The equations derived from this model [28] describe anatomical dead space (i.e., the volume down to the virtual square gas front) as a function of the constants K and a, which describe airway geometry (Fig. 3-4), and of breath-holding time. These equations fit dead space measurements reasonably well, using 0–5-second-periods of breath holding (see p. 53). Implications of the model for gas mixing in the lungs are discussed in Chapter 4.

UNEQUAL PATHWAY LENGTHS

The preceding section discussed one reason for the S shape of the expiratory N_2 curve after a breath of oxygen. This section deals with a morphological feature that can explain, at least in part, the same phenomenon. Study of human and dog lungs provides good evidence that pathway lengths from the trachea to the alveoli vary a great deal in different parts of the lungs. In the dog lung, Ross [26] found the shortest pathways (carina-alveoli) only about 2 cm long, and the longest about 14 cm. For the human lung, Weibel's data [37] on the distribution of airways of equal diameter also suggest a wide variability of pathway lengths. Most bronchi with an internal diameter of 2 mm belong to the 7th through 11th generations, with the total range varying from the 4th to the 13th. Pathway lengths for these, from the carina, vary from about 17 to 32 cm. The distribution of 0.5-mm diameter airways [37] suggests that total pathway lengths (carina-alveoli) may vary from roughly 22 to 40 cm (at 75% TLC). Since the volume of the common dead space (upper airway and trachea) is about 90 ml, and N_2 already begins to appear at the mouth after some 60 ml gas has been expired, unequal pathway lengths do not completely explain the S-shaped curves. To the extent that they account for part of it, airway models based solely on gas-transport mechanisms should underestimate the range of volumes over which the expired gas front is blurred when it arrives at the mouth during expiration.

STRATIFIED DEAD SPACE

The term stratified dead space has recently been proposed to designate that part of the conducting airways where diffusion is an important transport mode.[34] The delineation of this space is, unfortunately, not clear. The virtual boundary of the anatomical dead space is sharply defined by the position of the oxygen front in a model and by the Bohr equation in the experiment. The boundaries of stratified dead space are also virtual ones, and they can be defined only arbitrarily. Consider Figure 3-6: the stratified dead space might be the area between points A′ and B′, or one might choose points closer to or farther away from the 100 percent and c_0 limits. Strictly speaking, the limits are never reached but only approached asymptotically; so stratified dead space might be equal to total airway or even lung volume in this absolute sense. The concentration gradients in the diffusion zone around the front cannot be determined accurately. While the term stratified dead space implies a measurable volume with virtual but defined boundaries, such a space exists neither in theory nor in practice.

GAS TRANSPORT TIME

A bolus of CO injected into the trachea can be detected at the pleural surface by continuous monitoring for CO-hemoglobin with a photoelectric method. Wagner et al.[36] used this ingenious technique in anesthetized dogs to estimate the time it takes the CO bolus to travel from the trachea to the alveoli. The additional time needed for CO to diffuse across the alveolocapillary membrane and to bind to Hb is short compared to its transport time through the airways. During slow and fast inspirations, CO transport time was about 50 percent of the duration of inspiration. This corresponds well with Scherer's model (Fig. 3-5), in which the inspired gas front arrives in very small airways at about the midpoint of inspiration. However, the data obtained with Wagner et al.'s method do not allow firm conclusions concerning the modes of gas transport.[32]

FACTORS THAT MODIFY DEAD SPACE

Lung Volume

Airway caliber increases with lung distension,[16] and dead space volume therefore increases with lung volume. Since the increase is in the order of 2–3 ml per 100 ml increase in postexpiratory lung volume,[5] dead space should be measured as a function of lung volume.

Widdicombe [38] has pointed out that since about 50 percent of the dead space is in upper airways and trachea where little change in volume is expected, the intrapulmonary and particularly the small airways (bronchioles) may inflate much more in proportion with lung volume. For instance, his own data [38] indicate a total V_D of about 150 ml at a lung volume of 2 liters, and a V_D of about 250 ml at 5.5 liters—an overall increase of about 3 ml V_D per 100 ml increase in lung volume. If one assumes that x ml of dead space does not change with lung volume, and the remainder changes in proportion to lung volume, one has: $2000{:}5500=(150-x){:}(250-x)$, from which $x=93$ ml. This is close to Rohrer's value of 90 ml for the dead space of the extrathoracic airways and trachea.[24] The dead space of the bronchial tree increases from 57 to 157 ml with this lung volume increase, or 28.5 ml/liter.

Tidal Volume

The relation between dead space and tidal volume was the subject of the classical Haldane-Krogh controversy, reviewed elsewhere.[5] There is no evidence that tidal volume influences dead space in any way other than by increasing postinspiratory lung volume (see above).

Breath Holding

Even a few seconds' breath holding after inspiration of 100 percent O_2 lowers the dead space value [33] (Fig. 3-3). Breath holding for more than 5 seconds does not have much additional effect (Fig. 3-7). Scherer's model (see pp. 48–51) predicts the rapid decrease of V_D during the first few seconds, but after about 5 seconds the model and the data diverge. This results from the boundary conditions of the model; it assumes an infinite reservoir of alveolar gas. Therefore, diffusion in the model continues while in the lungs there is a finite amount of alveolar gas and hence a limit to the extent of diffusion. In intact man, the heartbeat may be an additional factor which promotes gas mixing during breath holding.[35a]

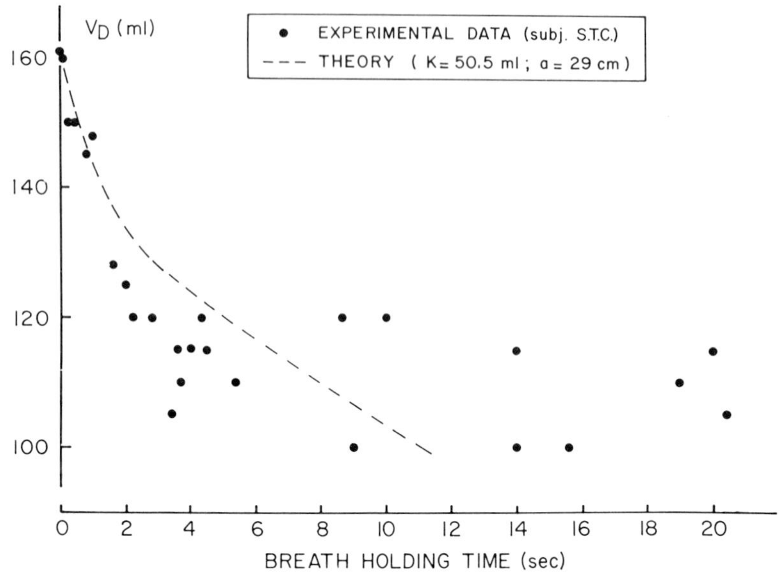

Fig. 3-7. Theoretical data for V_D as a function of breath-holding time are based on Scherer's model.[28, 29] Experimental data, on one subject, from Chiang, Snyder, and Bouhuys (unpublished).

Airflow Rates

Inspiratory flow rate has little effect on V_D if time and postinspiratory volume are kept constant (Chiang, Snyder, and Bouhuys, unpublished material). Also, expiratory flow rates varying from 1–5 liters/second had little influence on V_D in the same experiments (Fig. 3-8). This does not confirm an earlier report [2] of large decreases of dead space at high expiratory flow rates. By the time flow has reached

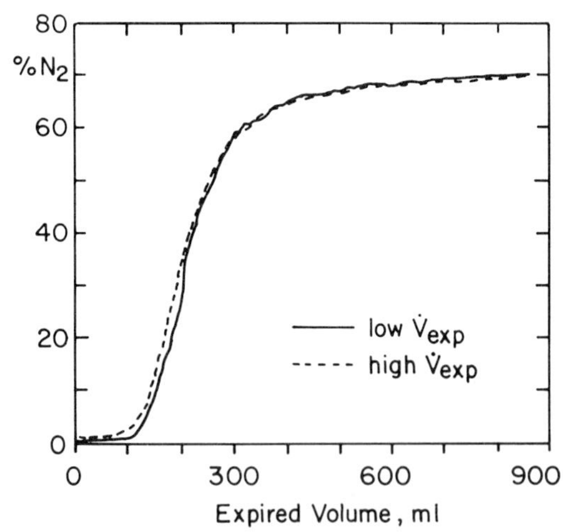

Fig. 3-8. Single-breath N_2 curve at different rates of expiratory flow (*drawn line:* $\dot{V} = 1.4$ liters/sec; *dashed line:* $\dot{V} = 5.7$ liters/sec) in healthy subject. Data from Chiang, Snyder, and Bouhuys (unpublished).

maximum values, the front has left small airways. Hence, differences in diffusion times due to the different duration of expiration should not affect dead space significantly. Decreasing dead space at high expiratory flows has been attributed to large airway compression,[2] but it is not clear how this would affect dead space.

Volume History

Froeb and Mead [11] demonstrated that in certain subjects anatomical dead space depends on volume history of the lungs. When dead space is measured after several expirations to residual volume, other parameters being equal, dead space is smaller than when the measurement is made after several inspirations to TLC. This phenomenon apparently varies individually. It was confirmed in some of the subjects of Chiang et al. (unpublished). The mechanisms of hysteresis of the dead space may be related to those which cause volume history dependence of airway resistance (Chap. 8). Temporary closure of airways at small lung volumes is probably an important factor.

Body Size

Hart et al.[14] determined dead space with the N_2 single-breath method in children, and Chiang et al. obtained similar data in children and adults. Their results are summarized in Figure 3-9. Dead space increases as a linear function of standing

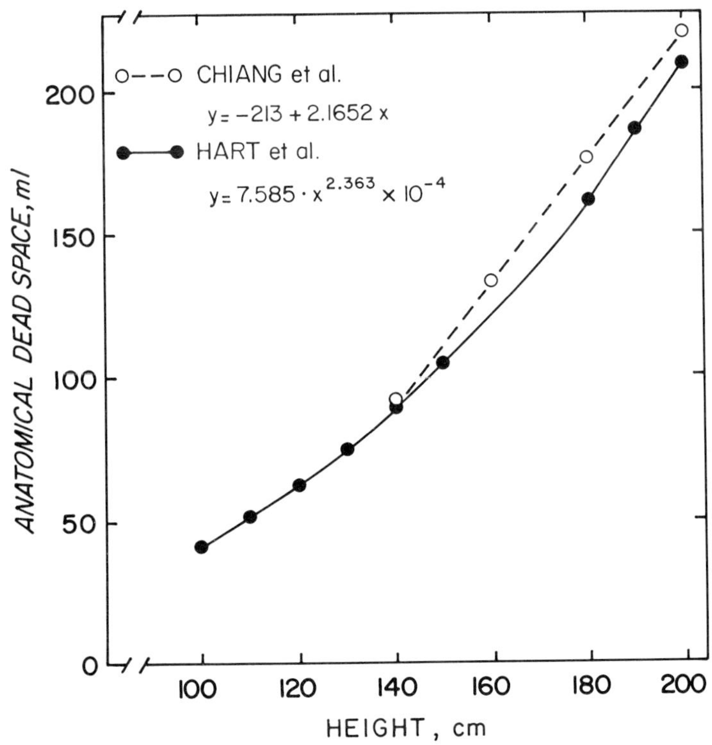

Fig. 3-9. Anatomical dead space as a function of standing height in two groups of subjects. The group of Hart et al.[14] included children; the group of Chiang et al. (unpublished) were healthy adults. Lines shown are regression lines fitted to experimental data.

body height, and also approximately in proportion to vital capacity and total lung capacity. In the 140-cm tall child, V_D is about 3.5% VC and 3% TLC, while in the 180-cm tall adult, these percentages are 3.4% VC and 2.4% TLC (see also Table 1-4, p. 20).

Effects of Drugs

In studies reviewed elsewhere,[5, 38] bronchodilator drugs increased dead space volume, while constrictor drugs decreased it. These responses have not been observed consistently.[8] In our laboratory, Chiang et al. (unpublished) found no consistent effect of isoproterenol inhalation, in doses known to decrease airway resistance, on dead space in healthy subjects (method as shown in Fig. 3-3). A large fraction of dead space is in upper airways and in the trachea, where major caliber changes induced by drugs are unlikely. In peripheral airways, more subject to caliber changes, other factors, such as airway closure and lung elastic recoil, also affect caliber. Thus, dead space measurements are not very suitable for the quantitative assessment of airway responses to drugs.

SUMMARY

The volume of conducting airways varies from about 150 to 300 ml, depending on the state of lung inflation. Although gas transport modes are complex and not completely defined, gas dilution methods (using an inert test gas) can measure this volume reasonably accurately in healthy men, using Bohr's equation. When lung ventilation is markedly nonhomogeneous, the definition of alveolar gas becomes arbitrary and the Bohr equation then does not measure dead space volume per se. Therefore, anatomical dead space is difficult to measure in many patients with lung disease.

Gas transport in the conducting airways can be studied with simplified mathematical models. Convection and diffusion are two important gas-transport modes. Unequal bronchial pathway lengths also influence the shape of the expiratory N_2 curve recorded at the mouth after oxygen inspiration. Gas-transport times from trachea to alveoli have been measured in animals but do not give insight into transport modes.

Dead space values measured in healthy persons are a function of body size, lung volume, the time course of the test maneuver, and, in some subjects, of lung volume history. Airflow rates have a minor effect, and changes induced by bronchoactive drugs are difficult to measure in the presence of the several other variables that influence anatomical dead space in vivo.

Appendix: Definitions of Dead Space

1. *Anatomical:*
   A. Morphological definition: the volume of the conducting airways, i.e., airways not lined with respiratory epithelium, measured from a cast of the bronchial tree. Most data exclude the supralaryngeal airways; the precise extent of the cast must be specified. This is a volume with "spatial boundaries identified by anatomical means."[12]

B. Functional definition: the volume of inspired gas that does not mix with alveolar gas, measured in vivo by gas-dilution methods as indicated by Fowler.[9] Synonymous term—series dead space.[8]

2. *Physiological:*
The volume of gas that is inspired and expired but takes no part in gas exchange in the alveoli, measured from V_{CO_2} and Pa_{CO_2} by assuming that PA_{CO_2} equals Pa_{CO_2} (Chap. 5).

3. *Alveolar:*
A volume of inspired gas that mixes with gas in alveolar spaces but takes no part in alveolar gas exchange, thus, a volume of gas in well-ventilated, non-perfused alveoli. Alveolar V_D=physiological V_D−anatomical V_D. Synonymous term—parallel dead space.[8]

4. *Instrumental or mechanical:*
The volume of mouthpiece, breathing valves, or other apparatus connected to the airways, in which inspired and expired gas are not separated. It is customary to subtract this volume from calculated dead-space volumes, but a more complex correction method is needed for calculation of physiological dead space.[33a]

5. *Personal:*
A term used to indicate the calculated dead-space volume, either physiological or anatomical V_D, minus instrumental dead-space volume.

6. *Respiratory:*
This general term needs qualification; the definitions 1–3 are more specific and, therefore, preferable.

REFERENCES

1. Bartels J, Severinghaus JW, Forster RE, Briscoe WA, Bates DV: The respiratory dead space measured by single breath analysis of oxygen, carbon dioxide, nitrogen or helium. J Clin Invest 33:41–48, 1954
2. Bashoff MA, Ingram RH Jr, Schilder DP: Effect of expiratory flow rate on the nitrogen concentration vs. volume relationship. J Appl Physiol 23:895–901, 1967
3. Birath G: Lung volume and ventilation efficiency. Change in collapse-treated and non-collapse-treated pulmonary tuberculosis and in pulmonectomy and lobectomy. Acta Med Scand 120 (suppl 154):1–168, 1944
4. Bohr C: Ueber die Lungenathmung. Skand Arch Physiol 2:236–268, 1891
5. Bouhuys A: Respiratory dead space, in Fenn WO, Rahn H (eds): Handbook of Physiology, Section 3: Respiration, vol. I. Washington, D.C., American Physiological Society, 1964, pp 699–714
6. Briscoe WA, Forster RE, Comroe JH Jr: Alveolar ventilation at very low tidal volumes. J Appl Physiol 7:27–30, 1954
7. Enghoff H: Volumen Inefficax. Bemerkungen zur Frage des schädlichen Raumes. Upsala Laekaref Foerh 44: 191–218, 1938
8. Folkow B, Pappenheimer JR: Components of the respiratory dead space and their variation with pressure breathing and with bronchoactive drugs. J Appl Physiol 8:102–110, 1955
9. Fowler WS: Lung function studies. II. The respiratory dead space. Am J Physiol 154:405–416, 1948
10. Fowler WS: Lung function studies. V. Respiratory dead space in old age and in pulmonary emphysema. J Clin Invest 29:1439–1444, 1950

11. Froeb HF, Mead J: Relative hysteresis of the dead space and lung in vivo. J Appl Physiol 25:244–248, 1968
12. Gray JS, Grodins FS, Carter ET: Alveolar and total ventilation and the dead space problem. J Appl Physiol 9:307–320, 1956
13. Gréhant N: Recherches physiques sur la respiration de l'homme. J Anat Physiol Homme Anim 1:523–55, 1864
14. Hart MC, Orzalesi MM, Cook CD: Relation between anatomic respiratory dead space and body size and lung volume. J Appl Physiol 18:519–522, 1963
15. Henderson Y, Chillingworth FP, Whitney JL: The respiratory dead space. Am J Physiol 38:1–19, 1915
16. Huizinga E: Ueber die Physiologie des Bronchialbaumes. Pflueger's Arch 238: 767–779, 1937
17. Loewy A: Ueber die Bestimmung der Grösse des "Schädlichen Luftraumes" im Thorax und der alveolaren Sauerstoffspannung. Arch Ges Physiol 58: 416–427, 1894
18. Mundt E, Schoedel W, Schwarz H: Ueber den effektiven schädlichen Raum der Atmung. Pflueger's Arch 244:107–119, 1940
19. Nunn JF, Campbell EJM, Peckett BW: Anatomical subdivisions of the volume of respiratory dead space and effect of position of the jaw. J Appl Physiol 14:174–176, 1959
20. Owen PR: Turbulent flow and particle deposition in the trachea, in Wolstenholme GEW, Knight J (eds): Circulatory and Respiratory Mass Transport. Boston, Little, Brown & Company, 1969, pp 236–252
21. Pappenheimer JR, Fishman AP, Borrero LM: New experimental methods for determination of effective alveolar gas composition and respiratory dead space, in the anesthetized dog and in man. J Appl Physiol 4:855–867, 1952
22. Radford E Jr: Ventilation standards for use in artificial respiration. J Appl Physiol 7:451–460, 1955
23. Robin ED, Corson JM, Dammin GJ: The respiratory dead space of the giraffe. Nature 186:24–26, 1960
24. Rohrer F: Der Strömungswiderstand in den menschlichen Atemwegen und der Einfluss der unregelmässigen Verzweigung des Bronchialsystems auf den Atmungsverlauf in verschiedenen Lungenbezirken. Pflueger's Arch 162:225–299, 1915
25. Rohrer F: Die Grösse des schädlichen Raumes der Atemwege. Pflueger's Arch 164:295–302, 1916
26. Ross BB: Influence of bronchial tree structure on ventilation in the dog's lung as inferred from measurements of a plastic cast. J Appl Physiol 10:1–14, 1957
27. Rossier PH, Bühlmann A: The respiratory dead space. Physiol Rev 35:860–876, 1955
28. Scherer PW: Modeling of the dispersion of gases in the human bronchial tree. PhD Thesis, Yale University, 1971
29. Scherer PW, Chiang ST, Bouhuys A: A quantitative model of anatomical dead space. Fed Proc 29:396, 1970
30. Scholander PF: Experimental investigations on the respiration in diving mammals and birds. Hvalraadets Skr Nr 22, Norske Vid Akad 1–131, 1940
31. Schroter RC, Sudlow MF: Flow patterns in models of the human bronchial airways. Respir Physiol 7:341–355, 1969
32. Shair FH: Pulmonary gas transport time. Science 165:823, 1969
33. Shepard RH, Campbell EJM, Martin HB, Enns T: Factors affecting the pulmonary dead space as determined by single breath analysis. J Appl Physiol 11:241–244, 1957
33a. Singleton GJ, Olsen CR, Smith RL: Correction for mechanical dead space in the calculation of physiological dead space. J Clin Invest 51:2768–2772, 1972
34. Strieder DJ, Barnes BA, Levine BW, Kazemi H: Stratified dead space in excised perfused lungs. J Appl Physiol 29:486–492, 1970
35. Vierordt K: Physiologie des Athmens, mit besonderer Rücksicht auf die Ausscheidung der Kohlensäure. Karlsruhe, Groos, 1845, pp 130–133
35a. Wagner PD, Gaines RA, Mazzone RW, West JB: Mechanism of intrapulmonary gas mixing during breathholding in man. Physiologist 15:295, 1972
36. Wagner WW Jr, Latham LP, Brinkman PD, Filley GF: Pulmonary gas transport time: Larynx to alveolus. Science 163: 1210–1211, 1969
37. Weibel ER: Morphometry of the Human Lung. Berlin, Springer–Verlag, 1963

38. Widdicombe JG: The regulation of bronchial calibre, in Caro CG (ed): Advances in Respiratory Physiology. Baltimore, Williams & Wilkins, 1966, pp 48–82

39. Wilson TA, Lin K–H: Convection and diffusion in the airways and the design of the bronchial tree, in Bouhuys A (ed): Airway Dynamics; Physiology and Pharmacology. Springfield, Ill, Charles C Thomas, 1970, pp 5–19

Chapter 4

Distribution of Inspired Gas

Effective ventilation of the alveoli requires mixing of inspired gas with alveolar gas. First, an adequate amount of inspired gas must reach the terminal lung units; this depends on bulk flow as the main transport mode. The amount of gas distributed to each unit is determined by gravity and structural factors (such as length of the airway, stiffness of the terminal unit). However, once inside terminal bronchioles and alveolar units where forward velocities of gas are nearly zero, gas travels primarily by diffusion rather than by bulk flow. The effectiveness of diffusion within the terminal units depends largely on their dimensions, which determine how far gas molecules must travel.

After inspiration, alveolar gas is not of equal composition throughout the lungs. This is because of (1) variations in dilution of alveolar gas with inspired gas, and (2) uneven lung blood flow and, hence, unequal exchange of O_2 and CO_2 in different lung parts. This chapter discusses only the first of these factors, nonuniform distribution of inspired gas, as a process independent of gas exchange. Chapters 5 and 6 deal with the second mechanism and with gas exchange itself.

MECHANISMS OF UNEVEN DISTRIBUTION

Several mechanisms contribute to uneven inspired gas distribution, but there is no comprehensive lung model that takes all of them into account. Hence, it is difficult to assess how much each mechanism contributes to the overall nonuniform distribution of inspired gas. The principal mechanisms are: (1) *regional* or *parallel ventilation differences,* which are related to unequal bronchial pathway lengths, unequal stress, and unequal compliance of lung tissue, and, under some conditions, to local airway resistance, especially at low lung volumes (airway closure); and (2) *series ventilation,* including stratification within terminal units, although this is probably not of practical significance in normal lungs. The first principal mechanism relates to the amount of inspired air delivered to each terminal unit, the second to the effectiveness of gas mixing in alveolar lung units.

Regional or Parallel Ventilation

The pathologist Tendeloo,[74] noting that tuberculosis and emphysema do not affect all parts of the lungs equally, thought this was due to unequal expansion of different lung regions. He attributed unequal ventilation to differences in tissue compliance (e.g., hilar versus peripheral parts) and uneven distribution of respiratory forces through the lungs. Physiological evidence for regional ventilation differences came much later when Martin and Young [53] measured the rate of N_2 washout (p. 72) in the right upper and lower lobes of human subjects. They concluded that the lower lobe is better ventilated (i.e., receives more ventilation per unit volume) than the upper lobe, a conclusion confirmed by radioactive gas techniques. For instance, when a small amount of radioactive xenon (^{133}Xe) is injected into the inspired airstream directly after a maximum expiration, most of the xenon is inspired into the lung tops (in the subject sitting upright; Fig. 4-1). When xenon is injected later during inspiration, most of it goes to lower lung zones and less to the lung tops. Thus, there are marked regional ventilation differences in healthy lungs, and these depend on lung volume.

EFFECT OF GRAVITY

The anatomical substrate for regional ventilation differences remained rather obscure until Glazier et al.[34] showed that when fixed in situ, alveoli in the top of the vertical dog lung are much larger than alveoli near the base of the lung. The difference in alveolar size suggested that lungs behave like a spring suspended at the top, with the upper coils distended much more than the lower ones, owing to the weight of the spring.[57] Other experiments have suggested that the distribution of pleural pressure around the lungs may be crucial. In isolated, perfused dog lungs, suspended vertically, inspired xenon is distributed uniformly, but when the same lungs are suspended in a foam which creates a hydrostatic pressure gradient around them, the nonuniform distribution pattern typical of vertical lungs in situ becomes apparent.[79]

With the radioactive gas methods, counting radioactivity externally over relatively large areas of the chest, one can estimate regional volume, as well as regional

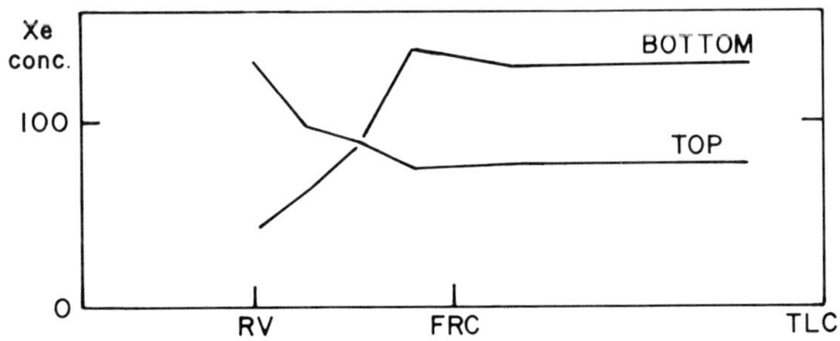

Fig. 4-1. Regional ventilation distribution determined with xenon. *Abscissa.* Lung volume at which Xe boli were injected into inspired airstream. *Ordinate.* Xe concentration as recorded with external counters over lung top and bottom, in percentage of value predicted if distribution were uniform. When inspired near RV, most Xe goes to the lung top; when inspired at or above FRC, most Xe goes to the bottom of the lungs. Average results in 5 young healthy subjects. Modified from reference 29.

expansion, relative to the volume of each counting zone at maximum inspiration.[17, 44, 57] The latter is called regional TLC (TLC_r), and regional volumes at lesser degrees of lung expansion are expressed as percentages of TLC_r.[57] Figure 4-2 is a diagram based on these measurements. Near the lung tops, regional FRC (FRC_r) is large, about two-thirds of TLC. In contrast, in the lower zones of the lungs of a seated person, FRC is only about one-third of TLC. Thus, these functional data in vivo in man agree with the data on alveolar size in dog lungs.[34]

Figure 4-3 is a different diagram based on similar data. If all lung regions expanded equally, regional volume everywhere would equal the same percentage of TLC, as indicated by the dotted lines in Figure 4-3. For instance, at residual volume (RV), regional volume would be about 25 percent of TLC_r for all lung zones. In fact, regional volume in the lung tops is always larger than the dotted line shows, and in bottom zones it is less. The difference is most marked near RV. Although Figure 4-3 is based on data obtained during conditions of zero airflow, it shows approximately how a tidal breath is distributed. A tidal breath inspired from FRC (VT_1) goes predominantly to the lower lung zones. Between FRC and TLC, the relations between regional and total lung volumes are linear (Fig. 4-3), and the distribution pattern is comparable with the effects of gravity discussed above—lower zones are better ventilated than lung tops. This is because the lung tops are more expanded than the lower zones and hence operate on a flatter portion of the static recoil curve (see Fig. 7-1, p. 150). Experiments on the human centrifuge[17] confirm the importance of gravity in determining regional expansion: increased acceleration leads to divergence of the regional expansion lines in Figure 4-3*B*. Above FRC, the uppermost lung areas are ventilated less than the dependent zones, irre-

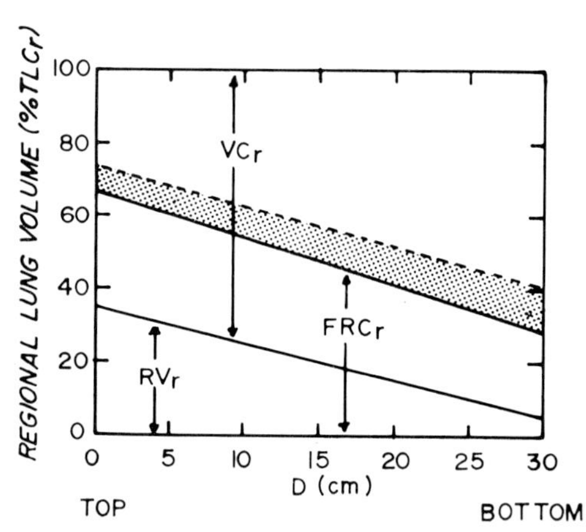

Fig. 4-2. *Ordinate.* Regional lung volume, as a percentage of regional TLC (TLC_r). *Abscissa.* Vertical distance, D, from lung top to lung bottom. At maximum inspiration, all lung regions are maximally expanded (100% on ordinate). At maximum expiration and at FRC, top regions are more expanded than lower ones. Regional VC is larger in lower zones than in the lung tops. *Shaded area.* Regional tidal volume, which is larger at the bottom than at the top. Modified from reference 57.

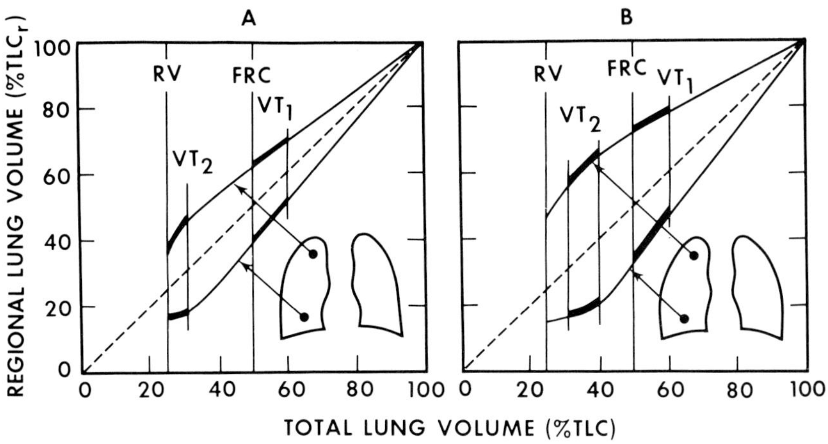

Fig. 4-3. *Ordinate.* Regional lung volume, in percentage of regional TLC_r. *Abscissa.* Total lung volume (% TLC). The dashed line of equality indicates regions which expand in proportion to total lung volume. The drawn line above the dashed line represents the expansion of an area in the top of a vertical lung, from RV to TLC; the lower drawn line represents the expansion of an area near the bottom of the lung. *A.* Control data; *B.* Data obtained during increased acceleration of gravity on human centrifuge. Heavy bars on lines indicate distribution of tidal volume above FRC (VT_1) and below FRC (VT_2). The slope of these bars indicates relative tidal volumes to each region. Particularly when gravity is increased, bottom zones receive little ventilation during tidals below FRC (bar nearly horizontal). Above FRC a larger fraction of VT goes to the bottom of the lungs (dependent region). Modified from reference 17.

spective of posture.[44] The difference is associated with the lungs' orientation in the gravity field and not with inherent properties of certain parts of the lungs.

Near RV, the lower lung zones are maximally deflated, because they are compressed by the lungs' own weight.[57, 77a, 79] Since this also impedes air entry into these zones, they receive little inspired air near RV (VT_2 in Fig. 4-3). Air entry into these dependent zones could be limited by alveolar collapse, closing of small airways, or closing of large airways. The exact mechanism is unclear, but since gas distribution near RV behaves as if airways in dependent zones were closed, the term airway closure is used to describe this mechanism. When gravity is increased (Fig. 4-3*B*), airway closure extends to a larger total lung volume. Posture also affects airway closure. If the alinear portions of the regional ventilation lines in Figure 4-3 are close to FRC, small postural changes can markedly influence gas distribution. For example, in the supine position FRC is moderately reduced, and the pattern of VT_1 might change into that of VT_2.

NONUNIFORMITY WITHIN LUNG LOBES

The external counters used to obtain the graphs of Figures 4-1–4-3 "see" radioactivity in large lung areas and do not detect ventilation differences within each area. These ventilation differences can be studied by passing catheters into large and small airways of one lobe to measure local N_2 clearance (p. 72). With this method, Suda et al.[73] found that inspired gas distribution within lobes and segments was markedly nonuniform. In fact, the differences within units as small as 20 ml were much greater than the ventilation differences between similar small units in the lung top and bottom. Since gravity effects must be negligible, they cannot explain nonuniform ventilation within such small lung segments. At least part of the ventilation inequalities in a 20-ml unit of lung must be due to unequal stress-strain relations or to unequal force distribution.[73] In such a unit, diffusion times (as calculated by Rauwerda, Table 4-1; p. 66) are too long to allow diffusion equilibration within the time span of a normal breath.

STRESS–STRAIN RELATIONS

Tendeloo [74] attributed unequal ventilation primarily to unequal distribution of the respiratory forces (stress) through lung tissue and unequal compliance of different lung parts. Later, physiologists proposed, by analogy with the theory of parallel electrical circuits, that the product of air flow resistance (R) and lung compliance (C) determines the rate of air entry into each lung region.[61] Regions where this product, the RC or time constant, is low should fill and empty faster than regions with a high RC constant. However, since peripheral airways have a very low resistance and hence a low time constant, RC constants in healthy lungs are probably too small to affect gas distribution.[56] Thus, bulk flow may largely be determined by elastic tissue properties and by stress distribution, rather than by airway resistance. Lung emptying patterns are influenced by expiratory flow rate,[43, 58] but this can be explained by local compliance variation as well as by the time constant theory.[78]

At small lung volumes, and also in older people or in patients with airway disease, regional airway-resistance differences are probably important in determining inspired gas distribution.[23, 29, 49] Increased airway muscle tone, as in asthma, increases nonuniform gas distribution (Chap. 12); again, changes in local airway resistance are the most likely determinant. At the end of the scale, airway closure (p. 63) in dependent lung zones and at low lung volumes implies infinitely high airway resistance to these zones and no air entry.

The difference between the top and bottom of a vertical lung is a good example of the importance of stress-strain relations. Since lung tissue in the top is stressed more, it is less distensible than lung tissue in the bottom zone. West has pointed out the consequences for lung pathology—emphysema is more common in the lung tops, and spontaneous pneumothorax due to rupture of lung tissue at the top occurs commonly in tall people.[77] These vulnerable regions, which may include the apical segment of the right lower lobe, may be under increased stress when lung volume decreases to near RV, as during shouting, laughter, or singing.

UNEQUAL PATHWAY LENGTHS

The varying length of bronchial pathways (p. 52) results in a sixfold range of transit times from the carina to the alveoli in the human lung.[40] The inspired gas front reaches the most proximal alveoli after 22 ml gas has passed the carina; 170 ml more must be inspired before the most distal alveoli are reached. This can account for a considerable degree of nonuniform gas distribution in normal lungs.[28, 40]

SEQUENTIAL FILLING AND EMPTYING

Fowler's sequential ventilation theory [31] continues to receive support.[75] It proposes that certain lung areas fill early in inspiration and expire late during expiration. For instance, when inspiring from RV (Fig. 4-3), the lung tops inspire first; the bottom zone receives a larger part of the inspired breath at higher volumes. During expiration, the bottom zones empty preferentially until airway closure occurs; the lung tops then contribute most of the remaining expired tidal volume. Thus, the area which fills first empties last. In contrast, the time-constant theory suggested a "first-in, first-out" sequence.[8] Both mechanisms may operate in the same lungs under different conditions. The first-in, first-out mechanism may predominate when time constants are increased, e.g., by airway obstruction. The "first-in, last-out" sequence may operate at low lung volumes and in other conditions when tidal volume overlaps with airway closing volume.

Series Ventilation

The mechanisms described above cause regional ventilation differences, or parallel nonuniformity, since the separate lobes, segments, and lobules are analogous to parallel elements in an electrical circuit. Alveoli, alveolar ducts, and larger airways are 'in series' elements, and if more inspired gas reaches terminal bronchioles than alveoli, there is series nonuniformity of ventilation. Parallel and series nonuniformity [64] are not mutually exclusive. The principal mechanisms of series ventilation are stratification in terminal units, collateral ventilation, redistribution of dead space gas, and pendelluft. None of these is quantitatively important in normal lungs, but each plays a role under abnormal conditions.

STRATIFICATION

According to Krogh and Lindhard: [46] ". . . the air in the airsacs (as well as in the atria) is not at the end of inspiration of the same composition throughout, because the inspired air is incompletely mixed with the air previously contained. The mixing takes place chiefly by diffusion and requires a certain time." This statement suggests a layering or stratified inhomogeneity of alveolar gas. Near the entrance to terminal units, gas composition would approach that of inspired gas; near the blood-air barrier, gas composition would be in equilibrium with blood. The opposite view is that diffusion within terminal lung spaces is fast enough for complete equilibration within the breathing cycle. Hence, any uneven composition of alveolar gas must be due to differences in regional ventilation.

Gas diffusion is no doubt an essential mode of transport in terminal airways and alveoli. The question is whether diffusion is a rate-limiting factor in gas-exchanging units. Since there is no precise anatomical delineation between conducting and gas-exchanging airways (see Fig. 2-2*B*), the debate on stratification is to some extent a matter of semantics. Two lines of evidence, from lung models and from gas exchange experiments, suggest that diffusional mixing in terminal lung units is rapid and that stratified inhomogeneity is minimal in normal lungs.

Rauwerda [63] used a 7-mm long cylindrical lung model to represent the diffusion path within a primary lobule. This distance is realistic in anatomical terms; according to Weibel's data (Table 2-1, p. 31), the average pathway length from the terminal respiratory bronchioles to the alveoli is less than 5 mm. In a 7-mm long cylinder, diffusion alone would decrease gas concentration differences to 16 percent of their initial value after 0.38 second.[63] Thus, diffusion appeared to be highly effective within the primary lobules. In larger units (lobules and lobes), diffusion times increase as the anatomical pathway lengths increase (Table 4-1). In his experiments, Rauwerda found that after an inspiration of oxygen, the early expired gas always contained more O_2 and less N_2 than gas expired later [63] (Fig. 4-4). When the breath was held before expiring, the difference between early and late samples decreased but did not disappear. Even after 60 seconds of breath holding, the early and late samples differed by about 2 percent O_2 and N_2. The first 30 seconds of breath holding appear to establish equilibrium in small lung units, where diffusion distances are short. However, even prolonged breath holding could not abolish concentration differences between lung regions that communicate via long pathways. Comparing these data to his model calculations (Table 4-1), Rauwerda concluded that (1) diffusion equilibrium would be reached in normal primary lobules within the duration of a normal inspiration, and (2) any concentration differences remaining after more than 30 seconds of breath holding should be attributed to regional ventilation differences between large units such as lung lobes. The dimensions Rauwerda chose for his lung model were anatomically realistic, but the model's cylindrical shape has been criticized.[24] However, more recent model computations largely confirm Rauwerda's conclusions.[48] A recent model of Cumming et al.,[27] which analyzes bulk flow and diffusion in alternating steps, yields little support for stratified inhomogeneity.

The present discussion may appear to contradict several studies with aerosols [59] and with heavy and light gases [25, 33, 62] which have confirmed that molecular weight and hence gas diffusivity markedly influence mixing of inspired gas in normal lungs. Heavy gases diffuse less and are expired first; lighter, more readily diffusible gases appear at the mouth only late during expiration [33] (*dashed line,* Fig. 4-5). Clearly, diffusion equilibrium is incomplete after a normal inspiration. However, these results show only that incomplete diffusion equilibrium occurs somewhere in the airways or in the alveoli; they offer no clues to the site of occurrence. Since stratified inhomogeneity is unlikely on the grounds discussed above, this site is

Table 4–1
Rauwerda's Diffusion Time Calculations

Part of the Lung	Diffusion Path (cm)	Diffusion Time § (sec)
Alveolar duct	0.05	0.002
Primary lobule	0.70	0.380
Lobule (small)	0.80 *	0.490
Lobule (large)	3.00 *	6.900
Lobe (small)	8.80 †	60.000
Lobe (large)	17.00 †	222.000
Lobe (small)	22.80 ‡	400.000
Lobe (large)	31.00 ‡	739.000

* From entrance of lobular bronchus to alveoli.
† Distance from carina to alveoli.
‡ Distance from trachea entrance to alveoli.
§ $t=(\alpha^2/D)\times 0.2$, where α=diffusion path length, and D=diffusion coefficient (0.260 cm^2/sec for O_2 into N_2 at 37° C). Data from Rauwerda.[63]

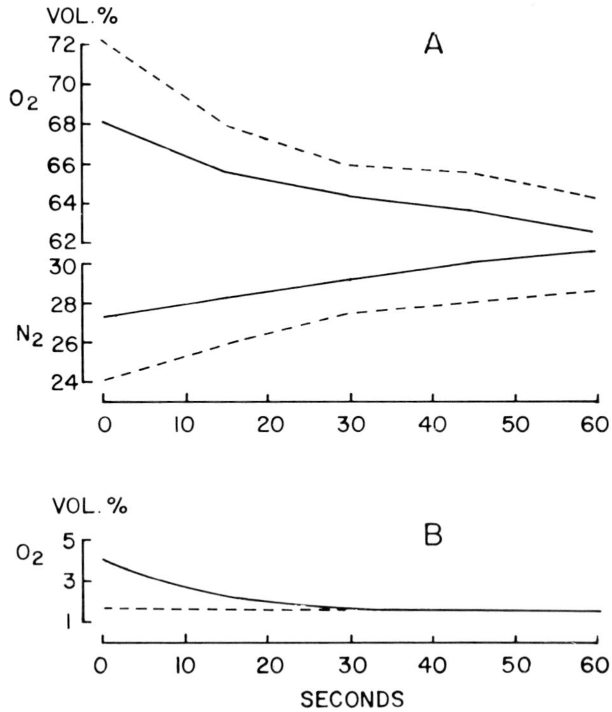

Fig. 4-4. Analysis of expired gas after inspiration of O_2 in a healthy subject. *A.* Lines drawn through points obtained in separate experiments with 0, 15, 30, 45, and 60 seconds' breath-holding. *Dashed lines.* Samples after 1-liter expiration. *Solid lines.* Samples after 2.5-liter expiration. The gas expired later contains less O_2 and more N_2. This difference decreases with breath holding, as indicated in *B* for O_2. *Abscissa.* Breath holding time. Modified from reference 63.

probably in conducting airways rather than in terminal lung units. This conclusion is in agreement with calculations based on a model in which bulk flow and diffusion operate simultaneously and continuously (Chap. 3, p. 50), calculations which suggest that diffusion in conducting airways can account for the effects of breath holding on dead space.

Another argument against stratified inhomogeneity is derived from experiments on gas exchange. If diffusional gas mixing influences gas concentrations adjacent to the alveolocapillary membrane, one would expect gases of high density to impede gas exchange. But even large increases in gas density do not impede gas exchange in man [68] or in dogs.[55] Only when dogs breathe hyperoxygenated liquid (with the density of water) does gas exchange become limited by diffusion in what used to be air spaces.[47]

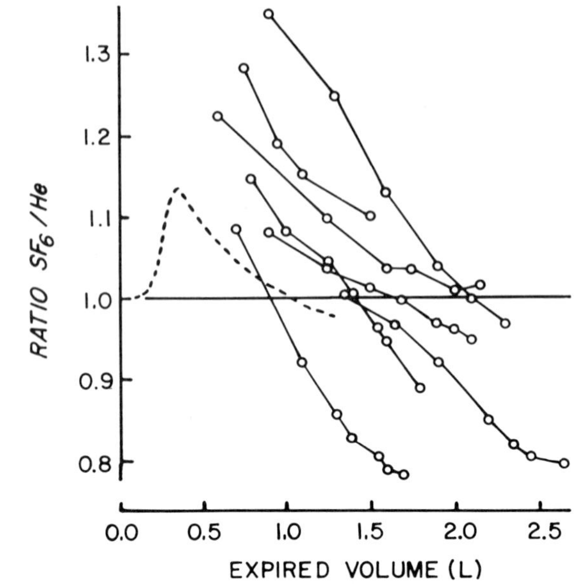

Fig. 4-5. Analysis of six successive samples of expired gas after inspiration of a gas mixture containing about 10% SF_6 and 30% He. *Dashed line.* Average data in 7 healthy subjects. *Solid lines.* Individual data in 7 patients with emphysema. Ratio $SF_6/He = 1.0$ when ratio in expired gas equals that in inspired mixture, i.e., 10/30. Early in expiration, the expired air is relatively rich in the heavy gas SF_6; later on, in the much lighter He. Reproduced from reference 33.

COLLATERAL VENTILATION

The passage of gas between adjacent alveoli (through alveolar pores) and between adjacent bronchioles (through connections between these structures) is called collateral ventilation.[51, 54] In human lungs, polystyrene spheres less than 60 μm in diameter can pass from one segment to another next to it.[38] In principle, collateral ventilation might promote equality of alveolar gas tensions in different lung regions. Actually, this effect is probably minimal, since the flow resistance of collateral pathways in human lungs is high.[39] However, collateral ventilation may be important in disease, where it may be the only means of ventilating lung regions behind occluded airways. Without collateral ventilation, these regions might collapse. With collateral ventilation, they are ventilated through other alveolar regions, i.e., in series with lung units with open bronchi.[38] Hence they become, in West's terminology, a parasitic space, which seriously affects gas exchange.[76] Histamine and histamine-releasing drugs (curare, 48/80) reduce collateral ventilation in dogs,[18] perhaps because smooth muscle contraction occludes connections between respiratory bronchioles. If bronchial pathways become occluded, lungs without collateral ventilation pathways are vulnerable to atelectasis. Local tissue damage as well as drugs used in anesthesia can release histamine, and this may promote postoperative atelectasis in surgical patients.

DISTRIBUTION OF DEAD SPACE GAS

A large part of the anatomical dead space—the trachea and upper airways—is common to all parts of the lungs. At the end of expiration, this space is filled with a mixture of alveolar gas from all lung regions. During inspiration, this gas is distributed throughout the lungs. Thus, the common dead space, acting as a mixing chamber in series with the alveoli, tends to equalize alveolar gas concentrations throughout the lungs.[11] If one breathes through a long tube, this mixing is sufficient to turn N_2 washout curves into single exponential functions (Fig. 4-6).

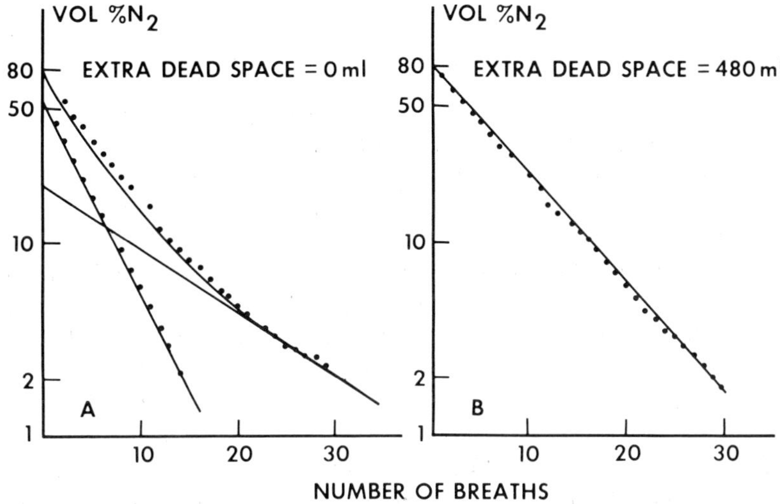

Fig. 4-6. Semilogarithmic plots of end-tidal N_2 concentration (log scale) versus number of breaths (linear scale) during O_2 breathing in a healthy subject. *A*. Control curve, analyzed as the sum of two exponential functions, each represented by a straight line. *B*. Washout curve from the same subject breathing through an extra dead space of 480 ml. Reproduced from reference 11.

PENDELLUFT

When different lung regions have grossly unequal time constants, one region may still inspire air while another region already expires. Thus, when ventilation is markedly asynchronous, alveolar gas may be shuttled back and forth (German: pendeln = to shuttle) between different lung regions, via the dead space. Pendelluft often contributes to ventilatory failure after severe chest injuries.[76]

MEASUREMENT OF NONUNIFORM DISTRIBUTION

Since inspired gas distribution is markedly uneven in obstructive lung disease, measurements of distribution are useful in diagnosing these conditions and in assessing treatment. Simple clinical tests (auscultation, percussion, and observation of chest movements) sometimes indicate regional lack of air entry, gross asynchrony or asymmetry of ventilatory movements, or decreased local air content. The chest x-ray film often provides similar qualitative information, and a more complex x-ray method (lung scanning after ^{133}Xe inhalation) can detect lung areas with poor or absent ventilation. However, the amount of ^{133}Xe seen on a scan cannot be related to the volume of each lung region. Thus, as usually applied, lung scanning provides qualitative, rather than quantitative, information.[57]

Here I shall discuss only quantitative methods, usually divided into single-breath and multiple-breath methods.[8, 14] Both use the principle of tracing a gaseous marker that undergoes little or no exchange with blood, i.e., a physiologically inert gas. Nitrogen is always available for this purpose; helium and radioactive xenon are also used. The marker can be traced by serial or continuous analysis of expired gas and, in the case of ^{133}Xe, by external counting as well.

Single-Breath Washout Curve

After 100 percent O_2 has been inspired, the N_2 concentration in expired gas increases rapidly as dead space gas is cleared (phases 1 and 2; Figs. 4-7 and 4-8). The concentration continues to rise slightly in phase 3 after dead space gas has been washed out, indicating nonuniform composition of alveolar gas. Several gas distribution tests use recordings of this type.[2, 22, 45] In healthy people, the slight slope of phase 3 may reflect a distribution of transit times[28] and some degree of sequential emptying.[75] Unequal $\dot{V}_A/\dot{Q}$ ratios (Chap. 5) contributes since all test gases are slightly soluble in blood; this can be eliminated by using two inert gases that are similarly affected by unequal perfusion.[30, 71]

In disease, several mechanisms may contribute to increased slopes of phase 3 (Fig. 4-7*B*). Stratified inhomogeneity may contribute when the lungs contain pathological spaces with large diffusion distances, as in emphysema. Time constant differences may be at fault when small airway narrowing is widespread, but unequally distributed, as in bronchitis or asthma. For clinical purposes, the percentage of N_2 difference between 750 and 1250 ml expired volume is used to quantitate phase 3 slopes.[22] The slopes are markedly influenced by lung volume,[42] flow

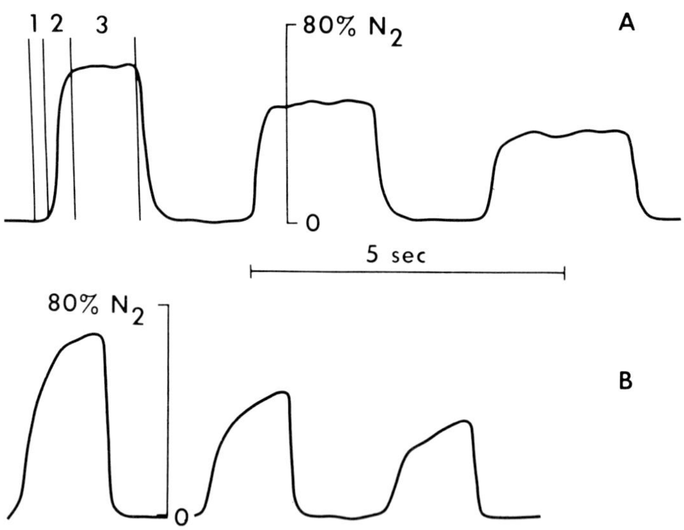

Fig. 4-7. Three breathing cycles from nitrogen washout curves during quiet breathing in a normal subject (*A*) and in a patient with emphysema (*B*). Washout of dead space gas (*1, 2*) followed by alveolar plateau (*3*). Phases 2 and 3 cannot be distinguished in emphysema, in which alveolar N_2% continues to increase throughout expiration.

rates,[43, 58] and posture.[3, 20] Therefore, standardized procedures are required for their use as a quantitative test. Gross abnormalities (e.g., the curves of Fig. 4-7*B*) are easily detected with any version of the test, but more subtle changes require careful assessment. Third phase slopes are more pronounced in healthy young adults than in healthy children, but do not increase beyond age 20.[2]

Expired gas and regional alveolar gas can be monitored simultaneously with the ^{133}Xe method. When inspired as a bolus at a volume close to RV, most Xe goes to the lung tops (Fig. 4-1). Figure 4-8 shows Xe concentration versus time

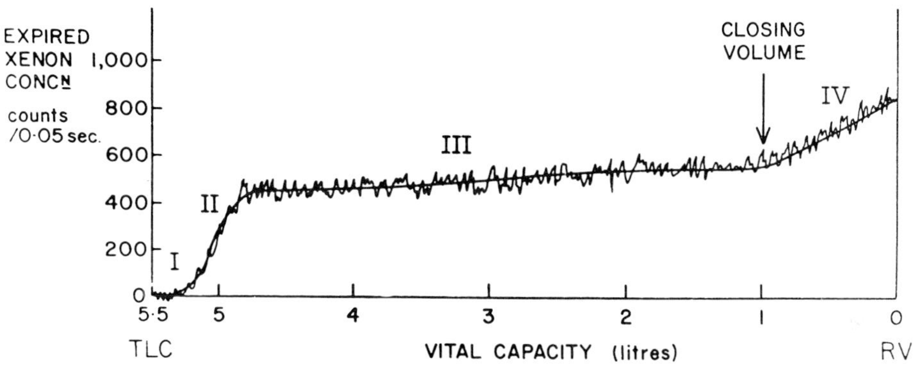

Fig. 4-8. Expired ^{133}Xe concentration (ordinate) as a function of lung volume, during a full VC expiration from TLC to RV. During the preceding inspiration, a bolus of ^{133}Xe was injected near RV. Phase 3 (alveolar plateau) and phase 4 (terminal rise) are indicated. Closing volume is about 1 liter above RV. Reproduced from reference 49.

in the next expiration. After phase 3, the curve shows a final rise (phase 4) at a volume close to RV. Dollfuss et al.[29] proposed that the high Xe levels in phase 4 show a large contribution of apical, Xe-rich zones to expired air. Lower zones appear to contribute progressively less to expired air, in phase 4, which agrees with the concept of airway closure in dependent lung zones (p. 63). The lung volume at which phase 4 begins is called airway closing volume (ACV).[2, 23, 49] In young adults, ACV is less than FRC, but in older persons with increased ACV some airways in dependent lung zones may be closed during quiet breathing.[49] Phase 4 can also be shown in N_2 single-breath curves if the subject expires to RV, then inspires O_2 to TLC, and holds his breath for 15–30 seconds before expiring to RV.[2] With the N_2 method, ACV was 10% of VC or less in children and young adults, and about 20 percent of VC in 40- to 50-year-old subjects.[2] The terminal rise (phase 4) in N_2 concentration was also increased in older persons.

Airway closing volume appears to rise with increasing expiratory flow.[43] Hyatt et al[41, 41a] reported that phase 4 begins when expiratory flow becomes limited by dynamic compression of intrathoracic airways (Fig. 4-9). These data suggest that airway closure in dependent lung zones is determined by dynamic compression of larger airways, rather than by alveolar collapse or closing of small airways. Thus, determination of ACV may have the same significance as measurement of flow rates at low lung volumes on MEFV curves (Chap. 9). That is, large closing volumes would correspond to low maximum flows. Several observations

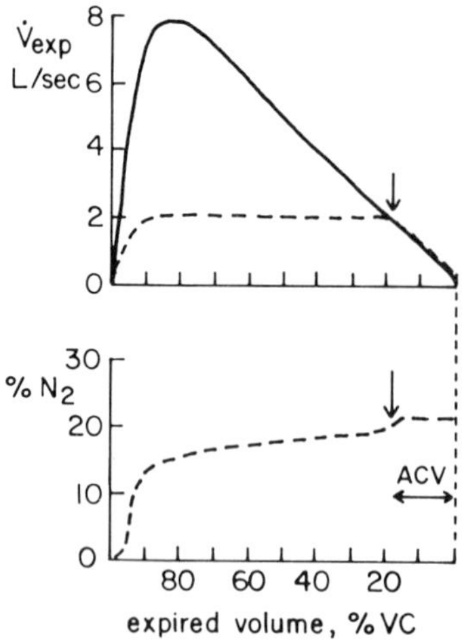

Fig. 4-9. *Top.* MEFV curve of a healthy person (*drawn line*). (See Chap. 9 for discussion of these curves.) *Dashed line.* Expired flow rates during N_2 single-breath curve recording. *Bottom.* N_2 single-breath curve. 100% O_2 inspired from RV during previous inspiration. At the arrow, expiration becomes flow-limited; i.e., flow reaches the maximum value indicated by the MEFV curve (*top graph*). At the same moment, N_2% rises to a phase 4 (*bottom graph*). Airway closing volume (ACV) is indicated; its value depends on expiratory flow during the single-breath curve and increases with increasing flow.[41, 43] Modified from reference 41a.

support this interpretation. For instance, increasing age and cigarette smoking are both associated with large ACV's [2, 49] and with decreased flow rates on MEFV curves (Chap. 9).

Multiple-Breath Inert Gas Washout

If a tidal volume of oxygen is distributed to all parts of the lungs in proportion to their volumes, alveolar N_2 concentrations decrease by the same factor everywhere. This dilution factor depends on lung volume, tidal volume, and dead space. If the dilution factor is constant from breath to breath, alveolar N_2 concentrations ($F_{A_{N_2}}$) decrease exponentially after successive breaths of O_2. Hence, a graph of log $F_{A_{N_2}}$ versus the number of breaths then yields a straight line. In healthy persons these graphs are sometimes linear (Fig. 4-10*A*), but frequently they are not (Fig. 4-6*A*). -This indicates nonuniform inspired gas distribution, which might be due to regional ventilation differences, or stratified inhomogeneity, or both. Since the curve does not provide information on mechanisms, it requires interpretation in conjunction with other data. The graph of Figure 4-6*A* changed into that of Figure 4-6*B* when the subject breathed through a long tube at the mouth—an example of the effect of redistribution of dead space gas (p. 69). The graph of Figure 4-10*A* changed into that of Figure 4-10*B* after inhalation of an airway-constricting drug—this probably reflects a variable increase of time constants in different lung regions, which changed the ventilation from a uniform pattern (*A*) to a nonuniform distribution (*B*).

Alinear N_2 clearance curves can be analyzed by a curve-stripping procedure (Figs. 4-6 and 4-10) into a sum of two or three exponential functions. Computer methods can eliminate observer bias from this procedure.[36] To quantitate nonuniform ventilation, several numerical indices, reviewed earlier,[8] are derived from clearance curves.[32, 64] New indices have been published more recently.[36, 60, 67] The accuracy of these procedures is limited by the accuracy of the experimental data, which may show considerable breath-to-breath variations (e.g., in Fig. 4-10*B*).

A simpler way of expressing N_2 washout data, independent of the shape of the clearance curve, is to calculate the lung clearance index [5]:

$$LCI = nV_T/V_L \tag{1}$$

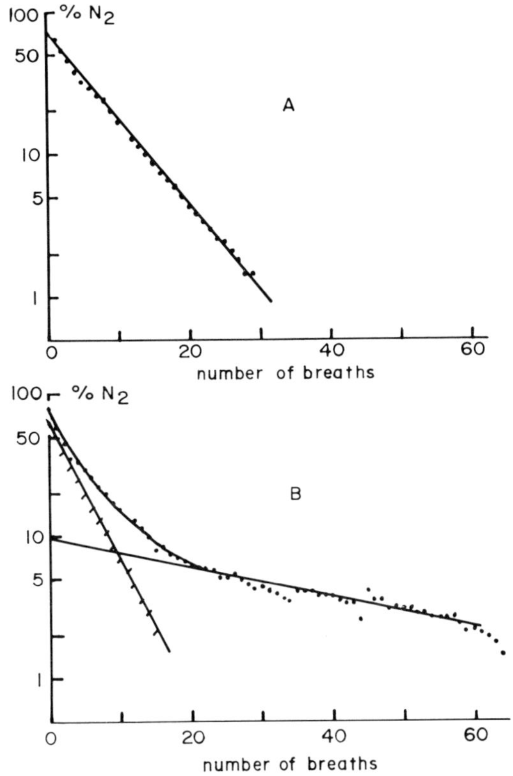

Fig. 4-10. Expired $N_2\%$ (log scale) versus number of breaths during N_2 washout. The points are end-tidal N_2 concentrations in successive expirations; the line through the points has been drawn freehand. The curve of *B* has been analyzed into two exponential components by curve-stripping. *A*. Control curve in healthy subject (LCI=7.5). *B*. Directly after inhalation of histamine aerosol (LCI=16.1). Histamine aerosol induces marked nonuniformity of ventilation. Reproduced from reference 10.

where LCI= lung clearance index, n=the total number of breaths during N_2 washout, V_T=tidal volume, and V_L=the lung volume that is being washed out. V_L=FRC when the washout is begun at the end of a normal expiration. Thus, LCI simply indicates the amount of ventilation required to eliminate N_2 during a clearance test, to a predetermined end-point, commonly $F_{A_{N_2}}=0.02$; this value ranges from 6–10 in healthy persons. LCI is related to the exponential functions which describe N_2 clearance, and this enables one to predict values for LCI as a function of tidal volume, at a fixed end-expiratory lung volume.[13] With tidal volumes greater than 600 ml, LCI is relatively independent of tidal volume. However, its experimental values are always higher than those predicted, even when N_2 clearance curves show a single exponential function.[13, 67] The actual values of LCI may reflect residual nonuniformity not detected by the analysis of exponential components. With tidal volumes less than about 600 ml, N_2 clearance is delayed because dead space is a large fraction of tidal volume, and LCI is increased.[13] This also happens when extra dead space is added at the mouth.[11] LCI increases because added ventilation is needed to clear the extra dead space volume. At the same time, N_2 clearance curves become linear (Fig. 4-6), because the dead space act as a mixing chamber (p. 69). Thus, LCI and clearance curves do not always change in the same direction.

N_2 clearance tests provide objective information about lung ventilation during quiet breathing, but their clinical potential (p. 75) has not been widely utilized because of technical complexity and the labor required for data analysis. Improved N_2 meters and electronic data processing may now increase their use. Some programs for curve analysis are already available.[66] New electronic circuits allow direct plotting of $F_{A_{N_2}}$ versus accumulated expired volume on semilogarithmic coordinates.[70] On-line computation of the amount of N_2 expired during each breath of the clearance test is feasible and allows rapid data analysis using the method of Fowler et al.[32]

PHYSIOLOGICAL FACTORS INFLUENCING DISTRIBUTION

Breathing Pattern and Lung Volume

Increases in tidal volume and in breathing rate have little effect on N_2 clearance.[13, 69] At small tidal volumes ($<$600 ml), N_2 clearance is delayed (see above). Lung volume may affect distribution if airway closing volume is close to FRC (p. 63). Incomplete mixing because of shortened diffusion times occurs at unphysiological breathing rates ($>$100/min).[65]

Age

Few data are available in newborns.[6] Older children ($<$12 yrs) nearly always have single exponential clearance curves; adolescents and adults have increasingly nonuniform distributions.[8, 19] Single-breath curves also vary with age (p. 71). The effects of age on regional ventilation differences have not been described in detail. Closing volume increases with age.[2, 49]

Posture

Regional ventilation patterns shift with posture, according to the direction of gravity.[44] Since closing volume is larger in the supine than in the upright position,[49] there is an overall increase in nonuniformity when supine.[15, 20]

Tissue N_2 Elimination

During O_2 breathing, N_2 is eliminated from tissue stores in the body. Unless a correction is made, this leads to overestimation of FRC, underestimation of LCI, and errors in N_2 clearance analysis.[7] Data on tissue N_2 elimination in man [50] and in dogs [35] can be used for approximate corrections.

Airway Smooth Muscle Tone

Histamine and other smooth-muscle-contracting substances increase nonuniform distribution[10] (Fig. 4-10). N_2 clearance is also prolonged after inhalation of textile dust or allergens (Chap. 12). Epinephrine, which relaxes airway smooth muscle, increases LCI in healthy subjects.[9, 15] This may suggest that normal muscle tone helps to minimize nonuniform distribution: when airway muscle tone is abolished with a relaxant drug, distribution becomes less uniform. The mechanisms controlling this adjustment of tone are unknown. The effect of constrictor drugs or dust on N_2 single-breath curves varies.[4, 21, 72] Severe airway obstruction is compatible with a normal phase 3 slope.[4, 72] The initial slope and its underlying mechanisms (e.g., sequential emptying or increased time constants) may affect the results and explain the variability.

INSPIRED GAS DISTRIBUTION IN DISEASE

N_2 clearance is often grossly delayed in asthma and chronic bronchitis. Clearance curves are markedly alinear, and LCI is increased. Slopes of phase 3 in single-breath curves are usually increased as well (Fig. 4-7*B*); in such instances it may be difficult to distinguish phase 3 and 4 and to determine airway closing volume (ACV).

Measurement of ACV has been suggested for early detection of *airway obstruction.*[49] An increase in ACV may be related to the decrease in maximum flow rates, which is also a sensitive test for airway obstruction (Chap. 9). When a patient with asthma is undergoing treatment, N_2 clearance may remain abnormal even though other tests ($FEV_{1.0}$, airway resistance) are normal.[52] Regional xenon distribution in asthma may be normal even when other indices (e.g., maximum midexpiratory flow) are low.[37] Nonuniformity in asthma is probably related to obstruction in intralobar or intralobular airways, and collateral ventilation (p. 68) may contribute to prolongation of N_2 washout.

In *emphysema,* gas distribution is highly nonuniform.[12, 16] Stratified inhomogeneity and collateral ventilation, as well as widespread airway obstruction, may contribute. The large concentration gradients which occur in these lungs when a SF_6-He mixture is inspired (Fig. 4-5)[33] suggest that diffusion distances are increased. Since infused xenon is not as effectively cleared from alveolar air as inhaled xenon,[1] the layers of gas close to blood vessels may have a slower turnover than layers closer to airways in connection with the atmosphere. Cumming et al.[26] have demonstrated dilated airway structures in different types of emphysema, and these provide an anatomical substrate for increased diffusion distances. Stratified inhomogeneity within such abnormal spaces can contribute considerably to the overall inefficiency of ventilation and to sloping third phases of single-breath curves.[14, 63]

The lungs are a nonuniform structure in which respiratory and gravity stresses are distributed unequally. Physiological tests of gas distribution can detect the consequences of these nonuniformities, especially when the tests maximize the effect of particular mechanisms of uneven distribution. Yet, many young and healthy adults have linear N_2 clearance graphs (Fig. 4-10*A*) and minimal phase 3 slopes (Fig. 4-7*A*). This indicates that their inspired tidal volume is distributed uniformly, or nearly so. Yet, such subjects do have regional ventilation inequalities as shown by radioactive gas methods. Although N_2 clearance may lack the sensitivity to show this inequality, it seems remarkable that gross regional ventilation differences might occur in persons with linear N_2 clearance graphs like the one of Figure 4-10*A*. Unfortunately, no comparison of regional studies with N_2 clearance graphs in the same subjects appears to have been made. It seems possible, however, that the effects of different factors leading to nonuniform distribution might cancel one another, or that there may be regulation processes which maintain uniform gas distribution. In any case, markedly nonuniform distribution of inspired gas, as defined by N_2 single- or multiple-breath tests, is found only in older persons and in patients with lung disease.

SUMMARY

Inspired air is distributed unequally to different regions in *normal lungs* because of regional or parallel ventilation differences, which include effects of unequal bronchial pathway lengths, unequal stress distribution, unequal lung compliance, and effects of the lungs' orientation in a gravity field. The latter leads to distortion of the lungs because of their weight, with relative overexpansion of alveoli in the lung top, while the lower zones are compressed and do not receive inspired gas near RV (airway closure).

In *diseased lungs,* increased airway resistance in obstructed airways, stratification of gas in enlarged alveolar spaces, collateral ventilation of lung regions behind occluded bronchi, and pendelluft cause increased nonuniform distribution of inspired gas.

Methods to quantitate unequal gas distribution in disease include single-and multiple-breath inert gas clearance tests. Single-breath curves (N_2 or ^{133}Xe) have phase 3 slopes that reflect unequal distribution, while their phase 4 reflects airway closure. Multiple-breath N_2 clearance is prolonged by unequal distribution; this can be quantitated by an analysis of exponential functions or by the lung clearance index.

Breathing patterns, age, posture, and airway smooth muscle tone are the principal physiological variables affecting inspired gas distribution. Gas distribution is often markedly unequal in asthma, bronchitis, and emphysema, or after severe chest injuries.

REFERENCES

1. Anthonisen NR, Bass H, Oriol A, Place REG, Bates DV: Regional lung function in patients with chronic bronchitis. Clin Sci 35:495–511, 1968
2. Anthonisen NR, Danson J, Robertson PC, Ross WRD: Airway closure as a function of age. Respir Physiol 8:58–65, 1969/1970
3. Anthonisen NR, Robertson PC, Ross WRD: Gravity-dependent sequential emptying of lung regions. J Appl Physiol 28:589–595, 1970
4. Arnoldsson H, Bouhuys A, Lindell SE: Byssinosis: Differential diagnosis from bronchial asthma and chronic bronchitis. Acta Med Scand 173:761–768, 1963

5. Becklake MR: A new index of the intrapulmonary mixture of inspired air. Thorax 7:111–116, 1952
6. Bolton DPG, Cross KW: Lung volume and mixing efficiency in the new-born infant. J Physiol (Lond) 208:25–26P, 1970
7. Bouhuys A: Influence of tissue nitrogen elimination on analysis of pulmonary nitrogen clearance curves. Acta Physiol Pharmacol Neerl 8:431–436, 1959
8. Bouhuys A: Distribution of inspired gas in the lungs, in Fenn WO, Rahn H (eds): Handbook of Physiology, Section 3: Respiration, vol I. Washington, D.C., American Physiological Society, 1964, pp 715–733
9. Bouhuys A, Jönsson R, Lichtneckert S, Lindell SE, Lundgren C, Lundin G: The effect of epinephrine and hexamethonium bromide on the pulmonary ventilation in man. Acta Physiol Pharmacol Neerl 8:437–446, 1959
10. Bouhuys A, Jönsson R, Lichtneckert S, Lindell SE, Lundgren C, Lundin G, Ringquist TR: Effects of histamine on pulmonary ventilation in man. Clin Sci 19:79–94, 1960
11. Bouhuys A, Jönsson R, Lundin G: Influence of added dead space on pulmonary ventilation. Acta Physiol Scand 39:105–120, 1957
12. Bouhuys A, Jönsson R, Lundin G: Nonuniformity of pulmonary ventilation in chronic diffuse obstructive emphysema. Acta Med Scand 162:29–46, 1958
13. Bouhuys A, Lichtneckert S, Lundgren C, Lundin G: Voluntary changes in breathing pattern and N_2 clearance from lungs. J Appl Physiol 16:1039–1042, 1961
14. Bouhuys A, Lundin G: Distribution of inspired gas in lungs. Physiol Rev 39: 731–750, 1959
15. Bouhuys A, van Lennep HJ: Effect of body posture on gas distribution in the lungs. J Appl Physiol 17:38–42, 1962
16. Briscoe WA, Cournand A: Uneven ventilation of normal and diseased lungs studied by an open-circuit method. J Appl Physiol 14:284–290, 1959
17. Bryan AC, Milic-Emili J, Pengelly D: Effect of gravity on the distribution of pulmonary ventilation. J Appl Physiol 21:778–784, 1966
18. Call EP Jr, Lindskog GE, Liebow AA: Some physiologic and pharmacologic aspects of collateral ventilation. J Thorac Cardiovasc Surg 49:1015–1025, 1965
19. Chiang ST, Wang BC, Chi YL, Hsieh YC: Ventilatory components of lungs in relation to sex and age. Am Rev Respir Dis 104:175–181, 1971
20. Clarke SW, Jones JG, Glaister DH: Change in pulmonary ventilation in different postures. Clin Sci 37:357–369, 1969
21. Colldahl H, Pegelow KO, Pokorny J: The single-breath nitrogen-elimination test for the registration of provocation tests in allergy diagnosis. Acta Allergol (Kbh) 22 (suppl 8):79–97, 1967
22. Comroe JH Jr, Fowler WS: Lung function studies. VI. Detection of uneven alveolar ventilation during a single breath of oxygen. Am J Med 10:408–413, 1951
23. Craig DB, Wahba WM, Don HF, Couture JG, Becklake MR: "Closing volume" and its relationship to gas exchange in seated and supine positions. J Appl Physiol 31:717–721, 1971
24. Cumming G, Crank J, Horsfield K, Parker I: Gaseous diffusion in the airways of the human lung. Respir Physiol 1:58–74, 1966
25. Cumming G, Horsfield K, Jones JG, Muir DCF: The influence of gaseous diffusion on the alveolar plateau at different lung volumes. Respir Physiol 2: 386–398, 1967
26. Cumming G, Horsfield K, Jones JG, Muir DCF: Inhomogeneity of ventilation in normal and abnormal lungs, in Cumming G, Hunt LB (eds): Form and Function in the Human Lung. Baltimore, Williams & Wilkins, 1968, pp 56–65
27. Cumming G, Horsfield K, Preston SB: Diffusion equilibrium in the lungs examined by nodal analysis. Respir Physiol 12:329–345, 1971
28. Davies AS: Gas transit times in the porcine lung. J Physiol (Lond) 222: 76p–77p, 1972
29. Dollfuss RE, Milic-Emili J, Bates DV: Regional ventilation of the lung, studied with boluses of ^{133}Xenon. Respir Physiol 2:234–246, 1967
30. Farhi LE: Diffusive and convective movement of gas in the lung, in Wolstenholme GEW, Knight J (eds): Ciba Foundation Symposium on Circulatory and Respiratory Mass Transport. Lon-

don, J & A Churchill Ltd, 1969, pp 277–293

31. Fowler WS: Intrapulmonary distribution of inspired gas. Physiol Rev 32: 1–20, 1952
32. Fowler WS, Cornish ER, Kety SS: Lung function studies. VIII. Analysis of alveolar ventilation by pulmonary N_2 clearance curves. J Clin Invest 31:40–50, 1952
33. Georg J, Lassen NA, Mellemgaard K, Vinther A: Diffusion in the gas phase of the lungs in normal and emphysematous subjects. Clin Sci 29:525–532, 1965
34. Glazier JB, Hughes JMB, Maloney JE, West JB: Vertical gradient of alveolar size in lungs of dogs frozen intact. J Appl Physiol 23:694–705, 1967
35. Groom AC, Morin R, Farhi LE: Determination of dissolved N_2 in blood and investigation of N_2 washout from the body. J Appl Physiol 23:706–712, 1967
36. Hashimoto T, Young AC, Martin CJ: Compartmental analysis of the distribution of gas in the lungs. J Appl Physiol 23:203–209, 1967
37. Heckscher T, Bass H, Oriol A, Rose B, Anthonisen NR, Bates DV: Regional lung function in patients with bronchial asthma. J Clin Invest 47:1063–1070, 1968
38. Henderson R, Horsfield K, Cumming G: Intersegmental collateral ventilation in the human lung. Respir Physiol 6:128–134, 1968–69
39. Hogg JC, Macklem PT, Thurlbeck WM: The resistance of collateral channels in excised human lungs. J Clin Invest 48: 421–431, 1969
40. Horsfield K, Cumming G: Functional consequences of airway morphology. J Appl Physiol 24:384–390, 1968
41. Hyatt RE, Okeson GC: Expiratory flow limitation, the cause of so-called "airway closure" or "closing volume." Physiologist 14:166, 1971

41a. Hyatt RE, Okeson GC, Rodarte JR: Influence of expiratory flow limitation on the pattern of lung emptying in normal man. J Appl Physiol 35:411–419, 1973

42. Jones JG: The effect of preinspiratory lung volume on the result of the single breath O_2 test. Respir Physiol 2:375–385, 1967
43. Jones JG, Clarke SW: The effect of expiratory flow rate on regional lung emptying. Clin Sci 37:343–356, 1969
44. Kaneko K, Milic-Emili J, Dolovich MB, Dawson A, Bates DV: Regional distribution of ventilation and perfusion as a function of body position. J Appl Physiol 21:767–777, 1966
45. Kjellmer I, Sandquist L, Berglund E: "Alveolar plateau" of the single breath nitrogen elimination curve in normal subjects. J Appl Physiol 14:105–108, 1959
46. Krogh A, Lindhard J: The volume of the dead space in breathing and the mixing of gases in the lungs of man. J Physiol 51:59–90, 1917
47. Kylstra JA, Paganelli CV, Lanphier EH: Pulmonary gas exchange in dogs ventilated with hyperbarically oxygenated liquid. J Appl Physiol 21:177–184, 1966
48. LaForce RC, Lewis BM: Diffusional transport in the human lung. J Appl Physiol 28:291–298, 1970
49. LeBlanc P, Ruff F, Milic-Emili J: Effects of age and body position on "airway closure" in man. J Appl Physiol 28:448–451, 1970
50. Lundin G: Nitrogen elimination during oxygen breathing. Acta Physiol Scand 30 (suppl 111):130–143, 1953
51. Macklem PT: Airway obstruction and collateral ventilation. Physiol Rev 51: 368–436, 1971
52. McFadden ER Jr, Lyons HA: Airway resistance and uneven ventilation in bronchial asthma. J Appl Physiol 25: 365–370, 1968
53. Martin CJ, Young AC: Lobar ventilation in man. Am Rev Tuberc Pulm Dis 73:330–337, 1956
54. Martin HB: Respiratory bronchioles as the pathway for collateral ventilation. J Appl Physiol 21:1443–1447, 1966
55. Martin RR, Anthonisen NR, Zutter M: Effect of increased gas density on respiratory gas exchange in the anesthetized dog. Physiologist 13:256,1970
56. Mead J: The distribution of gas flow in lungs, in Wolstenholme GEW, Knight J (eds): Ciba Foundation Symposium on Circulatory and Respiratory Mass Transport. London, J & A Churchill, Ltd, 1969, pp 204–209
57. Milic-Emili J, Henderson JAM, Dolovich MB, Trop D, Kaneko K: Regional distribution of inspired gas in the lung. J Appl Physiol 21:749–759, 1966

58. Millette B, Robertson PC, Ross WRD, Anthonisen NR: Effect of expiratory flow rate on emptying of lung regions. J Appl Physiol 27:587–591, 1969
59. Muir DCF: Distribution of aerosol particles in exhaled air. J Appl Physiol 23:210–214, 1967
60. Okubo T, Lenfant C: Distribution function of lung volume and ventilation determined by lung N_2 washout. J Appl Physiol 24:658–667, 1968
61. Otis AB, McKerrow CB, Bartlett RA, Mead J, McIlroy MB, Selverstone NJ, Radford EP Jr: Mechanical factors in distribution of pulmonary ventilation. J Appl Physiol 8:427–443, 1956
62. Power GG: Gaseous diffusion between airways and alveoli in the human lung. J Appl Physiol 27:701–709, 1969
63. Rauwerda PE: Unequal ventilation of different parts of the lung and the determination of cardiac output (Thesis). Groningen, The Netherlands, University of Groningen, 1946
64. Robertson JS, Siri WE, Jones HB: Lung ventilation patterns determined by analysis of nitrogen elimination rates; use of the mass spectrometer as a continuous gas analyzer. J Clin Invest 29: 577–590, 1950
65. Roos A, Dahlstrom H, Murphy JP: Distribution of inspired air in the lungs. J Appl Physiol 7:645–659, 1955
66. Rossing RG: Evaluation of a computer solution of exponential decay or washout curves. J Appl Physiol 21: 1907–1910, 1966
67. Rusher JL, Stoll PJ, Lenfant C: Exercise-induced hyperpnea and uniformity and efficiency of pulmonary ventilation. J Appl Physiol 28:63–69, 1970
68. Saltzman HA, Salzano JV, Blenkarn GD, Kylstra JA: Effects of pressure on ventilation and gas exchange in man. J Appl Physiol 30:443–449, 1971
69. Scheid P, Piiper J: Analysis of test gas washout from lungs with varying tidal volume: theory. J Appl Physiol 31: 292–295, 1971
70. Shinozaki T, Abajian JC Jr, Tabakin BS, Hanson JS: Theory and clinical application of a digital nitrogen washout computer. J Appl Physiol 21:202–208, 1966
71. Sikand R, Cerretelli P, Farhi LE: Effects of VA and VA/Q distribution and of time on the alveolar plateau. J Appl Physiol 21:1331–1337, 1966
72. Stanescu DC, Teculescu DB, Pacuraru R, Popa V: Effect of bronchoconstrictor aerosols on the alveolar plateau of the single breath O_2 test. Thorax 23:628–633, 1968
73. Suda Y, Martin CJ, Young AC: Regional dispersion of volume-to-ventilation ratios in the lung of man. J Appl Physiol 29:480–485, 1970
74. Tendeloo N Ph: Studien ueber die Ursachen der Lungenkrankheiten. Erster (Physiologischer) Teil. Wiesbaden, JF Bergmann, 1901
75. Tsunoda S, Young AC, Martin CJ: Emptying pattern of lung compartments in normal man. J Appl Physiol 32:644–649, 1972
76. West JB: Gas exchange when one lung region inspires from another. J Appl Physiol 30:479–487, 1971
77. West JB: Distribution of mechanical stress in the lung, a possible factor in localisation of pulmonary disease. Lancet 1:839–841, 1971
77a. West JB, Matthews FL: Stresses, strains, and surface pressures in the lung caused by its weight. J Appl Physiol 32:332–345, 1972
78. Young AC, Martin CJ, Pace WR: Effect of expiratory flow patterns on lung emptying. J Appl Physiol 18:47–50, 1963
79. Zardini P, West JB: Topographical distribution of ventilation in isolated lung. J Appl Physiol 21:794–802, 1966

Chapter 5

Distribution of Ventilation and Perfusion

Exchange of oxygen and carbon dioxide between alveolar air and the blood in pulmonary capillaries is the essential function of the lungs. The ultimate energy-exchanging reactions between oxygen and metabolic substrates take place in the mitochondrial membranes in cells.[11] To maintain these processes, the circulating blood transports oxygen and carbon dioxide, and gas exchange in the lungs maintains O_2 and CO_2 partial pressures at constant levels, adequate for tissue gas exchange. The amounts of gases exchanged in the lungs depend on the amount of ventilation reaching the alveoli per unit time ($\dot{V}_A$), and the amount of blood circulating through lung capillaries per unit time (perfusion of the lungs, $\dot{Q}$). Gas and blood do not reach individual alveolar units at equal rates. Hence, the ratio of ventilation to perfusion ($\dot{V}_A/\dot{Q}$ ratio) differs locally. Since the alveoli are ventilated only during inspiration, the $\dot{V}_A/\dot{Q}$ ratio also changes during the breathing cycle. The variations in $\dot{V}_A/\dot{Q}$ ratios give rise to differences in partial pressures of O_2, CO_2, and N_2 between alveolar gas and blood in the lung capillaries. The net effect of the distribution of $\dot{V}_A/\dot{Q}$ ratios throughout the lungs is that a fraction of inspired gas does not participate in gas exchange (physiological dead space), while a fraction of blood perfusing the lung does not alter its composition (venous admixture).

EXCHANGE OF INERT GASES

The exchange of O_2 and CO_2 is complicated by chemical reactions in the blood (Chap. 6). Hence, to focus on events in the lungs, we will first consider inert gases, i.e., those which do not react chemically with blood components. Their exchange depends on (1) alveolar ventilation, (2) perfusion of the lung capillaries with blood, (3) diffusivity through the pulmonary capillary membrane, and (4) solubility in blood. Diffusivity will be considered later; for present purposes we may assume that diffusion through the membrane does not limit gas exchange. The diagrams developed by Farhi[6] show the relationships between ventilation, perfusion, and solubility (Fig. 5-1*A, B*). The relative importance of ventilation

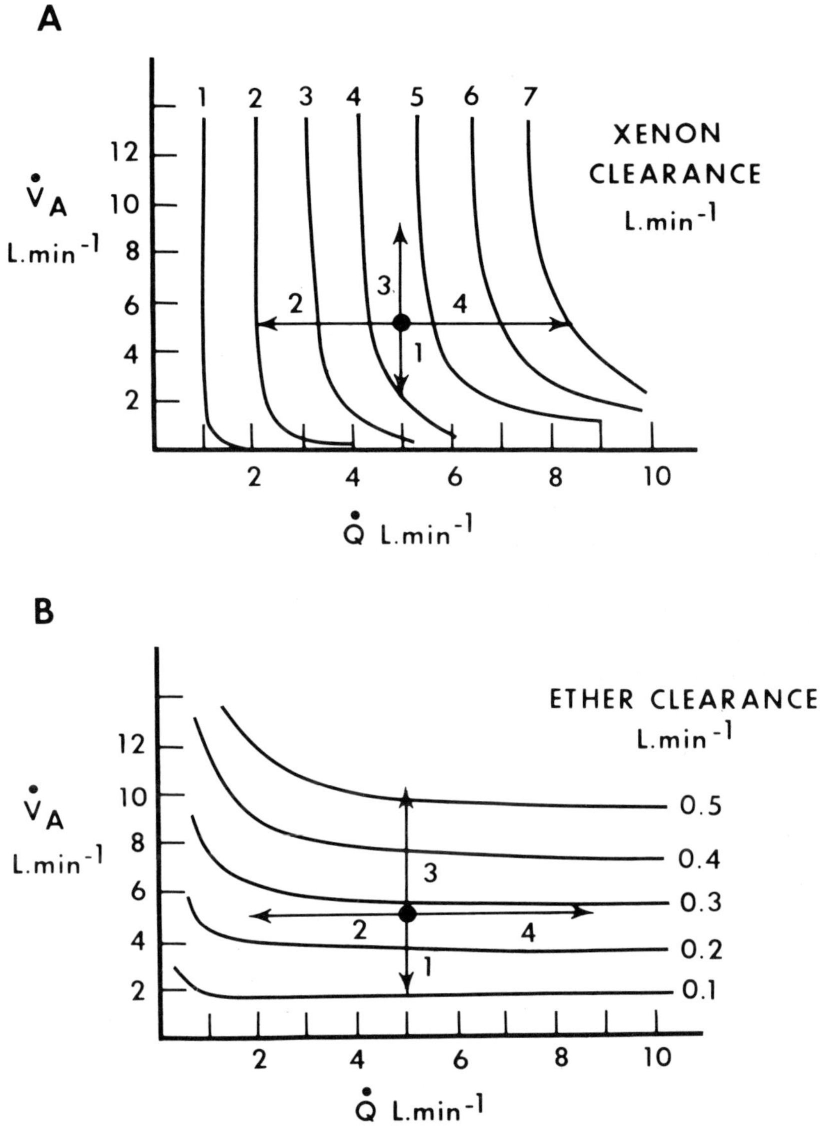

Fig. 5-1. Clearance of inert gases in the lungs. ● indicates clearance rates at normal average ventilation and perfusion rates ($\dot{V}_A = 5$ liters/min^{-1}; $\dot{Q} = 5$ liters/min^{-1}). Lines are isopleths of equal clearance rates for an insoluble (*A*, xenon) and a soluble (*B*, ether) gas. *A*. Xe clearance is largely determined by perfusion rate (*arrows* 2 and 4), and only slightly by ventilation rate (*arrows* 1 and 3). *B*. Ether clearance is largely determined by ventilation rate (*arrows* 1 and 3) and only slightly by perfusion rate (*arrows* 2 and 4). Modified from reference 6.

and perfusion in gas clearance depends on the solubility of the gas. Consider first xenon, a comparatively insoluble gas (Fig. 5-1*A*). At normal ventilation and perfusion rates (5 liters/min), dissolved xenon is cleared from blood at a rate of about 4.5 liters/min. This rate depends almost exclusively on perfusion of the lung capillaries; ventilation has little effect. Increasing or decreasing the rate of alveolar ventilation ($\dot{V}_A$), at constant perfusion rate, $\dot{Q}$, does not significantly alter xenon clearance (see arrows *1* and *3* in Fig. 5-1*A*). In contrast, decreasing perfusion ($\dot{Q}$) from 5 to 2 liters/min leads to a nearly equally large drop in xenon clearance, and an increase in $\dot{Q}$ from 5 to 8 liters/min leads to a proportionate increase in xenon clearance. Thus, the clearance of a relatively insoluble gas from blood depends mostly on how much of it reaches the gas-exchanging capillaries.

With a soluble gas, ethylether, the relations between ventilation and perfusion are different (Fig. 5-1*B*). Increasing $\dot{Q}$ fourfold from 2 to 8 liters/min at constant $\dot{V}_A$ (*2* and *4*) has only minimal effect on clearance, while a comparable increase in alveolar ventilation at constant $\dot{Q}$ (*1* and *3*) increases clearance about fivefold. These relations change when ventilation or blood flow are very low. With minimal alveolar ventilation (less than 0.5 liters/min), even large increases of perfusion cannot significantly increase xenon clearance; when perfusion is equally minimal, even large increases of ventilation cannot extract much more ether from blood.

Both alveolar ventilation and pulmonary blood flow are unevenly distributed throughout the lung.[19, 24] For instance, in the vertical lung, ventilation increases threefold from the lung top to the bottom (Chap. 4), and blood flow is even more dependent on gravity. According to West's calculations, blood flow increases from 0.07 liters/min in the top 7 percent of the lung volume to 1.29 liters/min in the bottom 13 percent.[24] Hence, the ratio of ventilation to perfusion ($\dot{V}_A/\dot{Q}$ ratio) decreases from 3.3 to 0.63 from the top to the bottom of the vertical lung. Although they receive little inspired air, the top alveoli are still overventilated in relation to blood flow since they receive almost no blood, and the bottom zones are relatively underventilated even though they receive a larger share of the inspired air.

The ratio between ventilation and perfusion has a pronounced effect on gas exchange. For inert gases, the partial pressures in alveolar gas depend solely on three variables: mixed venous partial pressure, solubility, and the $\dot{V}_A/\dot{Q}$ ratio. Figure 5-2 indicates the ratio between alveolar and mixed venous gas pressures as a function of solubility and the $\dot{V}_A/\dot{Q}$ ratio.[7] Relatively soluble gases (*1* and *3*) have alveolar pressures that nearly equal those in mixed venous blood at $\dot{V}_A/\dot{Q}$ ratios <1.0. The less soluble gas (*2*) always has an alveolar pressure much less than that in mixed venous blood, even when $\dot{V}_A/\dot{Q}$ is very low.

Figure 5-3 compares the behavior of an insoluble and a more soluble gas (i.e., gases *1* and *2* in Figure 5-2) by plotting their relative alveolar pressures against one another at different values of $\dot{V}_A/\dot{Q}$. At each value of $\dot{V}_A/\dot{Q}$, the insoluble gas (*2*) has a lower alveolar pressure, relative to mixed venous pressure, than the more soluble gas (*1*). Farhi and Yokoyama[7] have pointed out that the drawn curve in Figure 5-3 is a $\dot{V}_A/\dot{Q}$ line: the locus of all possible combinations of alveolar pressures of the two gases at given values of $\dot{V}_A/\dot{Q}$ ratios. The diagram considers the two gases in terms of their elimination from blood passing through the lungs. However, the basic relationships are similar whether one deals with

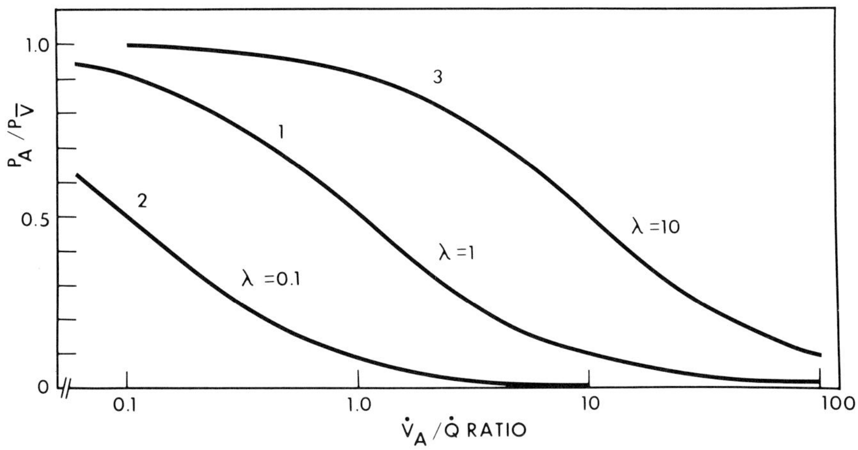

Fig. 5-2. Alveolar pressure (as a fraction of mixed venous pressure; $P_A/P_{\bar{V}}$ ratio) as a function of $\dot{V}_A/\dot{Q}$ ratio, for gases of increasing solubility (partition coefficient, $\lambda =$ 0.1, 1, and 10). At all values of $\dot{V}_A/\dot{Q}$, the relative alveolar pressure is higher for soluble than for insoluble gases. O_2 behaves approximately as gas *2*, CO_2 as gas *1* (See Fig. 5-3). After reference 6.

elimination or uptake, as Farhi and Yokoyama emphasized by constructing appropriate coordinates for CO_2 and O_2 partial pressures in the diagram of Figure 5-3. Thus, the physiological exchange of oxygen and carbon dioxide appears to follow rules similar to those for inert gases. Oxygen behaves as a relatively insoluble gas, and CO_2 as a soluble gas, with a ratio of partition coefficients of about 1:10.

EXCHANGE OF O_2 AND CO_2 IN ALVEOLI

The uptake of O_2 and the production of CO_2 are determined by the body's metabolic needs. Ventilation and blood flow adapt, through complex control systems, to restore altered O_2 and CO_2 pressures to normal. This results in adequate transfer of O_2 and CO_2 between the tissues and atmospheric air. Because of the chemical nature of the metabolic substrates, more O_2 is consumed than CO_2 is produced in the tissues. Thus, the respiratory quotient ($R = \dot{V}_{CO_2}/\dot{V}_{O_2}$) is usually less than 1. This means that less CO_2 is exchanged in the lungs than O_2, per unit time, unless the tissues release or store these gases. The total amount of O_2 and CO_2 exchanged by the body can be determined by measuring the amounts added or removed from inspired air. Thus, O_2 uptake and CO_2 production are measured from the amount of air ventilated and the concentrations, or partial pressures, of O_2 and CO_2 in the inspired and expired air. Since ventilation is the same for O_2 and CO_2, this cancels out when $\dot{V}_{O_2}$ is divided into $\dot{V}_{CO_2}$; therefore, R can be determined solely from the gas tensions. The equations relating R to the inspired and alveolar partial pressures of O_2 and CO_2 are described by Rahn and Fenn.[18] Figure 5-4 shows them graphically in an O_2 versus CO_2 diagram. If $R = 1$, equal amounts of O_2 and CO_2 are exchanged, and the decrease in partial pressure of O_2 in alveolar gas equals the increase in the partial pressure of CO_2.

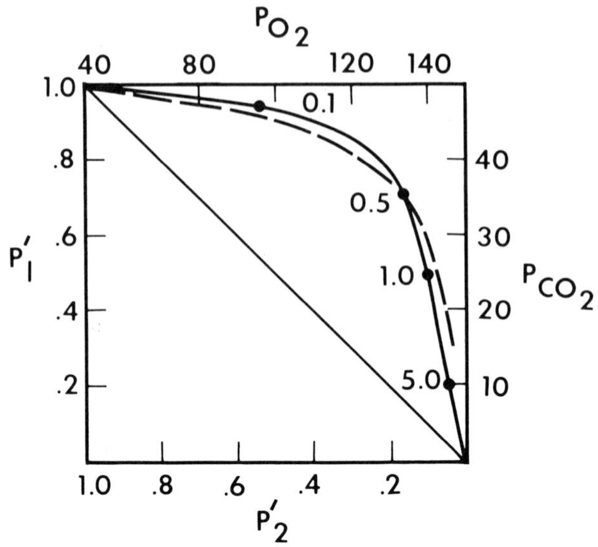

Fig. 5-3. *Abscissa.* $P_A/P_{\bar{v}}$ ratio for insoluble gas *2* from Figure 5-2 (P'_2). *Ordinate.* $P_A/P_{\bar{v}}$ ratio for soluble gas *1* (P'_1). The higher relative alveolar pressure of the more soluble gas *1* appears from the fact that all points that relate the two $P_A/P_{\bar{v}}$ ratios to one another are situated to the right of the diagonal line of equality, on the curved drawn line. Values for the $\dot{V}_A/\dot{Q}$ ratio can be placed on this line by reading $\dot{V}_A/\dot{Q}$ values from Figure 5-2. For instance, at $\dot{V}_A/\dot{Q}=1.0$; $P'_2=0.1$, and $P'_1=0.5$. Points for $\dot{V}_A/\dot{Q}=0.1$, 0.5, 1.0, and 5.0 are indicated on the curve. The dashed curve is the $\dot{V}_A/\dot{Q}$ line for O_2-CO_2 exchange (see text). Modified from reference 7.

In Figure 5-4, *I* represents the composition of inspired air: $P_{O_2}=150$ mm Hg; $P_{CO_2}=0$. A_1 is one possible composition of alveolar gas when $R=1$. At that point, oxygen tension has decreased 40 mm Hg (from 150 to 110) and P_{CO_2} has increased from 0 to 40 mm Hg. When R is less than 1, the influx of CO_2 into the alveolar gas is less than the efflux of O_2 into the blood; hence, the sum of P_{O_2} and P_{CO_2} decreases. The total pressure of alveolar gas, of course, remains the same; the balance is made up by N_2. The solid line for $R=0.8$ shows that, at any point, the sum of P_{O_2} and P_{CO_2} is less than their sum in inspired air (150 mm). For example, at *A,* which represents one possible composition of alveolar gas, this sum is $102+40=142$ mm Hg. Thus, the composition of inspired gas changes into that of alveolar air along the pathway IA_1 or *IA,* depending on the value of *R*. The solid and dashed lines in Figure 5-4 represent all possible compositions of alveolar gas when $R=0.8$ or $R=1$, respectively. Lines for $R<0.8$ lie to the left of the drawn line; lines for $R>1$ lie to the right of the dashed line.

Where is the alveolar point located on the *R* line? This depends on the supply of inspired air (alveolar ventilation) and the uptake of O_2 (or output of CO_2) in or from blood. The equations developed by Rahn and Fenn[18] show that the ratios $\dot{V}_A/\dot{V}_{O_2}$ and $\dot{V}_A/\dot{V}_{CO_2}$ are the determining factors. Two values of the $\dot{V}_A/\dot{V}_{O_2}$

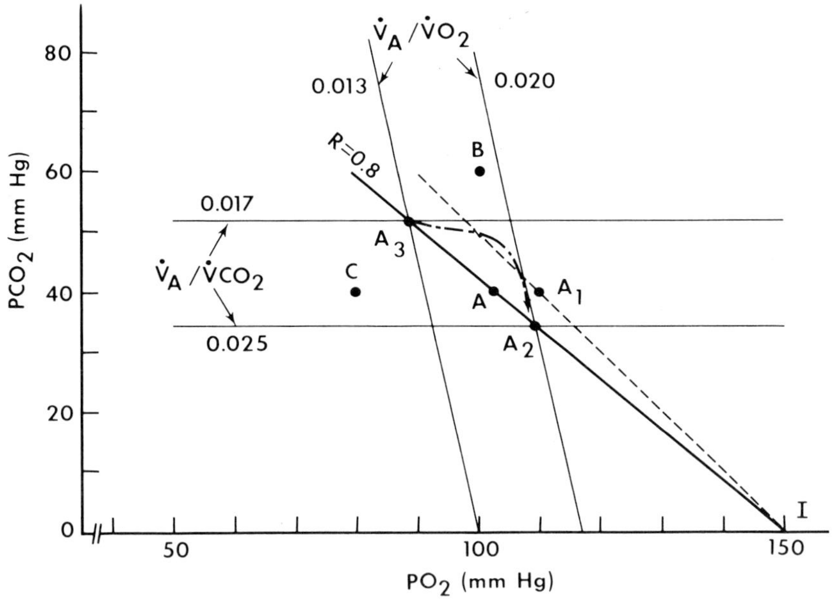

Fig. 5-4. O_2-CO_2 diagram.[17] Dashed line at 45° indicates $R=1$ ($P_{O_2}+P_{CO_2}=150$ mm Hg$=PI_{O_2}$). Heavy drawn line for $R=0.8$. $\dot{V}_A/\dot{V}_{CO_2}$ and $\dot{V}_A/\dot{V}_{O_2}$ lines and individual data points are discussed in text. I = inspired gas point. Alveolar point A is identical to point A in Figure 5-5. Units ($\dot{V}_A$ in liters/min; $\dot{V}_{O_2}$ in ml/min) are those used by Rahn and Fenn.[18] See also text footnote.

ratio are shown in Figure 5-4. The line marked .020 is the locus of all alveolar points consistent with a $\dot{V}_A/\dot{V}_{O_2}$ ratio$=0.020$. For instance, $\dot{V}_A$ might be 6 liters/min BTPS* and $\dot{V}_{O_2}$ might be 300 ml/min STPD. Alveolar point A_2 lies on this line and also on the $R=0.8$ line; it is the only point consistent with both conditions. If, during light exercise, $\dot{V}_{O_2}$ increases from 300 to 460 ml/min while $\dot{V}_A$ remains constant at 6 liters/min, $\dot{V}_A/\dot{V}_{O_2}$ decreases to $6/460=0.013$. If R remains at 0.8, the only alveolar point consistent with the exercise conditions is A_3, the intersection of the $R=0.8$ line with a $\dot{V}_A/\dot{V}_{O_2}=0.013$ line. Thus, a small increase in O_2 uptake substantially changes the composition of alveolar gas if ventilation does not change. At A_3, P_{CO_2} is 18 mm Hg higher, and P_{O_2} is 20 mm Hg lower, than at A_2. Obviously, alveolar ventilation must be precisely controlled if the composition of alveolar air is to remain constant (Chap. 10). To maintain the alveolar point at A_2, $\dot{V}_A$ must increase in proportion to $\dot{V}_{O_2}$, i.e., from 6 to 9.2 liters/min, so that the $\dot{V}_A/\dot{V}_{O_2}$ ratio remains at 0.020.

Since R is the ratio of CO_2 production and O_2 uptake, each alveolar point must correspond to a level of CO_2 production consistent with R and $\dot{V}_A/\dot{V}_{O_2}$. For instance, if $\dot{V}_{O_2}=300$ ml/min and $R=0.8$, $\dot{V}_{CO_2}$ must be 240 ml/min. Thus, if

* This choice of units is convenient since ventilation is commonly expressed in terms of the physical condition of alveolar air (BTPS = body temperature, ambient pressure, saturated with water vapor), while O_2 uptake and CO_2 output are measured in STPD conditions (0°C, 760 mm Hg, dry).

at A_2, $\dot{V}_A = 6$ liters/min and $\dot{V}_{O_2} = 300$ ml/min, $\dot{V}_A/\dot{V}_{CO_2}$ must be $6/240 = 0.025$. In the absence of CO_2 in inspired air, the ratio $\dot{V}_A/\dot{V}_{CO_2}$ is independent of P_{O_2}, and hence the lines for this ratio run parallel with the abscissa in Figure 5-4. The values for the ratio $\dot{V}_A/\dot{V}_{CO_2}$ decrease as P_{CO_2} increases. Thus, if $\dot{V}_A$ remains constant, the amount of CO_2 excreted can only increase if alveolar P_{CO_2} increases concomitantly. Each unit of expired alveolar gas then contains more CO_2 and total excretion increases. Similarly, if oxygen uptake increases while $\dot{V}_A$ is constant, alveolar O_2 tension decreases; more O_2 is extracted from each volume unit inspired gas.

The terms *hypoventilation* and *hyperventilation* indicate ventilation levels that result in abnormal alveolar gas tensions. They do not refer to set levels of 'normal' minute volumes of ventilation. Hypoventilation results in elevated P_{CO_2} and decreased P_{O_2} values (e.g., point A_3 in Fig. 5-4); hyperventilation decreases P_{CO_2} and raises P_{O_2}. During changes in ventilation levels, alveolar gas composition does not change as predicted by the R line between A_2 and A_3. For instance, during recovery from hypoventilation (A_3), extra CO_2 must be eliminated and extra O_2 taken up to reestablish equilibrium at the new alveolar gas composition, A_2. In steady-state conditions, alveolar gas tensions correspond to certain levels of CO_2 and O_2 which are stored in blood and in body tissues. The stores for CO_2 are considerably greater than those for O_2. Therefore, when a change in $\dot{V}_A$ leads to a change in alveolar gas composition, the oxygen stores assume the new level quicker than the CO_2 stores. As a consequence, alveolar P_{O_2} reaches its new steady-state value more rapidly than P_{CO_2}, and the pathway followed by alveolar gas describes a half loop (dashed arrow in Fig. 5-4).[18] Thus R does not remain constant but is temporarily elevated during the transition. A half loop in the reverse direction is followed when $\dot{V}_A$ decreases.

The management of patients with respiratory insufficiency, a condition which leads to hypoventilation and often severe hypoxia (low P_{O_2}) and hypercapnia (high P_{CO_2}), is often based on arterial blood gas data (p. 115). Determinations of R require expired gas collections, which is usually not feasible at the bedside. However, in a steady state, R should be less than 1 and therefore the sum of alveolar P_{O_2} and P_{CO_2} should be less than the inspired P_{O_2} (p. 84). This should also be true for arterial P_{O_2} and P_{CO_2}, since arterial P_{O_2} is usually at least several mm Hg lower than alveolar P_{O_2}, and arterial P_{CO_2} is close to alveolar P_{CO_2}. Hence, if arterial P_{O_2} plus arterial P_{CO_2} exceeds inspired P_{O_2}, one must suspect a technical error or a markedly unsteady state. The two can be distinguished if ventilation data are obtained at the time of blood sampling. To calculate $\dot{V}_A$ from total ventilation rate, one may assume an average value for anatomical dead space (Chap. 3), and with approximate data for $\dot{V}_{O_2}$ (from metabolic tables) one can estimate the $\dot{V}_A/\dot{V}_{O_2}$ ratio. This can be used to test the validity of arterial blood gas data. For instance, a $\dot{V}_A/\dot{V}_{O_2}$ ratio of 0.013 would be incompatible with an arterial $P_{O_2} = 100$ mm Hg and a $P_{CO_2} = 60$ mm Hg (Fig. 5-4*B*). However, because of the alveolar-arterial P_{O_2} difference, it would be compatible with an arterial blood point C ($P_{O_2} = 80$ mm Hg; $P_{CO_2} = 40$ mm Hg). Since alveolar gas can be sampled directly with rapid gas analyzers, it is possible to define alveolar points in persons in whom alveolar gas composition is fairly homogeneous. This is unfortunately not the case in most patients with respiratory insufficiency.

COMPOSITION OF ALVEOLAR GAS

Alveolar gas composition is not uniform throughout the lungs (Chap. 4); Figure 5-4 presents an idealized perspective. Additional elements of uncertainty concerning alveolar gas composition, not yet discussed in Chapter 4, include (1) variations during the breathing cycle, and (2) variations resulting from nonuniform perfusion of lung capillaries. The latter are discussed in relation to ventilation rates, i.e., as one determinant of $\dot{V}_A/\dot{Q}$ ratios.

Variations During the Breathing Cycle

Expiration is breath holding with a decreasing lung volume; CO_2 production continues into the contracting lung and hence alveolar P_{CO_2} increases. O_2 extraction also continues, with a resulting decrease in P_{O_2}. At the beginning of inspiration, dead space gas with a high CO_2 content is inspired into the alveoli; hence P_{CO_2} increases further in the first moment of inspiration, whereas P_{O_2} drops to a minimum. Then, fresh inspired air dilutes the alveolar gas; P_{O_2} rises and P_{CO_2} decreases until expiration starts again. The composition of alveolar air during a breathing cycle describes a loop on an O_2 versus CO_2 diagram; [4] the loop's excursions are normally small—some 2 mm Hg for P_{CO_2} and 3 mm Hg for P_{O_2}. Yet, even this slight deviation has implications for gas exchange.[16] Normally, peak flow rates occur early in expiration, after about one-third of its total duration.[2] If peak flow occurred later, the air would contain more CO_2, and more CO_2 would be transported in the same expired volume. With a late peak flow, the same gas exchange rate could be maintained with 6 percent less alveolar ventilation.[16] Thus, gas can be exchanged with less ventilation by delaying expiration and also by hastening inspiration. In Nye's model analysis the two together resulted in further economy of breathing. The combination is a gasping type of breathing called apneustic breathing (Chap. 10). Experiments in dogs have confirmed that this pattern can increase breathing efficiency. Arterial P_{O_2} increased within 30 seconds after altering the breathing pattern, while total ventilation, breathing rate, and tidal volume were unchanged.[12] This finding should be taken into account in selecting an optimal airflow pattern for artificial ventilation.

Ventilation-Perfusion Ratio

The $\dot{V}_A/\dot{Q}$ ratio has been discussed for inert gases (p. 83), and the concept of a $\dot{V}_A/\dot{Q}$ line was presented in Figure 5–3. In order to apply the ratio to O_2 and CO_2, perfusion must be introduced into the O_2 versus CO_2 diagram. This complicates matters because the relations between partial pressures and contents of O_2 and CO_2 in blood are not linear. In a steady state, gas exchange between tissues, blood, and lung air proceeds at the same average rate; that is, R must be the same for all exchanges. Obviously, the R for blood ($\dot{V}_{CO_2}/\dot{V}_{O_2}$) is determined by the contents of O_2 and CO_2 in arterial and venous blood. These contents can be related to corresponding partial pressures by referring to dissociation curves for O_2 and CO_2.[18] This enables one to plot combinations of P_{O_2} and P_{CO_2} that are consistent with given values of R. Figure 5–5 includes four such "blood R lines," all of which originate at the mixed venous point $\overline{V}$ and intersect the R lines for

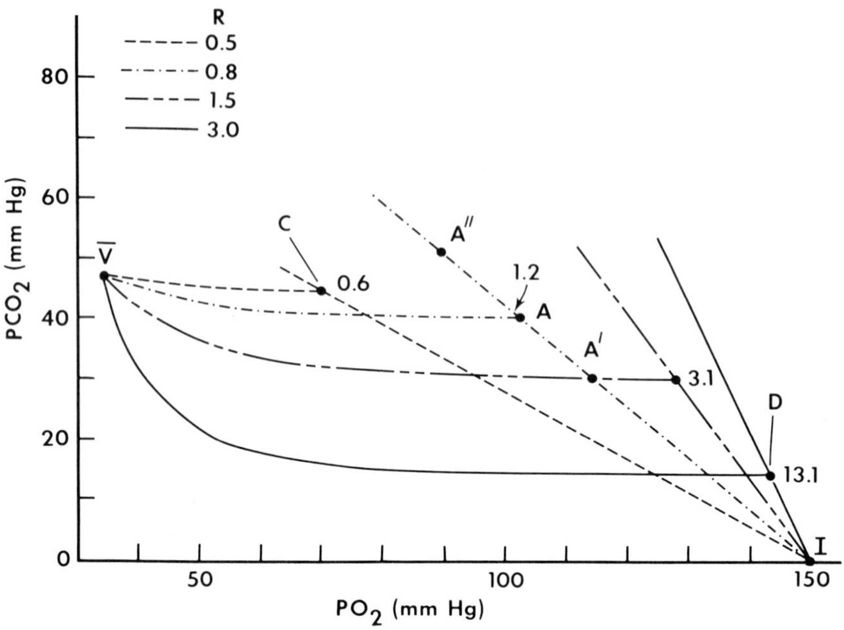

Fig. 5-5. *R* lines for blood and gas in an O_2-CO_2 diagram. I=inspired gas point; $\bar{V}$=mixed venous blood point. Gas *R* lines originate at *I*, blood *R* lines at $\bar{V}$. Alveolar point *A* is identical to *A* in Figure 5-4. Alveolar points *A*, *A'*, and *A''* are all situated on the $R = 0.8$ line for gas; only *A* is situated on the $R = 0.8$ line for blood. Hence, *A* represents the only composition of alveolar gas at which blood and gas can exchange O_2 and CO_2 at $R=0.8$, for the chosen values of *I* and $\bar{V}$. Points *C* and *D* explained in text. Values of $\dot{V}_A/\dot{Q}$ ratios indicated at each intersection of blood and gas *R* lines (0.6, 1.2, 3.1, and 13.1).

The O_2 and CO_2 pressures of mixed venous blood ($\bar{V}$) correspond to gas contents of about 129 ml/liter O_2 and 540 ml/liter CO_2, according to standard dissociation curves.[18] Arterialization of this blood at $R = 0.8$ might add 40 ml/liter O_2 and eliminate $0.8 \times 40 = 32$ ml/liter CO_2. The gas contents of the arterialized blood would then be $129 + 40 = 169$ ml/liter O_2 and $540 - 32 = 508$ ml/liter CO_2. Referring again to standard dissociation curves, these contents correspond to a P_{O_2} of 52 mm Hg and a P_{CO_2} of 43 mm Hg. This is a point on the $R=0.8$ line for blood. Other points on the same line are obtained by assuming different values for O_2 uptake and CO_2 elimination. Points on other blood *R* lines are obtained by performing similar calculations with the appropriate *R* value, always starting with the composition of mixed venous blood. For details see reference 18.

alveolar gas. For instance, point *A* indicates the only possible composition of alveolar air compatible with steady-state gas exchange at $R=0.8$ for given values of points *I* and $\bar{V}$, the compositions of inspired air and of mixed venous blood. Point *A* also corresponds to a fixed value of the $\dot{V}_A/\dot{Q}$ ratio, just as the points on the curve of Figure 5–3 indicate $\dot{V}_A/\dot{Q}$ values derived from the exchange ratios of inert gases. For point *A*, $\dot{V}_A/\dot{Q}=1.2$ (Eq. 21 in reference 18).

Each of the intersections of blood and gas *R* lines in Figure 5–5 indicates blood and gas exchanging CO_2 and O_2 at a particular value of $\dot{V}_A/\dot{Q}$ (0.6, 1.2, 3.1, and 13.1). If a line is drawn through the mixed venous and inspired points as well as through the intersections of blood and gas R lines, the $\dot{V}_A/\dot{Q}$ line results (Fig. 5–6). Since $\bar{V}$ represents blood as it arrives in the lungs, unchanged by gas exchange, its $\dot{V}_A$ is zero, and its $\dot{V}_A/\dot{Q}=0$. In contrast, I represents inspired air unchanged by gas exchange; its $\dot{Q}$ is zero, and hence it stands for $\dot{V}_A/\dot{Q}=\infty$. Thus, $\dot{V}_A/\dot{Q}$ increases from zero to infinity along the $\dot{V}_A/\dot{Q}$ line, from $\bar{V}$ to I.

If ventilation and perfusion were uniformly distributed throughout the lungs, their ratio would be the same everywhere, and the composition of alveolar air would be constant at values consistent with one particular $\dot{V}_A/\dot{Q}$ ratio. In fact, neither ventilation nor $\dot{Q}$ is uniformly distributed and hence $\dot{V}_A/\dot{Q}$ varies locally and in time. In a vertical human lung, $\dot{V}_A/\dot{Q}$ varies from about 0.6 at the bottom to more than 3 in the lung top.[23, 24] That is, alveolar O_2 tensions vary from about 70 to 130 mm Hg, and P_{CO_2} from 45 to less than 30 mm Hg (see Fig. 5–6 and its legend). Since ventilation distribution is nonuniform even in small portions of the lungs (p. 63), some degree of $\dot{V}_A/\dot{Q}$ nonuniformity probably exists within subsegments and lobules. In addition, ventilation and blood flow in a single alveolar unit may be nonuniform. Thus, it is very unlikely that alveolar air ever has an ideally uniform composition. Yet, in healthy lungs the expired O_2 and CO_2 concentrations vary much less than one would expect from the wide range of alveolar tensions consistent with $\dot{V}_A/\dot{Q}$ ratios between 0.6 and 3 in the vertical lung. This is partly because areas with a low $\dot{V}_A/\dot{Q}$ contribute little to the expired

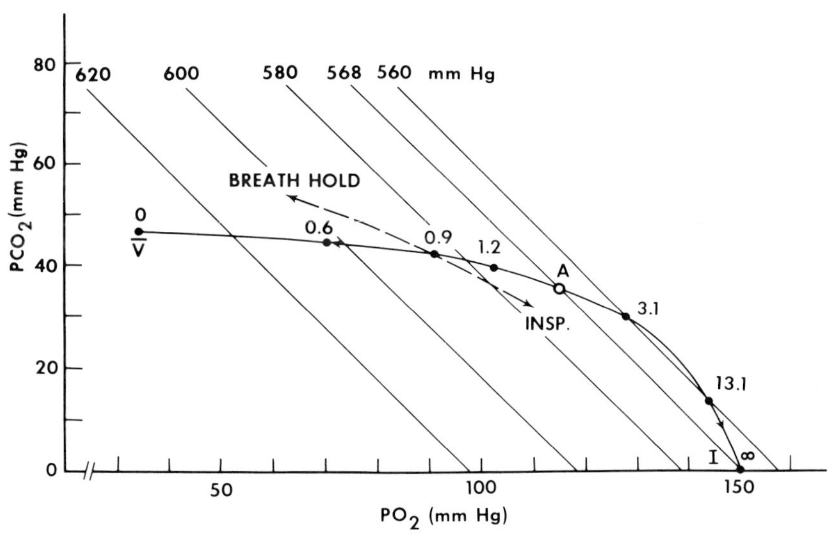

Fig. 5-6. $\dot{V}_A/\dot{Q}$ line in an O_2-CO_2 diagram. Inspired gas point, I; mixed venous blood point, $\bar{V}$. Numbers indicate $\dot{V}_A/\dot{Q}$ ratio at different points (from 0 at $\bar{V}$ to ∞ at I). In a vertical lung, $\dot{V}_A/\dot{Q}$ ratio varies from about 0.6 at the top to over 3.0 at the bottom. The graph indicates the wide range of alveolar O_2 and CO_2 tensions consistent with this range of $\dot{V}_A/\dot{Q}$ values. Dashed arrows indicate changes of alveolar gas composition during breath holding and during rapid inspiration, both starting at an alveolar point where $\dot{V}_A/\dot{Q} = 0.9$. A decrease of $\dot{V}_A/\dot{Q}$ from 0.9 to 0.6 (*arrow*) leads to a lower PA_{O_2} but little change in PA_{CO_2}. At high $\dot{V}_A/\dot{Q}$ ratios, a further increase in ventilation (*arrow near I*) decreases PA_{CO_2} while PA_{O_2} increases little. Diagonal lines are isopleths of alveolar P_{N_2} (see text). At A, $PA_{N_2} = PI_{N_2}$ (see also Fig. 5-7).

air; also, the dead space functions as a mixing chamber, which tends to equalize alveolar gas tensions (p. 69). Expired air, therefore, is a mixed gas weighted toward the composition of gas in high $\dot{V}_A/\dot{Q}$ areas. In contrast, the composition of arterial blood is determined largely by contributions from areas with a large blood flow, i.e., a low $\dot{V}_A/\dot{Q}$ ratio.

During breath holding alveolar P_{O_2} decreases much more than P_{CO_2} increases. This is partly because CO_2 is much more soluble in blood and tissues (including lung tissue [5]) than O_2 and partly because of the shape of the $\dot{V}_A/\dot{Q}$ line. During breath holding, alveolar ventilation stops, and hence gas exchange proceeds at a rapidly decreasing $\dot{V}_A/\dot{Q}$ ratio. On the other hand, after a rapid and deep inspiration, alveolar gas composition changes toward higher $\dot{V}_A/\dot{Q}$ values.[4] The dashed arrows in Figure 5-6 indicate the direction of these changes; these arrows deviate from the $\dot{V}_A/\dot{Q}$ line. Shifts of the mixed venous point are one reason for the deviation. Even within one circulation time, systemic circuits with short circulation times contribute blood with higher P_{CO_2} and lower P_{O_2} to mixed venous blood during breath holding. Also, cardiac output changes during breath holding, and this, too, affects the mixed venous point, since the arteriovenous O_2 and CO_2 differences are inversely related to cardiac output. The direction of alveolar gas changes during inspiration is also uncertain. As a result of dead space gas distribution, the composition of inspired air is not uniform in all lung areas (p. 64).[22] Thus, alveolar gas composition varies with inspiration and expiration, with time during breath holding, and with location in the lungs according to the $\dot{V}_A/\dot{Q}$ ratio. In addition, its exact value at any time is influenced by the position of the mixed venous point and of the inspired point for a given lung area. Because of these inherent uncertainties, it is difficult to reproduce a $\dot{V}_A/\dot{Q}$ line experimentally. However, in principle, this concept is well established and provides many important insights that can be confirmed by experimental data. Normally, $\dot{V}_A/\dot{Q}$ is between 0.8 and 1.0 in large parts of the lung. Increased perfusion leads to lower $\dot{V}_A/\dot{Q}$ ratios and decreases the alveolar P_{O_2}; increased ventilation leads to decreased P_{CO_2} tensions but has less effect on P_{O_2} (see Fig. 5-6 and its legend). Hence, in terms of total blood and gas flow, gas exchange is optimal when $\dot{V}_A/\dot{Q}$ ratios are about 0.8–1.0.

The principles described for the exchange of inert gases (p. 80) have been used to determine the distribution of $\dot{V}_A/\dot{Q}$ ratios in lungs of healthy persons and of patients with lung disease.[25, 26] The method requires intravenous administration of six inert gases with different solubilities, ranging from sulfur hexafluoride (SF_6) as the least soluble to acetone as the most soluble gas. The concentration of each gas is measured in arterial blood, mixed venous blood and mixed expired gas, during a steady state of gas exchange. If the solubility of each gas is also known, one can obtain graphs of ventilation and of blood flow in function of the $\dot{V}_A/\dot{Q}$ ratio. The distribution of ventilation and of blood flow is log-normal with respect to $\dot{V}_A/\dot{Q}$, showing little dispersion of $\dot{V}_A/\dot{Q}$ ratios. In older healthy persons, the dispersion of $\dot{V}_A/\dot{Q}$ is larger, and more blood flow goes to areas with low $\dot{V}_A/\dot{Q}$ ratios. The results obtained under a variety of conditions were consistent with the values of dead space and of the (A-a) DO_2 (see below) in the same subjects. Thus, conclusions about $\dot{V}_A/\dot{Q}$ distribution previously drawn from measurements of alveolar-arterial gas pressure differences or dead space can now be tested with an independent method which indicates the distribution of $\dot{V}_A/\dot{Q}$ ratios.

A-a PARTIAL-PRESSURE DIFFERENCES

Alveolar and arterial gas pressures would be equal if gas exchange in the lungs led to complete equilibration and if all arterial blood passed through the lungs. Neither is true. Arterial blood receives small contributions of venous blood through connections in the heart and from bronchial veins; a small amount of pulmonary blood flow may pass through unventilated zones ($\dot{V}_A/\dot{Q}=0$) or through arteriovenous anastomoses in the lung circulation. These result in a venous admixture in arterial blood, which reduces its P_{O_2} and slightly raises its P_{CO_2}. In addition, diffusion limits alveolocapillary equilibration for O_2 (Chap. 6); thus, even if all parts of the lungs exchanged gas at the same $\dot{V}_A/\dot{Q}$ ratio, alveolar and arterial gas tensions would differ. This alveolar-arterial difference is not the same for O_2, CO_2, and N_2. The (A-a)DO_2, or alveolar-arterial P_{O_2} difference, is determined partly by diffusion limitation, but mostly by the distribution of $\dot{V}_A/\dot{Q}$ ratios. The P_{O_2} of arterial blood is weighted in favor of high perfusion, low $\dot{V}_A/\dot{Q}$ areas, while the P_{O_2} of mixed alveolar air is weighted in favor of well-ventilated alveoli, i.e., gas from high $\dot{V}_A/\dot{Q}$ areas. Figure 5-6 shows that, if alveolar gas tensions are close to the point where $\dot{V}_A/\dot{Q}=1.2$, and arterial gas tensions close to that for $\dot{V}_A/\dot{Q}=0.9$, this alone accounts for an (A-a)DO_2 of 12.5 mm Hg. The alinearity of the HbO_2 dissociation curve contributes to the (A-a)DO_2 in particular when O_2 tensions lie on the curved portion of that curve. The (A-a)DCO_2 has long been believed to equal zero. There is indeed no diffusion limitation for CO_2, but a distribution of $\dot{V}_A/\dot{Q}$ ratios can cause an (a-A) DCO_2 even though it is usually minimal. In particular, when there are substantial areas with a high $\dot{V}_A/\dot{Q}$ ratio, the P_{CO_2} of expired alveolar gas may be much lower than the P_{CO_2} of arterial blood. In contrast, areas with low $\dot{V}_A/\dot{Q}$ ratios do little to increase arterial blood P_{CO_2}; e.g., when $\dot{V}_A/\dot{Q}$ decreases from 0.9 to 0.6 (Fig. 5-6), P_{CO_2} increases only 2.5 mm. Changes in P_{CO_2} are much greater at the right-hand side of the $\dot{V}_A/\dot{Q}$ line where the ratios are high. Thus, a measurable (a-A)DCO_2 usually indicates the presence of lung areas with a high $\dot{V}_A/\dot{Q}$ ratio. This is the basis for its use as a diagnostic tool in pulmonary embolism, in which regional vascular occlusion causes part of the lungs to have a high $\dot{V}_A/\dot{Q}$ ratio. However, the difficulty in defining an acceptable value for alveolar P_{CO_2} limits its practical use. Temporary hyperventilation may decrease alveolar P_{CO_2} before blood P_{CO_2} follows, and the variations of P_{CO_2} in the normal breathing cycle (p. 87) are a substantial fraction of the venoarterial P_{CO_2} difference. In clinical settings, arterial blood is seldom collected under conditions approaching a steady state, and this alone makes refined interpretations of arterial and alveolar CO_2 tensions hazardous.

The A-a Nitrogen Difference

Blood leaving the alveoli contains N_2 in direct proportion to the alveolar P_{N_2}. The latter depends on the O_2-CO_2 exchange ratio, R. For instance, in Figure 5-5, the sum of O_2 and CO_2 tensions at point C ($R=0.5$) is 115 mm Hg, and at point D ($R=13.1$) 158 mm Hg. At both points, the sum of all partial pressures is atmospheric (disregarding alveolar pressures needed for airflow; Chap. 8). Thus, alveolar N_2 tension is $765-47-115=603$ mm Hg at point C and

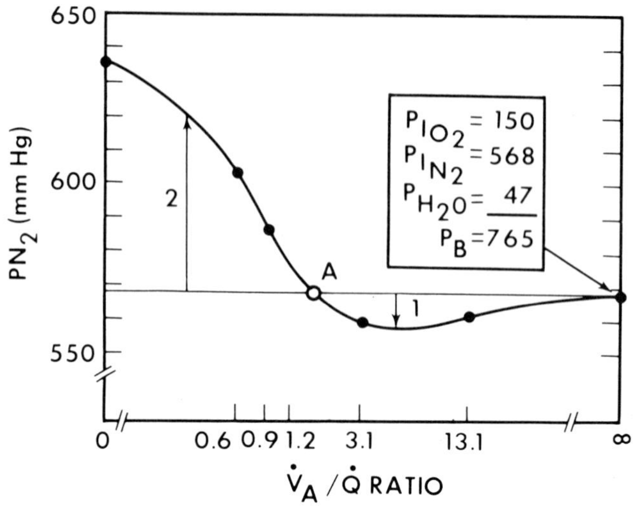

Fig. 5-7. Alveolar P_{N_2} (*ordinate*) as a function of $\dot{V}_A/\dot{Q}$ ratio (*abscissa*). At *A*, $PA_{N_2}=PI_{N_2}$ (see Fig. 5-6). Composition of inspired air in box. Arrows explained in text. Adapted from reference 19.

$765-47-158=560$ mm Hg at *D*. Blood leaving alveoli corresponding to *C* and *D* has a P_{N_2} of 603 and of 560 mm Hg, respectively. Isopleths for P_{N_2}, included in the $\dot{V}_A/\dot{Q}$ diagram of Figure 5-6, show that there is only one point (*A*) on the $\dot{V}_A/\dot{Q}$ line where $PA_{N_2}=PI_{N_2}$. At higher $\dot{V}_A/\dot{Q}$ values, PA_{N_2} is less; as the $\dot{V}_A/\dot{Q}$ ratio decreases, PA_{N_2} increases.[8, 19]

The arterial blood P_{N_2} reflects a mixture of blood with P_{N_2} values which vary as a function of $\dot{V}_A/\dot{Q}$. The average is weighted in favor of low $\dot{V}_A/\dot{Q}$ areas, since these contribute more to arterial blood than areas where $\dot{V}_A$ is high and $\dot{Q}$ is low. Also, as Figure 5-7 shows, alveolar P_{N_2} increases greatly in low $\dot{V}_A/\dot{Q}$ areas (*arrow* 2), while it decreases only slightly in high $\dot{V}_A/\dot{Q}$ areas (*arrow* 1). The point where $PA_{N_2}=PI_{N_2}$ is indicated by *A* (identical with *A* in Fig. 5-6). Hence, when significant areas in the lungs have low $\dot{V}_A/\dot{Q}$ ratios, arterial P_{N_2} will be relatively high. At the same time, expired alveolar gas reflects areas with higher $\dot{V}_A/\dot{Q}$ ratios and therefore has a P_{N_2} much closer to that of inspired gas. Hence, there will be an (a-A) P_{N_2} difference, which indicates the presence of areas with low $\dot{V}_A/\dot{Q}$ ratios in the lungs.[8]

Although alveolar P_{N_2} varies as a function of the $\dot{V}_A/\dot{Q}$ ratio throughout the lungs, no net exchange of N_2 between gas and blood takes place because the body tissues are saturated with N_2 during breathing of atmospheric air. In areas where PA_{N_2} is high, N_2 passes from alveolar air to blood; where it is lower, N_2 passes from blood to air. The amounts exchanged in either direction are equal and no net exchange occurs. Since there is no exchange of nitrogen in the tissues, arterial and mixed venous N_2 pressures are equal. Hence, the (a-A) P_{N_2} difference is not influenced by shunts.

Many clinical conditions lead to hypoventilation of certain portions of the lung, for instance, prolonged bedrest, accumulation of secretions after general anesthesia, and inadequate aeration of the newborn's lungs. Thus, a method for detecting the presence of lung areas with low $\dot{V}_A/\dot{Q}$ ratios is clinically important. Since all body fluids are in equilibrium with arterial blood, as far as N_2 exchange is concerned, it is not even necessary to determine the arterial P_{N_2}; analysis of a urine sample (collected anaerobically) is sufficient. With this method, Abernethy et al.[1] found that recumbency at night, in healthy persons, increases the urinary-alveolar $(U\text{-}A)_{N_2}$ pressure difference; it was much lower during the day. The average P_{N_2} difference, 3.7 mm Hg before lying down, increased significantly, to 8.7 mm Hg 1 hour after lying down.[1] Therefore, recumbency increased non-uniform $\dot{V}_A/\dot{Q}$ distribution with a preponderance of low $\dot{V}_A/\dot{Q}$ areas. Healthy newborns have a normal $(U\text{-}A)P_{N_2}$ difference less than 10 mm Hg, but gradients up to 39 mm Hg were measured in infants with pneumonia.[13] The principal difficulty with the method is technical: it is extremely difficult to measure small variations in N_2 partial pressures. When the $(a\text{-}A)_{N_2}$ difference is 30 mm Hg (a highly abnormal value), arterial or urinary P_{N_2} is about 600 mm Hg, and the alveolar P_{N_2} about 570 mm Hg. A 1 percent error in the P_{N_2} measurement introduces an uncertainty of 6 mm Hg, 20 percent of the a-A difference. The analytical requirements have so far limited this method to small-scale research studies. As collection and analytical methods improve, this potentially important technique may be applied routinely.

In summary, A-a partial pressure differences can be measured for O_2, CO_2, and N_2. The presence of an abnormally high $(A\text{-}a)P_{O_2}$ difference indicates an abnormally wide range of $\dot{V}_A/\dot{Q}$ ratios in the lungs, including contributions of diffusion limitation and venous admixture. An $(a\text{-}A)P_{CO_2}$ difference indicates the presence of areas with high $\dot{V}_A/\dot{Q}$ ratios (hyperventilated, underperfused areas), while an abnormally large $(a\text{-}A)P_{N_2}$ difference suggests the presence of areas with low $\dot{V}_A/\dot{Q}$ ratios (hypoventilated, overperfused areas).

PHYSIOLOGICAL DEAD SPACE

Chapter 3 discussed the anatomical dead space, the volume of the airways without gas exchange function. Another definition of dead space is the ventilated airway and lung volume which does not participate in gas exchange (p. 57), the physiological dead space. It includes the anatomical dead space and any alveolar spaces that are not perfused via the pulmonary circulation. Physiological dead space is determined from the Bohr equation (p. 44) by substituting measurements of O_2 or CO_2 for those of the inert gases discussed in Chapter 3. Rahn [17] gave a graphical solution for the Bohr equation which illustrates several of its problems (Fig. 5-8). For CO_2, Eq. (3) on p. 45 can be rewritten by substituting partial pressures, which are proportional to gas concentrations, and by introducing measurements from Figure 5-8 (for the alveolar gas point A and expired air point E)

$$\frac{V_D}{V_E}=\frac{F_A-F_E}{F_A}=\frac{P_A-P_E}{P_A}=\frac{AB-DB}{AB}=\frac{AD}{AB} \tag{1}$$

A similar solution for O_2 yields

$$\frac{V_D}{V_E}=\frac{AF}{AC} \tag{2}$$

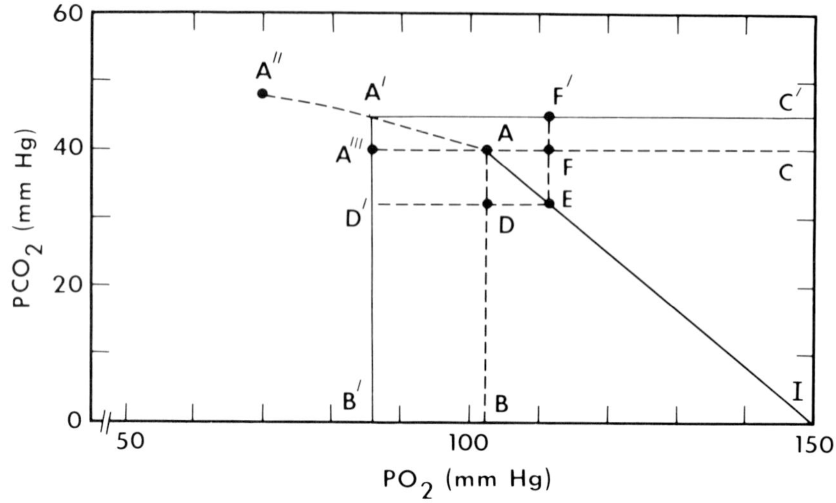

Fig. 5-8. Graphical solution of the Bohr equation in the O_2-CO_2 diagram (after Rahn[17]). See equations (1) and (2) in text. The true dead space for CO_2 is obtained from: $V_D/V_E = AD/AB = A''' \; D'/A''' \; B'$. The dead space for CO_2 obtained with the Haldane-Priestley method is given by: $V_D/V_E = A' \; D'/A' \; B'$, which is larger than $A'''D'/A'''B'$. Similarly, the dead space for O_2 is obtained from AF/AC which equals AD/AB. The Haldane-Priestley method yields a much larger value, indicated by $A'F'/A'C'$. See also text.

Since $AF/AC = AD/AB$, the dead space for O_2 equals that for CO_2. This graphical solution of the Bohr equation is feasible because the composition of expired air, a mixture of alveolar air with inspired air retained in the dead space, must be somewhere between points A and I on the diagram (Fig. 5-8). The smaller the dead space, the more the expired air point, E, approaches A. The larger the dead space, the more inspired air is mixed with the alveolar air, and the closer E will be to the inspired point, I. Eqs. (1) and (2) reflect these relations quantitatively.

As with anatomical dead space, the crux of the problem is the validity of alveolar air samples. The classical method is to collect the air last expired, at the end of a forced expiration (Haldane-Priestley method). However, no ventilation occurs during this forced expiration and hence alveolar gas composition changes as predicted from the breath-hold line in Figure 5-6. Depending on the depth and duration of expiration, the measured alveolar air composition might be that of point A′ or A″ in Figure 5-8. Expired air, on the other hand, is collected independently during quiet breathing. Thus, with the Haldane-Priestley procedure one may find alveolar air at A′ and expired air at E. Applying Eq. (1), one finds a dead space for CO_2 which equals $A'D'/A'B'$, and for O_2, $A'F'/A'C'$. This results in a larger dead space than would be obtained if the true alveolar gas composition during quiet breathing (point A) could be measured. $A'F'/A'C'$ is larger than $A'D'/A'B'$; hence one measures a larger dead space for O_2 than for CO_2, because A' deviates from the line AI, a consequence of the shape of the $\dot{V}_A/\dot{Q}$ line. Figure 5-8 can explain why Haldane's method gave large values for dead space. During exercise, the increased O_2 consumption would lead to a more rapid movement of point *A* along the breath-hold line, so that the error in determining alveolar gas composition increases. Thus, Haldane found that dead space increased greatly during exercise.[9] However, anatomical dead space only increases in proportion to end-tidal inspiratory volume, and Haldane's results during exercise do not allow conclusions about the size of the anatomical dead space (see also review of Haldane-Krogh controversy in reference 3). Early studies[10] suggested that the difference between O_2 and CO_2 dead space resulted from excretion of CO_2 in airways as well as in alveoli, while O_2 is taken up only in alveoli. There is no evidence for this; the difference between O_2 and CO_2 dead space with the Haldane method can be fully explained by changes in alveolar gas during prolonged expirations.

There is no satisfactory solution for the alveolar gas sampling problem. End-tidal samples eliminate the breath-holding effect of Figure 5-8 but include uncertainties related to timing and unequal distribution of $\dot{V}_A/\dot{Q}$ ratios; they are weighted in favor of relatively well-ventilated areas. Another weighting procedure is introduced if one collects arterial blood and uses its P_{CO_2} to represent alveolar P_{CO_2}. The assumption that there is no (a-A)P_{CO_2} difference is not always valid (p.). Moreover, using the circulatory system as an averaging circuit means that the P_{CO_2} value is weighted in favor of lung areas with high perfusion rates. If blood flow is not uniform, high flow areas (such as the bases of the vertical lungs) contribute more to the arterial P_{CO_2} than low flow areas, such as the lung tops.

In healthy persons, anatomical and physiological dead space are nearly equal; that is, there are no ventilated, unperfused areas that can be measured with these methods. In lung disease, physiological dead space is often much larger than anatomical dead space, which suggests the presence of large ventilated but unperfused areas in the lungs. Some studies have shown that man's physiological V_D increases when he goes from the supine to the standing position; this is consistent with the development of underperfusion in the lung tops. The difference between physiological and anatomical dead space is called the alveolar dead space. This is the volume of a virtual space with a $\dot{V}_A/\dot{Q} = \infty$, which represents the effect of all gas-exchanging areas with a higher than average $\dot{V}_A/\dot{Q}$ ratio. The term indicates a non-gas-exchanging alveolar space. Like other dead space volumes, alveolar dead space is a virtual volume, since no sharp gas fronts separate inspired and alveolar gas (p. 50). In addition, even unperfused alveoli receive some CO_2 by inspiring gas from the common dead space. Calculations of alveolar dead space can be corrected for this rebreathing effect.[22] In practice, the importance of alveolar dead space is that it indicates an abnormally large degree of nonuniformity in $\dot{V}_A/\dot{Q}$ ratios throughout the lungs.

Physiological dead space [using arterial P_{CO_2} in Eq. (1)] increases with end-tidal inspiratory lung volume to an extent comparable to anatomical V_D. It also increases with tidal volume and breathing rate and is largest when both are high. In older persons, physiological dead space may range up to 350 ml at normal tidal volumes and breathing rates.[14]

VENOUS ADMIXTURE

The concepts of venous admixture and physiological dead space are used in a comprehensive model of alveolar gas exchange developed by Riley.[20, 21] Rather than describing gas exchange in terms of a continuous distribution of $\dot{V}_A/\dot{Q}$ ratios, it treats alveolar gas and arterial blood composition as the net result of (1) gas exchange in alveoli with a normal or ideal alveolar air composition; (2) dead space ventilation; and (3) venous admixture. The latter is the virtual amount of venous blood that, if admixed with blood oxygenated to complete equilibrium with ideal alveolar air, would account for the actual gas pressures in arterial blood. Thus, venous admixture is a concept similar to that of dead space. Apart from the venous blood contributed by direct shunts to the arterial side of the systemic circulation, and by venoarterial shunts in the pulmonary circulation, venous admixture reflects the distribution of $\dot{V}_A/\dot{Q}$ ratios. It is as if arterial blood were a mixture of blood in equilibrium with alveolar air at the average $\dot{V}_A/\dot{Q}$ ratio, and blood coming from shunts or lung areas where $\dot{V}_A/\dot{Q}$ is zero. For clinical applications, therefore, nonuniform distribution of $\dot{V}_A$ and $\dot{Q}$ can be expressed in two simple numbers—dead space and venous admixture.

CLINICAL APPLICATIONS

Many lung diseases lead to nonuniform distribution of $\dot{V}_A/\dot{Q}$ ratios in the lungs. Areas with obstructed airways have diminished alveolar ventilation but may still have a normal pulmonary blood flow; their $\dot{V}_A/\dot{Q}$ ratio is low. Areas with obstructed blood vessels have diminished perfusion but their alveolar ventilation may be normal; their $\dot{V}_A/\dot{Q}$ ratio is high. Whenever one lung area has a $\dot{V}_A/\dot{Q}$ higher than the average, another area must have a lower than average $\dot{V}_A/\dot{Q}$ ratio. Hence, areas with high and low $\dot{V}_A/\dot{Q}$ ratios coexist in the same diseased lung, as well as in the healthy vertical lung (p. 89). The resulting wide dispersion of $\dot{V}_A/\dot{Q}$ ratios can be recognized by measuring A-a partial-pressure differences, physiological dead space, and venous admixture. Many clinical studies using these methods have shown that nonuniform distribution of ventilation and perfusion is the main cause of arterial hypoxia and hypercapnia in lung diseases. In obstructive lung disease, nonuniform $\dot{V}_A/\dot{Q}$ ratios may increase even when ventilatory tests show relatively little abnormality. For instance, a recent study of hemp workers with byssinosis showed a marked decrease in arterial P_{O_2} during dust exposure that caused only a small decrease in $FEV_{1.0}$[15] (see also Chap. 12). Theoretical and technical problems associated with measuring alveolar gas tensions in steady-state conditions limit the clinical use of A-a partial pressure differences. Furthermore, little specific diagnostic information is derived from knowing the distribution of $\dot{V}_A/\dot{Q}$ ratios. Since arterial puncture is needed, the methods are not suitable for routine use in the early detection of functional abnormalities in lung disease. For the clinical management of patients with ventilatory failure, it is essential to know the causes (e.g., airway obstruction) and effects (hypoxemia, hypercapnia) of gas exchange disturbances. Although detailed studies of $\dot{V}_A/\dot{Q}$ distribution increase understanding of the disease process, they are usually not required for decisions on treatment.

SUMMARY

The exchange of O_2 and CO_2 in the lungs is determined by the ratio between alveolar ventilation ($\dot{V}_A$) and pulmonary blood flow ($\dot{Q}$), by the gas tensions in inspired air and in mixed venous blood, and by chemical binding processes in blood. Since the latter do not occur with inert gases, their exchange illustrates the fundamental relations between $\dot{V}_A/\dot{Q}$ ratios and lung gas exchange without the complexities introduced by chemical binding of O_2 and CO_2.

The composition of alveolar gas varies throughout the lungs and during the breathing cycle and is markedly altered during breath holding and forced-breathing maneuvers. These variations occur as a function of the $\dot{V}_A/\dot{Q}$ ratio and can be illustrated graphically with gas and blood R lines, isoventilation ($\dot{V}_A/\dot{V}_{O_2}$ and $\dot{V}_A/\dot{V}_{CO_2}$) lines, and the $\dot{V}_A/\dot{Q}$ line in O_2-CO_2 diagrams.

The O_2 and CO_2 partial pressures in arterial blood are largely determined by the distribution of $\dot{V}_A/\dot{Q}$ ratios in the lungs, which can be assessed by measuring alveolar-arterial partial-pressure differences, physiological dead space, and venous admixture. An alveolar dead space and an (a-A)P_{CO_2} difference indicate areas with abnormally high $\dot{V}_A/\dot{Q}$ ratios. An abnormally large (a-A) or (U-A) (urinary-alveolar) P_{N_2} difference suggests the presence of areas with low $\dot{V}_A/\dot{Q}$ areas. Venous admixture includes the effects of low $\dot{V}_A/\dot{Q}$ areas and of lung blood flow shunts. The concepts and measurements discussed in this chapter have clinical applications in disorders of gas exchange (hypoventilation, hyperventilation, airway obstruction, pulmonary embolism) and in the interpretation of arterial blood gas data.

REFERENCES

1. Abernethy JD, Maurizi JJ, Farhi LE: Diurnal variations in urinary-alveolar N_2 difference and effects of recumbency. J Appl Physiol 23:875–879, 1967
2. Bouhuys A: Pneumotachography. Thesis, University of Amsterdam, (Assen, The Netherlands, Van Gorcum & Co.), 1956
3. Bouhuys A: Respiratory dead space, in Fenn WO, Rahn H (eds): Handbook of Physiology, Section 3: Respiration, vol I. Washington, D.C., American Physiological Society, 1964, pp 699–714
4. DuBois AB: Alveolar CO_2 and O_2 during breath holding, expiration, and inspiration. J Appl Physiol 5:1–12, 1952
5. DuBois AB, Fenn WO, Britt AG: CO_2 dissociation curve of lung tissue. J Appl Physiol 5:13–16, 1952
6. Farhi LE: Elimination of inert gas by the lung. Respir Physiol 3:1–11, 1967
7. Farhi LE, Yokoyama T: Effects of ventilation-perfusion inequality on elimination of inert gases. Respir Physiol 3:12–20, 1967
8. Farhi LE: Ventilation-perfusion relationship and its role in alveolar gas exchange, in Caro CG (ed): Advances in Respiratory Physiology. Baltimore, Williams & Wilkins, 1966, pp 148–197
9. Haldane JS: The variations in the effective dead space in breathing. Am J Physiol 38:20–28, 1915
10. Henderson Y, Chillingworth FP, Whitney JL: The respiratory dead space. Am J Physiol 38:1–19, 1915
11. Jöbsis FF: Basic processes in cellular respiration, in Fenn WO, Rahn H (eds): Handbook of Physiology, Section 3: Respiration, vol I. Washington D.C., American Physiological Society, 1964, pp 63–124
12. Knelson JH, Howatt WF, DeMuth GR: Effect of respiratory pattern on alveolar gas exchange. J Appl Physiol 29:328–331, 1970
13. Krauss AN, Soodalter JA, Auld PAM: Adjustment of ventilation and perfusion in the full-term normal and distressed neonate as determined by urinary alveolar nitrogen gradients. Pediatrics 47: 865–869, 1971
14. Lifshay A, Fast CW, Glazier JB: Effects of changes in respiratory pattern on physiological dead space. J Appl

Physiol 31:478–483, 1971
15. Lopez Merino V, Llopis Lombart R, Flores Marco R, Barbero Carnicero A, Gomez Guillen F, Bouhuys A: Arterial blood gas tensions and lung function during acute responses to hemp dust. Am Rev Respir Dis 107:809–815, 1973
16. Nye RE: Influence of the cyclical pattern of ventilatory flow on pulmonary gas exchange. Respir Physiol 10:321–337, 1970
17. Rahn H: A concept of mean alveolar air and the ventilation-bloodflow relationships during pulmonary gas exchange. Am J Physiol 158:21–30, 1949
18. Rahn H, Fenn WO: A graphical analysis of the respiratory gas exchange; the O_2–CO_2 diagram. Washington D.C. American Physiological Society, 1955
19. Rahn H, Farhi LE: Ventilation, perfusion, and gas exchange—the $\dot{V}_A/\dot{Q}$ concept, in Fenn WO, Rahn H (eds): Handbook of Physiology, Section 3: Respiration, vol I. Washington, D.C., American Physiological Society, 1964, pp 735–766
20. Riley RL, Cournand A: "Ideal" alveolar air and the analysis of ventilation-perfusion relationships in the lungs. J Appl Physiol 1:825–847, 1949
21. Riley RL: Pulmonary gas exchange. Am J Med 10:210–220, 1951
22. Ross BB, Farhi LE: Dead-space ventilation as a determinant in the ventilation-perfusion concept. J Appl Physiol 15: 363–371, 1960
23. West JB: Regional differences in gas exchange in the lung of erect man. J Appl Physiol 17:893–898, 1962
24. West JB: Ventilation, Blood Flow and Gas Exchange, ed 2. Philadelphia, FA Davis Co, 1970
25. Wagner PD, Laravuso RB, Uhl RR, West JB: Continuous distributions of ventilation-perfusion ratios in normal subjects breathing air and 100% O_2. J Clin Invest 54:54–68, 1974
26. West JB: New advances in pulmonary gas exchange. Anesth Analg 54:409–418, 1975

Chapter 6

Oxygen and Carbon Dioxide Transport

OXYGEN TRANSPORT

Oxygen is transported from points of higher to points of lower partial pressure. Figure 6-1 indicates its pathways from inspired to alveolar air, via the alveolo-capillary membrane to arterial blood, and on to tissues and venous blood. From the atmosphere to the alveoli, and again from the lung capillaries to the tissue capillaries, O_2 is transported largely by bulk flow. Transport by diffusion occurs within the alveolar gas (p. 65), between alveolar gas and lung capillaries, and from peripheral capillaries into the tissues and the cells. Transport between air, blood, and tissue occurs via membranes, and therefore diffusivity (a constant depending on molecular weight) and solubility in membrane media determine the transport rates. O_2 never moves against the dirction of partial-pressure gradients, and no active transport mechanisms are involved. Thus, O_2 exchange is governed by physical laws of diffusion and gas solubility. The application of these laws, however, is complicated by the thickness and heterogeneity of the membranes, the varying lengths of the diffusion pathways, and the nonlinear characteristics of the chemical binding process of O_2 in red blood cells. O_2 transport can be impeded at several sites in the transport pathways and by diverse mechanisms. These factors are discussed in this chapter.

GAS DIFFUSION IN THE LUNGS

The Alveolocapillary Diffusion Barrier

Oxygen must pass several layers of heterogeneous material on its path from alveolar gas to the interior of the red blood cell (Fig. 6-2). The length of this diffusion path varies from less than 0.5 μm to more than 2 μm. The membrane surface area available for diffusion is limited by the total epithelial surface of the alveoli. However, often only a portion of the membrane functions in gas exchange (Fig. 6-3). When perfusion pressure is low, as in the top of the vertical lung (Fig.

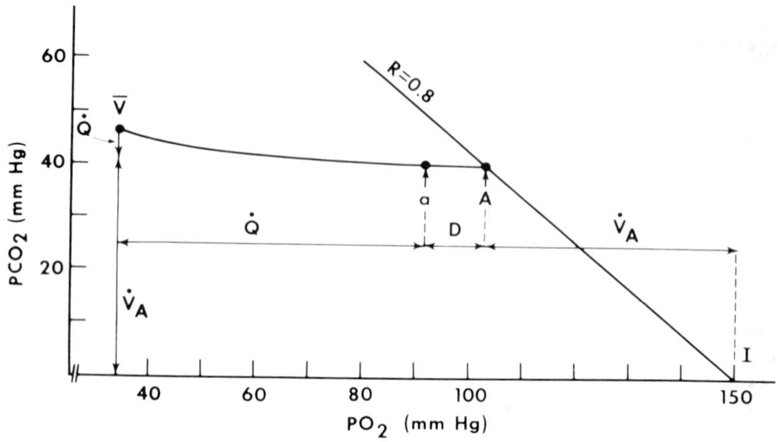

Fig. 6-1. The O_2-CO_2 diagram illustrates the relative importance of alveolar ventilation and lung blood flow for the transport of O_2 and CO_2. From the inspired point *I*, P_{O_2} decreases to its value at *A* by mixing of inspired and alveolar gas and further to a, owing to the (A-a) P_{O_2} difference. The largest P_{O_2} drop is from *a* to $\bar{V}$. Thus blood flow, $\dot{Q}$, accounts for the largest part of the decrease of P_{O_2} from *I* to $\bar{V}$. In contrast, P_{CO_2} drops only a few millimeters from $\bar{V}$ to *A*; CO_2 elimination is largely effected by alveolar ventilation $\dot{V}_A$. The relative importance of alveolar ventilation, diffusion, and cardiac output for gas transport is indicated by the relative lengths of the horizontal arrowes labeled $\dot{V}_A$, *D*, and $\dot{Q}$ for O_2, and of the vertical arrows $\dot{V}_A$ and $\dot{Q}$ for CO_2.

6-3*A*), or when lung capillary blood volume is decreased by high inflation pressures (Fig. 6-3*C*), only a small fraction of the membrane is in contact with red blood cells in the capillaries.[42] With higher perfusion pressure, lower inflation pressure, or both, more capillaries are filled with red cells and most of the membrane surface area can then be active in gas exchange (Fig. 6-3*B*).

Diffusion Coefficient and Diffusion Capacity

The partial-pressure difference between points on either side of the interface between alveolar gas and capillary blood can be measured indirectly. However, the length of the diffusion pathway and the surface area of the diffusion membrane cannot be measured in the intact lung. Hence, the *diffusion coefficient* (a physical constant—the amount of gas transported per unit time, per unit surface area, per unit partial-pressure gradient along the diffusion pathway) cannot be determined. Since the diffusion characteristics of individual wall components (membranes, cytoplasm, cell nuclei) vary considerably, it is difficult, if not impossible, to calculate the average diffusion properties of the total pathway.

Nevertheless, the overall diffusion characteristics of the interface can be assessed from the *diffusion capacity* of the lungs (D_L). In a small fraction, *i*, of the interface, the amount of gas transferred, $\dot{V}$, equals

$$\dot{V} = \frac{d_i \times s_i}{l_i} \tag{1}$$

where d_i is the diffusion coefficient of the interface, s_i is its surface area, and l_i is its

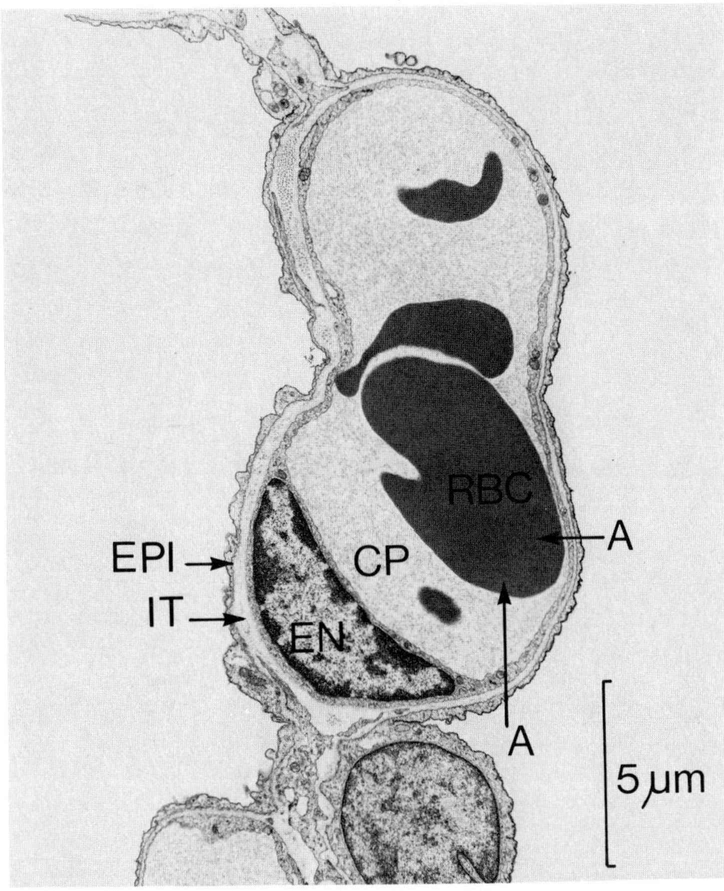

Fig. 6-2. Electron micrograph of alveolar capillary lined by endothelial cell (EN). A short and a longer diffusion pathway from alveolar air (A) to interior of red blood cell (RBC), via alveolar epithelium (EPI), interstitial tissue (IT), capillary endothelium (EN), and plasma in the capillary (CP) are indicated by arrows. From reference 102.

length. $\dot{V}$ is the rate of gas transfer per unit time and per unit A-a partial-pressure difference. By adding transfer rates in all parts of the interface, one obtains the overall transfer rate, or diffusion capacity

$$D_L = \sum \frac{d_i \times s_i}{l_i} \tag{2}$$

where i has values from 1 to n, the total number of diffusion pathways. D_L can be calculated from the total rate of transfer, $\dot{V}$, of CO or O_2 and its A-a partial-pressure difference

$$D_L = \frac{\dot{V}_{(CO,O_2)}}{PA_{(CO,O_2)} - P\bar{c}_{(CO,O_2)}} \tag{3}$$

where PA and $P\bar{c}$ are the alveolar and the mean capillary partial pressures of O_2 or CO. As an expression of overall gas transfer, D_L is determined by several un-

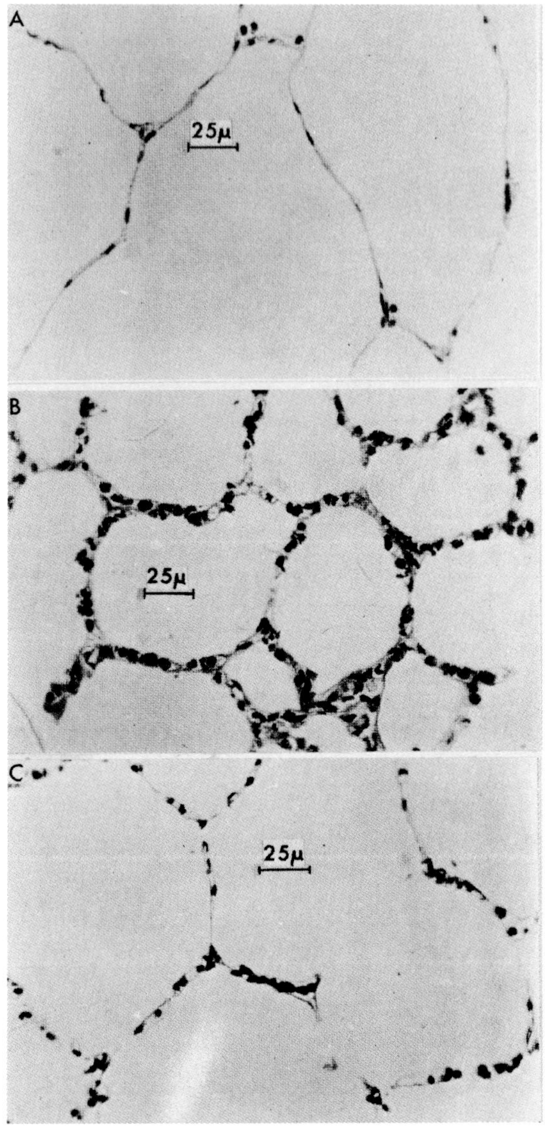

Fig. 6-3. 2-μm thick lung sections from greyhound dogs, prepared after freezing isolated lungs under different conditions. *A.* Top of a lung frozen in vertical position. Only a fraction of the alveolocapillary membrane is active in gas exchange because capillary blood flow is minimal (inflation pressure = 10 cm H_2O). *B.* Lower down in a lung prepared similarly. More capillaries are perfused, and most of the membrane is in contact with red blood cells (inflation pressure = 10 cm H_2O). *C.* Same preparation and location as in *B,* but with inflation pressure raised to 25 cm H_2O. This decreases blood flow and therefore the membrane surface area available for gas exchange. Drawn from micrographs of Glazier et al.[42]

knowns including the diffusion coefficient, the membrane's surface area, the length of the diffusion pathway, and gas solubility in the membrane substance. D_L is expressed in units of ml gas STPD/min/mm Hg (see footnote, p. 85).

D_L and $\dot{V}_A/\dot{Q}$ Distribution

Figure 6-3 suggests that $D_{L_{O_2}}$ may depend more on the extent of contact between alveolar gas and red blood cells than on the inherent properties of the alveolocapillary membrane. Obviously, no gas transfer takes place in areas where either $\dot{V}_A$ or $\dot{Q}$ is zero. The discussion in Chapter 5 showed that gas transfer is optimal in terms of total gas and blood flow when local $\dot{V}_A/\dot{Q}$ ratios do not differ much from the average value for the lungs as a whole (p. 90). In high $\dot{V}_A/\dot{Q}$ areas, ventilation is wasted; in low $\dot{V}_A/\dot{Q}$ areas, perfusion is wasted and little or no O_2 is transferred in spite of an intact transfer surface. These areas are, in effect, lost in the calculation of D_L, with a resultant decrease in D_L for the lungs as a whole.

The effect of nonuniform $\dot{V}_A/\dot{Q}$ ratios on D_L depends on whether O_2 or CO is used for its measurement. When blood flows slowly in a lung region, little O_2 is taken up since its transfer is negligible once all hemoglobin is saturated. Hence, high $\dot{V}_A/\dot{Q}$ areas decrease $D_{L_{O_2}}$. This effect is minimal with the CO breath-holding method, since CO is used in small quantities and capillary Hb is not saturated even when blood flow stagnates. Both $D_{L_{O_2}}$ and $D_{L_{CO}}$ are affected by uneven distribution of inspired gas, in particular when D_L is measured during tidal breathing (steady-state method): in poorly ventilated units gas transfer is limited by ventilation and not by alveolocapillary diffusion. This effect is less with the single-breath or rebreathing techniques (see below), which can be used for approximate prediction of diffusion limitations during exercise.[52,71]

Thus, a low value of D_L does not necessarily indicate a defect in the alveolocapillary diffusion of gases. With complex graphical techniques, one can distinguish some patients in whom diffusion disturbances are more important than $\dot{V}_A/\dot{Q}$ ratio nonuniformity,[1] but in many instances a low D_L indicates primarily that gas and blood do not meet efficiently.[34, 46]

Rationale for D_L Measurements

The validity of D_L as a lung function test has been questioned.[13] If diffusion capacity does not measure diffusion, why measure it at all? However, D_L is valuable as a measure of overall transport between inspired gas and arterial blood, a fact better reflected by the term transfer factor T_L[21] than by diffusion capacity. A low D_L value often indicates lung disease, and D_L may be decreased in conditions where other test results are normal. For instance, a low D_L is often an early sign of asbestosis (Chap. 12) when lung volumes still remain normal. In patients treated with bleomycin (an anticancer agent), D_L may decrease before lung volumes change.[77] In other cases, slight degrees of interstitial lung edema may decrease diffusion capacity while leaving other function tests unchanged.[1] Therefore, decreased D_L values frequently have clinical significance. Convenient and reproducible test techniques, in particular the single-breath method for $D_{L_{CO}}$, provide objective data about gas transfer without arterial puncture.

Measurement of D_L

To solve Eq. (3), one needs to measure (1) the uptake of a gas from inspired gas into blood, and, simultaneously, (2) the partial-pressure difference between alveolar gas and capillary blood for the same gas. This is feasible for only two gases—O_2 and CO; in practice, the latter is now used almost exclusively.

DIFFUSION CAPACITY FOR O_2

Measurement of D_L for O_2 is too complex to be practical. O_2 uptake can be measured by collecting and analyzing expired gas, and the alveolar P_{O_2} can be determined, subject to the uncertainties discussed in Chapter 5. However, the mean capillary partial pressure of O_2 is difficult to measure. In normal persons, a measurable alveolocapillary gradient at the end of the capillary exists only when the subject breathes a hypoxic gas mixture. The arterial P_{O_2} does not equal $P\bar{c}_{O_2}$ in Eq. (3) because of contributions of venoarterial shunts. In addition, the P_{O_2} of blood passing through pulmonary capillaries does not increase in proportion to the distance along the path of contact with alveolar gas. The mean capillary O_2 tension ($P\bar{c}_{O_2}$) must be calculated by a complex integration procedure. The interpretation of D_L values is complex regardless of the gas used. For these reasons, simpler techniques such as the CO method are preferable.

DIFFUSION CAPACITY FOR CO

This measurement is based on the high affinity of hemoglobin for binding with carbon monoxide. When one briefly breathes a gas with small amounts of CO, all CO taken up in blood is mopped up by Hb. The value of $P\bar{c}_{O_2}$ [Eq. (3)] remains so near zero that it can be neglected for practical purposes, and only alveolar CO pressure must be measured. The amount of CO inhaled during a single test is insignificant in terms of CO toxicity. D_L for CO can be measured with different procedures.[37,38] The single-breath or breath-holding method ($D_{L_{CO}}$ SB) is most practical for measurements at rest; either the breath-holding or the steady-state method ($D_{L_{CO}}$ SS) may be used for exercise studies.

Single-breath method ($D_{L_{CO}}$ SB). The test gas for this method commonly consists of 0.2%–0.3% CO, 21% O_2, and a suitable amount of helium (He) or neon (Ne), with N_2 as the balance. After a single inspiration of this gas mixture, from residual volume to TLC, the subject holds his breath for approximately 10 seconds. Then he expires rapidly, and a sample of expired air collected after at least 1000 ml of expiration is analyzed. This sample contains less CO and less He or Ne than the inspired mixture. The inert gas concentration drops because the inspirate is diluted with alveolar gas. If CO were not taken up in blood, its concentration would decrease by the same factor as the inert gas concentration. In fact, PA_{CO} is lower than that; the excess CO which disappeared is the amount taken up in blood. The inspired gas mixture may not be distributed evenly in the lungs, and this affects CO concentrations to the same degree as the He or Ne concentrations one measures. By calculating the alveolar CO pressure from the dilution of He or Ne, one corrects PA_{CO} for nonuniform gas distribution. Since the breathholding time is much longer than the duration of a quiet inspiration, the inspired gas has time to mix, by diffusion, even into spaces where it would barely penetrate during quiet breathing. Consequently, the value for

$D_{L_{CO}}$ SB may overestimate gas transfer during quiet breathing. Another factor that works in this direction is that the breath is held at close to maximum inspiratory lung volume. Hence, $D_{L_{CO}}$ SB reflects the surface area of the gas-exchanging membrane available at that volume; the surface area at lung volumes near FRC may be considerably smaller.[71] Both factors may explain, in part, why the single-breath methods yield higher values in healthy people than the steady-state method (which uses the spontaneous breathing pattern at lung volumes near FRC).

$D_{L_{CO}}$ depends on the inspired O_2 concentration. O_2 and CO compete for binding with hemoglobin, with the odds increasingly favorable to O_2 the higher its partial pressure. Hence, the higher the PA_{O_2}, the less CO is taken up and the lower the $D_{L_{CO}}$. This relation is used in partitioning D_L (see below).

Rebreathing method.[59,66] This method is similar to the previous one but eliminates the need for breath holding and is technically more complex. In one version, the subject rebreathes a mixture containing CO, neon, acetylene, and O_2.[62] Successive expired gas samples are collected automatically.[61] The expirates are analyzed in a gas chromatograph (Fig. 6-4) and reflect (1) dilution of inspired gas in alveolar

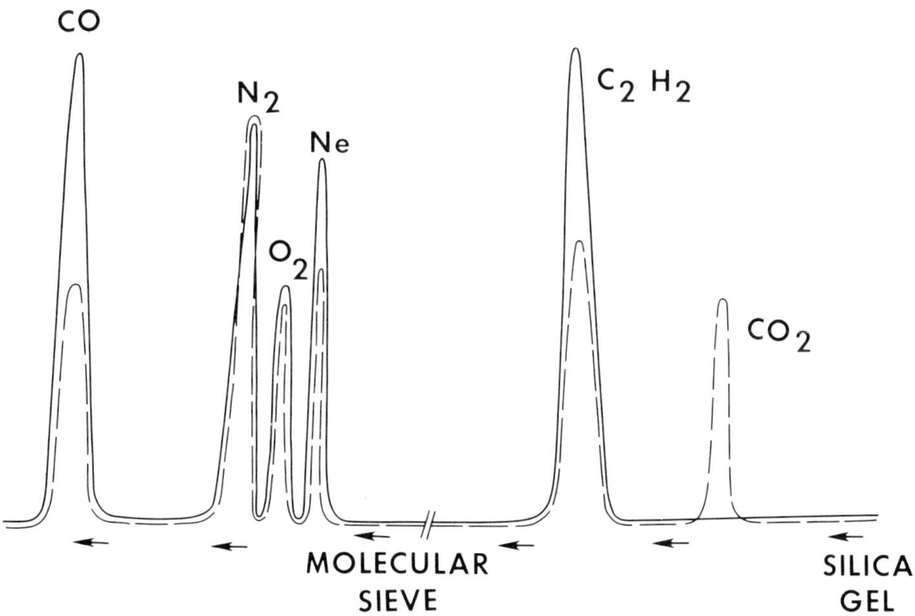

Fig. 6-4. Gas chromatographic analysis of inspired gas (*solid line*) and expired alveolar gas (*dashed line*) for determination of $D_{L_{CO}}$, lung volume, and $\dot{Q}$ with rebreathing method (see text). Composition of inspired gas = 0.5% CO, 0.5% C_2H_2, 0.5% Ne, balance air. The gas passes through a silica gel and a molecular sieve column. The decrease in C_2H_2 concentration in expired gas reflects its absorption into blood and is used for calculation of $\dot{Q}$. The decrease in Ne % in expired gas reflects dilution of alveolar with inspired gas and is used to calculate lung volume and alveolar P_{CO} [for use in Eq. (3)]. The relative decrease of alveolar CO concentration is much larger than that of the Ne concentration, reflecting CO uptake in blood. The inspired and expired P_{CO} values are used to calculate CO uptake [$\dot{V}_{CO}$ in (Eq. 3)]. Curves recorded by A.C. DeGraff and P. Snyder, Yale University Lung Research Center.

gas, measured from the dilution of Ne; (2) diffusion of CO; (3) disappearance of a soluble gas, acetylene, which is used to measure cardiac output. Disappearance curves during rebreathing are plotted for each of the three tracer gases, and this allows calculation of $D_{L_{CO}}$ and cardiac output.

Steady-state method ($D_{L_{CO}}$ *SS*). With this method, CO uptake is measured during spontaneous breathing, at rest, or during exercise. The subject breathes a CO-air mixture (e.g., 0.1 percent CO) during several minutes.* When a steady state has been reached, expired gas is collected for CO uptake measurement, and PA_{CO} is determined simultaneously. End-tidal sampling gives satisfactory PA_{CO} data in healthy persons, but not in patients with nonuniform gas distribution or in patients who breathe rapidly with small tidal volumes. In these patients PA_{CO} can be estimated with the Bohr equation (p. 44), using arterial P_{CO_2} values to calculate the physiological dead space. This method[32] can be applied in most patients but does not solve the distribution problem when physiological dead space is large—which it is in many patients in whom one would like to use this method. Physiological dead space then includes the volume of ventilated but unperfused alveoli where no gas exchange occurs, and when this is the case, $D_{L_{CO}}$ SS is low. Hence, regardless of how one estimates PA_{CO}, $D_{L_{CO}}$ SS is low whenever the lungs are ventilated nonuniformly. Small degrees of nonuniformity, as after administering small doses of histamine aerosol to healthy subjects,[15] are enough to decrease $D_{L_{CO}}$ SS. Since the single-breath or rebreathing methods are less influenced by nonuniform distribution of inspired gas, they are preferred. The steady-state method requires corrections for back pressure of CO in blood, because the subject takes up much more CO than with the single-breath method. This correction is always necessary in smokers (Chap. 12)

PARTITIONING OF D_L

Diffusion is a gas flow per unit pressure difference; hence, D_L is a conductance and its reciprocal, $1/D_L$, is a resistance. Using electric circuit theory, one might say there are several resistance elements in series which together make up the total resistance, $1/D_L$, of the diffusion barrier between gas and the red cell interior (alveolar gas; alveolar and capillary endothelial cells and their basement membranes and interstitial spaces; blood plasma in the capillaries; and red cells). Of these elements, the resistance of the red cell can be measured separately, with red cells in a well-stirred fluid. The resistance depends largely on the time required for O_2 or CO to bind with Hb. The total conductance of the red cells in lung capillaries equals θ, the rate of gas uptake per milliliter of blood, measured in vitro, times the blood volume in gas-exchanging capillaries, Vc. The resistance of this part of the diffusion pathway is $1/\theta Vc$. The sum of all resistances equals $1/D_L$. Thus, D_L can be partitioned into two conductances[92] according to

$$1/D_L = 1/D_M + 1/\theta Vc \tag{4}$$

* A protocol recommended for exercise studies includes the sequence: 0–2 min—exercise while breathing room air; 2–4 min—continue exercise; switch to 0.1 percent CO in inspired air; 4–7 min—collect expired gas; 5–6 min—collect arterial blood. (Unpublished committee report on standards of common measurements of lung function in interstitial lung disease for use in SCOR grant programs, National Heart and Lung Institute, 1972.)

where D_M is the diffusion capacity of all parts of the pathway between the alveolar gas and the wall of the red cell. Since it includes diffusion through the plasma layer, the term membrane diffusion capacity for D_M should not be taken literally.

Eq. (4) contains three unknowns. θ can be measured in vitro, which leaves two unknowns. A solution is feasible because the higher the PA_{O_2}, the lower the $D_{L_{CO}}$ (p. 105). Determination of $D_{L_{CO}}$ at a normal and a high inspired P_{O_2} yields two values for D_L that can be substituted in Eq. (4). If one knows θ at the same alveolar P_{O_2} values, D_M and Vc can be calculated. Normal values for D_M average about 57 ml/min/mm Hg; Vc is about 90 to 110 ml. In disease, D_M and Vc often but not always change in the same direction. In interpreting the results one should keep in mind that they depend critically on the value of θ. It is not certain that values for θ measured in vitro apply in vivo: gas exchange conditions for red cells in narrow capillaries may differ from those for red cells suspended in dilute solutions in vitro. Moreover, the kinetics of the reaction between CO and HbO_2 are more complex than has been assumed,[97] and hence improved values for θ are needed.

Using morphometric methods (p. 30), Weibel and his coworkers[102] have calculated maximum values for diffusion capacity from measurements of alveolar surface, barrier thickness, capillary surface area, and capillary blood and erythrocyte volume in sections of lung tissue. The values obtained with this method are larger than those obtained with the physiological techniques discussed above. In part, the discrepancy may be caused by the uncertainty concerning the physical constants, including θ, to be used in the calculations. For another part, the difference may be realistic: the morphometrist can include all potential gas-exchanging surfaces, whereas the physiologist measures the end result with indirect methods, several of which include systematic errors that tend to decrease D_L.

Physiological Variables That Affect D_L

In healthy persons, D_L increases with height, decreases with age, and is larger in men than in women. A comprehensive review of normal values in healthy men and women is available.[22] D_L SB increases with lung volume. Posture also affects D_L, probably chiefly because it changes regional perfusion. For instance, D_L is smaller in the sitting position (in which the lung tops receive little perfusion) than in the supine. During exercise, many factors increase D_L—increased cardiac output, increased capillary volume, and flow redistribution with opening of previously unperfused capillaries. The increase of D_L during exercise occurs in erect but not in supine subjects.[44] In the latter, capillary blood volume may already be maximal at rest; in the former, there is considerable scope for exercise-induced increases of perfusion, capillary blood volume, and effective gas-exchange surface area in the lung tops. Athletes commonly have a large D_L, probably because of a combination of age, physique, selection, and training. A high D_L seems to be one determinant of athletic prowess.

Newcomers to high-altitude areas do not experience increases in D_L;[58] even a 6-week stay at 3100 meters (Leadville, Col.) did not induce increases of D_L in sea-level residents.[24] However, highlanders (natives and long-term residents at high altitudes) have significantly higher values for D_L, D_M, and Vc than sea-level residents.[24, 88] Their TLC is also larger than expected. Increased lung size and increased D_L may be adaptive responses under the stress of long-term altitude hypoxia. Yet, these findings may also be explained by selection—persons with small lungs or low diffusion capacities, or both, may not tolerate high-altitude residence and move away. The older Leadville natives had well-preserved D_L values, which again may represent adaptation or merely selection of the fittest.

Clinical Significance of D_L Measurements[39]

A low D_L value indicates a decreased gas transport capacity of the lungs. This may be a consequence of (1) small lungs or lesions that decrease the amount of functioning lung tissue, e.g., pneumonectomy; (2) obstructive lung disease leading to nonuniform $\dot{V}_A/\dot{Q}$ distribution; (3) interstitial lung disease with decreased ventilation, perfusion, and diffusion in many areas; or (4) emphysema with a decrease of gas-exchanging surface area. The test result does not discriminate within this group of varied lung lesions. Lung disease affects different components of alveolar walls, e.g., by thickening of basement membranes, by accumulation of water or fibrous tissue in the interstitial space, or by hyperplasia of type II alveolar cells. All of these can contribute to low D_L values. A normal D_L value, on the other hand, is strong evidence against major degrees of alveolar destruction and hence practically rules out emphysema. However, obstructive airway disease and emphysema often coexist; thus a low D_L value often reflects obstruction (with nonuniform $\dot{V}_A/\dot{Q}$ ratio distribution) as well as emphysematous alveolar tissue destruction.

In interstitial lung disease, including sarcoidosis, asbestosis, silicosis, beryllium lung disease, and other forms of disseminated granulomatous or fibrous disease, D_L is a rough guide to the extent of parenchymal involvement. Decreased diffusion surface area, abnormal $\dot{V}_A/\dot{Q}$ distribution, and, perhaps to some degree, thickening of the alveolocapillary diffusion barrier, all contribute to a reduced D_L in these diseases. In some instances, D_L decreases while other tests remain normal (e.g., early asbestosis; p. 313). In the management of patients with interstitial lung disease, measurements of D_L at regular intervals can help assess the effectiveness of therapy.

OXYGEN TRANSPORT IN BLOOD

Oxygen is carried in blood and is dissolved in plasma as well as bound to hemoglobin (Hb). The amount dissolved is small but crucial for the transfer of O_2 between air and Hb and between Hb and tissues. The O_2 carried "in bulk" within the red cells is bound to the iron atom of Hb. The capacity of Hb to bind with oxygen and unload it depends on a minute change in the radius of its iron atom, which occurs when O_2 is bound or given off, and which leads to changes in the stereochemical structure of Hb.[80–82] The relation between the structure of Hb and its physiological function is now largely understood. However, the red cell is more than a simple package of Hb since other chemical processes within the red cell affect their oxygen-carrying function.

Oxygen-Binding Pigments

In the human body, only Hb and myoglobin (Mb) play a role. Each consists of an iron-porphyrin compound (heme) and a protein. Each Fe atom in heme binds one O_2 molecule. If the reaction were a simple one between two molecules, the law of mass action predicts that the relation between the O_2 pressure and the degree of oxygenation (the dissociation curve) would be a hyperbola. This is true for Mb but not for Hb (Fig. 6-5). The Mb molecule has one heme group; its reaction with O_2 is bimolecular. The dissociation curve for Hb is not as simple; its explanation has required many years of research, reviewed by Barcroft in 1928,[5] by Roughton in 1964,[91] and most recently by Perutz.[80–82]

Hb Oxygenation

The molecular weight of Hb is 64,500. Its protein (globin) consists of two α chains (with 141 amino acids) and two β chains (146 amino acids each). Portions of each chain are coiled up in α-helical forms. Together, the peptide chains form a tetrahedral molecule (tetramer) in which the four subunits are held together by bonds between positive and negative ions (salt bridges, hydrogen bonds, and van der Waals forces). Each polypeptide chain is folded to form a pocket on the surface of Hb, in which the heme group fits, easily accessible to O_2 from outside. The position of the heme groups in such pockets explains why the volume of the Hb molecule does not increase when O_2 is bound to it.[30] The Fe atom is bound to a nearby site on the globin chain as well as to heme. When O_2 binds to the Fe atom, the small change in the radius of the Fe atom leads to a slight movement of the helical chains. These changes are associated with (1) changes in the position of peptide chains near the heme pocket and (2) disruption of the salt bridges between the chains and weakening of the bonding between the molecule's four subunits. Consequently, the quaternary structure of the molecule is changed consider-

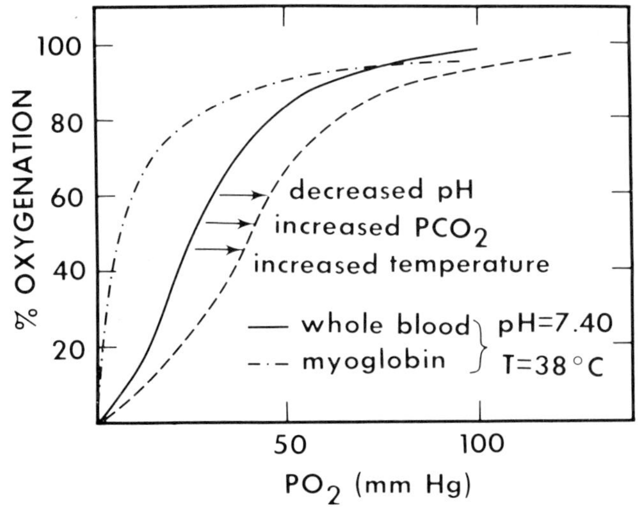

Fig. 6-5. O_2 dissociation curves for Hb and Mb. *Ordinate.* Percentage oxygenation (100% = full saturation of Hb or Mb with O_2). *Drawn line.* Typical curve for blood with normal Hb (HbA) under physiological conditions. Arrows indicate direction of change in position of curve as a function of pH, P_{CO_2}, and temperature. See also text. Modified from reference 91.

ably by slight displacements and rotations of amino acid groups near the heme pockets, because of oxygenation of one residue.

The four heme groups in Hb bind O_2 successively rather than simultaneously. Oxygenation of the first two or three heme groups of the tetramer leads to conformational changes about the heme pockets in the remaining chains and to disruption of the salt bridges between the molecule's four subunits. This increases the O_2 affinity of the chains with unoxygenated hemes. The shape of the dissociation curve reflects these successive binding reactions. O_2 binding to the first α chain is a bimolecular reaction.[93] After the first heme group is oxygenated, the O_2 affinity of the others increases and the dissociation curve slopes steeply upward. When three out of four heme groups have bound O_2, the rest of the binding process is again a bimolecular reaction. Therefore, the top parts of the dissociation curves of Mb and of Hb (if the effect of organic phosphate is removed; see below) coincide (Fig. 6-6).[9] The effect of oxygenation of one heme group on the O_2 affinity of the others, called *heme-heme interaction,*[82] ensures that, once the Hb molecule begins to unload O_2 in the tissues, the process proceeds rapidly because removing one O_2 molecule facilitates unloading the other three.

Bohr Effect

The Bohr effect also ensures adequate O_2 delivery to the tissues. Lowering the pH decreases the affinity of Hb for O_2, which promotes unloading of O_2 in the tissues, a consequence of binding of H^+ ions in the salt bridges that keep the Hb molecule in the deoxy strands.[82] At a lower pH, these do not split apart as easily, making O_2 binding more difficult. The binding of H^+ ions to the salt bridges also increases the capacity of Hb to bind CO_2. Hence, deoxygenated Hb binds more CO_2 than HbO_2 (Haldane effect). The Bohr and Haldane effects, which facilitate gas exchange in tissues, therefore depend on similar changes in the Hb molecule. In terms of the dissociation curve, a lower pH causes a shift to the right (Fig. 6-5).

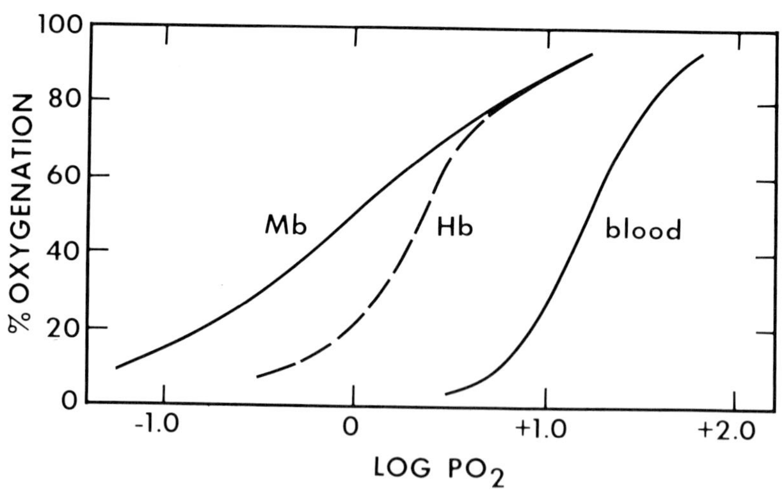

Fig. 6-6. Dissociation curves of myoglobin (Mb), stripped hemoglobin (Hb), and whole blood; P_{O_2} on log scale. After Benesch and Benesch.[9]

This is a graphical expression of the decreased O_2 affinity—at similar O_2 pressures, a smaller percentage of Hb is bound to oxygen.

2, 3-Diphosphoglycerate (2,3-DPG)

Although pH, P_{CO_2}, and temperature affect the affinity of Hb for O_2, these variables are close to constant in healthy persons. Therefore, a standard dissociation curve [25] has been widely used to study O_2 transport. But recent evidence suggests that metabolic mechanisms control O_2 binding. Changes in the O_2 affinity of Hb are important in several conditions, and standard Hb dissociation curves are not suitable to deal with these.

Organic phosphates in red cells, in particular 2,3-DPG, profoundly affect the Hb dissociation curve (Fig. 6-6). When all extraneous material is removed from the Hb molecule ("stripped Hb"), its O_2 affinity increases tenfold, and its dissociation curve approaches that of Mb. Addition of 2,3-DPG, which binds to the intact Hb molecule, moves the curve to the right and can return it to that of Hb in normal red cells. One molecule of 2,3-DPG may be bound per molecule of deoxyhemoglobin, probably to the β chains in the molecule's central cavity; under physiological conditions DPG is not significantly bound to oxyhemoglobin.[10, 82] The binding of DPG appears to stabilize the deoxy form of Hb. When the molecule is oxygenated, the central cavity becomes smaller and DPG is expelled. Adenosine triphosphate (ATP) acts similarly, but less effectively than 2,3-DPG.

2,3-DPG is formed as a by-product of glycolysis in the red cell. Factors, such as increased intracellular pH, which stimulate glycolysis tend to elevate the levels of 2,3-DPG. This compound's formation is also subject to a feedback mechanism. Increased levels of 2,3-DPG in the red cell inhibit its further formation by inhibiting the enzyme that forms 2,3-DPG from its precursors.[17] When 2,3-DPG is bound to Hb, the pool of free DPG diminishes and its formation is stimulated. This could explain why glycolysis increases when red cells are incubated under nitrogen—all Hb is in the deoxy form and binds DPG.[3] On the other hand, inhibiting glycolysis with chemical agents lowers red cell DPG content and increases the O_2 affinity of Hb. Thus, it is conceivable that DPG levels regulate O_2 binding by Hb under physiological conditions or in disease.[9, 17]

One instance where this regulatory role may be important is in adaptation to high altitude. The Hb dissociation curve of healthy humans shifts to the right within 24 to 36 hours after arrival at high altitudes (3000 or 4600 meters), an effect associated with an increased level of 2,3-DPG in the red cells.[63, 64] The process reverses on return to sea level. When long-term high-altitude residents are brought to sea level, their red cells and Hb also undergo the reverse change—DPG levels decrease and O_2 affinity of Hb increases. Hypoxia appears to induce DPG formation as part of an adaptive response to high altitude which promotes the unloading of oxygen from Hb and hence increases the oxygen availability to the body tissues. However, decreased affinity of Hb for O_2 is a two-edged sword: it may also decrease oxygenation of Hb in the lungs. This undesirable effect may become important at extremely high altitudes, where arterial P_{O_2} is decreased and a right-shift of the Hb dissociation curve may lead to considerable decreases of arterial O_2 saturation. In fact, under such conditions (at 9.180 meters) rats were able to survive only when their Hb affinity for O_2 was artificially increased, i.e., their Hb dissociation curve displaced to the left.[28]

Oxygenation of Mb, Fetal Hb, and Hb Variants

Myoglobin. At partial pressures less than about 60 mm Hg, Mb binds more O_2 than Hb (Fig. 6-5). Thus, in muscle tissue, which contains Mb, hemoglobin can unload O_2 at a given P_{O_2} of, for example, 20 mm Hg, while Mb stores it. This oxygen-storage mechanism probably plays a role in increasing a man's total work output during intermittent exercise.[4]

Fetal hemoglobin (HbF). Small changes in the composition of the amino acid chains distinguish HbF from adult Hb (HbA). In blood, HbF has a higher O_2 affinity than HbA (Fig. 6-7).[78] "Stripped" HbF has a lower Hb affinity than HbA. Fetal blood is exposed to O_2 only after it has passed an additional diffusion barrier in the placenta. However, the diffusion capacity of the placenta is sufficient to ensure complete equilibration of maternal and fetal O_2 partial pressures. Nevertheless, the P_{O_2} in the arterialized fetal blood (in the umbilical vein) is lower than the maternal arterial P_{O_2}, probably to a large extent because of uneven distribution of blood flow in the placenta. Because umbilical vein blood is mixed with fetal venous blood before it reaches the heart, fetal arterial P_{O_2} is lower still, about 25 mm Hg.[72] The high O_2 affinity of HbF insures adequate oxygenation of fetal blood despite lower partial pressures of O_2. That it also slightly inhibits unloading of O_2 in the tissues apparently does not bother the fetus, whose intrauterine movements constitute only light exercise. The fetus' metabolic demands are much less subject to rapid and large changes than those of animals after birth.

Hb variants. There are many genetic variants of Hb in man—some lead to disease (sickle cell anemia, Cooley's anemia); others are rare traits discovered only

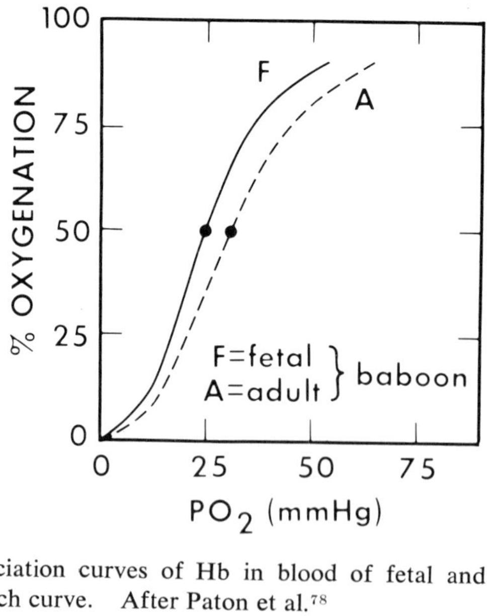

Fig. 6-7. Dissociation curves of Hb in blood of fetal and adult baboons. P50 indicated by dot on each curve. After Paton et al.[78]

by laboratory tests. They differ from HbA in the composition of the amino acid chains. In several variants, only a single amino acid residue is replaced by another. Yet, these changes are sufficient to alter the configuration of the Hb molecule, and especially the size and shape of the heme pocket. For many variants, the relation between stereochemical structure and physiological properties has been elucidated.[74] For example, Hb Zürich has an arginine group where HbA has a histidine group. The arginine residue is too large to fit in the heme pocket, and as a result, the heme pocket is wide open and O_2 is bound much easier than in HbA. Other Hb variants are less stable structures than HbA; they easily break apart into the four subunits. This, too, increases O_2 affinity.

Many Hb variants have a much higher or lower affinity to O_2 than HbA (Fig. 6-8).[98] Fortunately, there are compensatory changes in O_2 capacity: in general, the higher the O_2 affinity of the Hb variant, the larger the O_2 capacity. Hence, persons with a high O_2-affinity Hb variant, e.g., Hb Rainier, have a higher than normal O_2 capacity; persons with a low O_2-affinity variant, e.g., Hb Seattle, have a lower one.[76] Without this compensatory mechanism, persons with high O_2-affinity Hb variants where O_2 unloading is effective only at low O_2 tensions would suffer from O_2 deficiency in the tissues. Figure 6-8*B* shows how the changes in O_2 capacity normalize oxygen transport. With an arteriovenous O_2 difference of 4.5 vol%, mixed venous O_2 pressures vary only within a 10-mm Hg range in spite of the differences in O_2 affinity. The increased or decreased O_2 capacity allows O_2 transport over portions of the dissociation curve where the slopes are similar.

These differences in O_2 capacity suggest that Hb production is controlled to meet the demands of oxygen transport. There is indeed evidence that venous O_2

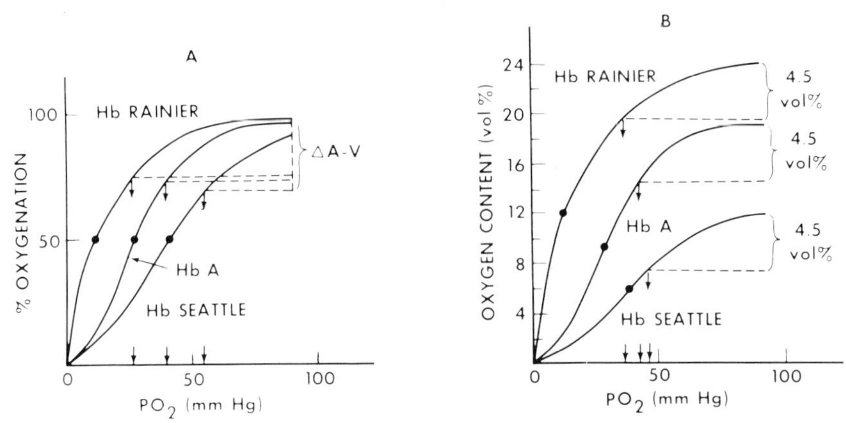

Fig. 6-8. A. Dissociation curves (% oxygenation scale) of blood with high affinity (Hb Rainier) and low affinity (Hb Seattle) hemoglobin variants, compared with blood with normal adult hemoglobin (HbA). ΔAV = Arteriovenous O_2 saturation difference (%). Arrows indicate mixed venous P_{O_2} of each blood for the same Pa_{O_2} and the same ΔAV. • indicates P50. B. Dissociation curves for same bloods as in *A*, with O_2 content of blood on ordinate. Normal blood (HbA) has O_2 capacity (=100% oxygenation) of 20 vol%; blood samples with Hb Rainier and Hb Seattle have a 20% higher and a 40% lower O_2 capacity, respectively. Because of the compensatory O_2 capacity changes, mixed venous P_{O_2} (*arrows*) is similar for blood with these variants when the arteriovenous O_2-content difference is the same (4.5 vol%). After Parer.[76]

tension influences the production of erythropoietin,[101] a hormone that regulates red cell production. When the number of red cells is drastically reduced by bloodletting, persons with Hb Rainier respond with a larger production of erythropoietin than persons with HbA. Because this compensatory mechanism involves production of new red cells, it takes time and is therefore useless under conditions involving acute changes in O_2 affinity of Hb.

OXYGEN TRANSPORT IN TISSUES

Oxygen molecules move along a gradient of decreasing partial pressure, from the red cell interior via blood plasma, through the capillary wall and the extracellular fluid, and through the cell membrane to the mitochondrial cristae. Electron transfers with the cytochrome chain of respiratory enzymes at the mitochondrial cristae are responsible for up to 90% of the cells' total O_2 consumption. Even within single cells, O_2 molecules are not distributed randomly. Also, there must be partial-pressure gradients, decreasing as one moves away from a capillary, in every tissue. For these reasons, the search for an average O_2 tension in tissues is not meaningful. But it is important to know what O_2 tensions must exist in capillary blood to insure adequate O_2 transfer to all cells.

With isolated mitochondria, a minimum O_2 tension of 0.5 mm Hg is required, and the critical intracellular P_{O_2} for intact cells is estimated at 3.5 mm Hg.[51] These are lower limits. Because of the partial-pressure gradients within a tissue, the capillary O_2 tension must be considerably higher to maintain these minimal values even in cells at a distance from the capillary or near its venous end where O_2 tension is low. The exact critical level is difficult to determine; one would need subtle indices of cell damage that could be related to capillary O_2 tensions.[105] Consciousness is lost when the internal jugular venous P_{O_2} falls below about 18 mm Hg (McDowell, quoted in ref. 55). A capillary oxygen tension of about 20 mm Hg is probably close to the lower limit that will prevent significant tissue hypoxia under most conditions and in most tissues.

Facilitation of Diffusion

Oxygen diffuses more rapidly in a layer of blood or Hb solution than in an equally thick layer of water. The presence of Hb or Mb in solutions appears to speed diffusion because the bound as well as the free O_2 can move by diffusion. For diffusion in red cells, experimental and theoretical results show that facilitation is not of great importance,[60] and Kreuzer[57] has concluded that the physiological importance of facilitated diffusion by Hb as well as Mb remains speculative. It is difficult to conceive how Hb could improve diffusion within the interior of red cells, where Hb molecules are tightly packed. In muscle tissue, facilitation of O_2 diffusion by myoglobin might make sense, but there is no evidence that it occurs.

OXYGEN TRANSPORT IN DISEASE

In disease, circulatory adaptations, blood viscosity, and many other factors outside the scope of this discussion are crucial for oxygen transport.[33] However, some clinical aspects of O_2 transport are particularly pertinent.

Although arterial O_2 and CO_2 tensions are often measured in patients with lung or heart diseases, they are rarely interpreted with accurate data on ventilation, cardiac output, and O_2 capacity of the blood. In extreme cases, a low arterial P_{O_2} clearly indicates inadequate O_2 transport. However, oxygen transport need not be normal when arterial P_{O_2} is within normal limits. The oxygen tensions in tissues are more nearly in equilibrium with venous than with arterial oxygen tensions. Low venous O_2 tensions can result from a large arteriovenous P_{O_2} difference, even if the arterial P_{O_2} is normal. This occurs when cardiac output is low and the tissues extract more O_2 from arterial blood to meet their metabolic demands. In patients with pulmonary edema, mixed venous O_2 tensions were lower than in bronchitic patients with ventilatory insufficiency, even though the latter had significantly lower arterial P_{O_2} tensions.[35] The bronchitics' larger cardiac output preserved tissue oxygenation in spite of a low arterial P_{O_2}. In the brain and the heart, where adequate oxygenation is particularly important, regional venous O_2 tensions are lower than the mixed venous value.[86] Thus, mixed venous O_2 tensions should always be well above critical levels to protect these hypoxia-sensitive tissues.

Improved interpretations of blood gas and associated data are feasible with computer programs that solve the alinear relations between ventilation, perfusion, and the characteristics of hemoglobin. Two groups of investigators have published their results from such programs in computer-produced tables [55] and nomograms [75] that allow calculations independent of any single standard dissociation curve and facilitate more complete interpretation of blood gas data. Kelman and Nunn's book [55] includes tables to calculate venous P_{O_2} if arterial P_{O_2}, arterial and venous O_2 content, temperature, and pH are known. Olszowska et al.[75] give examples to show the wide range of O_2 and CO_2 contents that may be associated with given values of P_{O_2} and P_{CO_2} in arterial blood, depending on O_2 capacity and the acid-base balance.

The principal causes of tissue hypoxia—inadequate arterial O_2 tension, anemia, and CO poisoning—indicate several important points for the clinical management of hypoxia.

ARTERIAL HYPOXEMIA

When arterial P_{O_2} decreases from 100 to 60 mm Hg, and the arteriovenous O_2 difference remains the same, the mixed venous P_{O_2} decreases only slightly (6 mm Hg; compare 1-1 and 2-2 in Fig. 6-9). This is because the mixed venous point is on the steep portion of the dissociation curve, where O_2 saturation changes considerably for each millimeter decrease of P_{O_2}. When the arterial point also reaches the steep portion of the curve, mixed venous P_{O_2} decreases almost as much as the arterial P_{O_2}, since both points are then on a nearly linear portion of the curve. However, this relationship holds only when the arteriovenous difference remains constant. If a slight arterial hypoxemia combines with a low cardiac output, the mixed venous point may drop to a dangerously low level. For instance, the person with an arterial P_{O_2} of 80 mm Hg and an arteriovenous difference of 7.5 vol% O_2 (corresponding to a 40 percent decrease in cardiac output) has a lower mixed venous O_2 tension than the person with an arterial P_{O_2} of 60 mm Hg and a normal cardiac output (compare 3-3 and 2-2 in Fig. 6-9).

Arterial hypoxemia in lung disease usually results from hypoventilation or

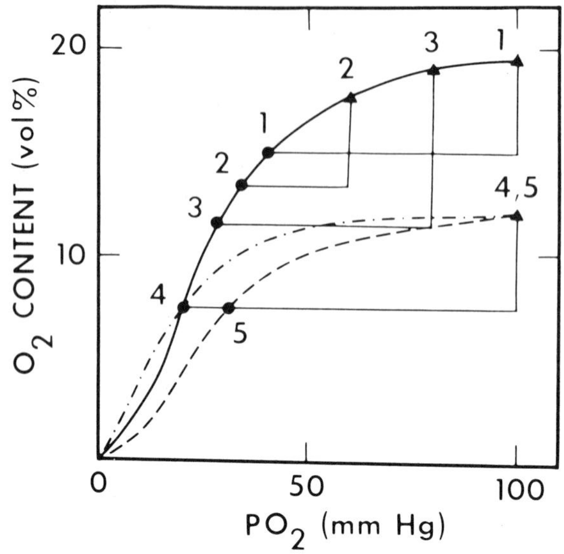

Fig. 6-9. Dissociation curves for blood with normal O_2 capacity (20 vol%, *solid line*) and low O_2 capacity (12 vol%, *dash-dot* and *dashed line*). Five different O_2 transport conditions (1-1 through 5-5) are shown. For each, the vertical line with arrow indicates the arteriovenous O_2-content difference (4.5 vol% for 1, 2, 4, and 5; 7.5 vol% for 3); the black circles on the dissociation curve indicate the corresponding mixed venous P_{O_2} values. Arterial P_{O_2} = 100 mm Hg (1, 4, and 5), 80 mm Hg (3), and 60 mm Hg (2). 4-4. O_2 transport in CO poisoning; 5-5. O_2 transport in anemia. See text for discussion. After reference 91.

nonuniform $\dot{V}_A/\dot{Q}$ ratios, or both. Since the relation between alveolar ventilation and alveolar P_{O_2} is nonlinear,[55] small changes in $\dot{V}_A$ can affect arterial P_{O_2} levels critically. For instance, under resting conditions a decrease of $\dot{V}_A$ from 5 to 4 liters/min may drop the alveolar P_{O_2} from 100 to 90 mm Hg, while a 1 liter/min decrease from 3 to 2 liters/min would decrease P_{O_2} from about 75 to 40 mm Hg.

Determination of mixed venous oxygen tensions may prove helpful in assessing tissue oxygenation in disease. Sampling via a pulmonary artery catheter is feasible but not always warranted; [35] a rebreathing method is also available.[18] Low values of mixed venous P_{O_2} indicate insufficient oxygenation, but normal values do not exclude oxygen deficiency in some tissues.

ANEMIA

Tissue hypoxia becomes a significant problem only when anemia is severe. In the example in Figure 6-9, a 40 percent loss of O_2 capacity is associated with a decrease of the mixed venous P_{O_2} from 40 to 32 mm Hg (compare 5-5 and 1-1 in Fig. 6-9). A compensatory increase in cardiac output often decreases the arteriovenous O_2 difference, so that the actual mixed venous P_{O_2} may remain normal.

CO POISONING

The shape of the O_2 dissociation curve in CO poisoning differs significantly from that in anemia.[91] It is placed to the left of the curve that corresponds to the same loss of O_2-binding capacity in anemia (compare 4-4 and 5-5 in Fig. 6-9). This displacement of the curve may be related to inhibition of 2,3-DPG synthesis [3] and results in low venous P_{O_2} values,[36] which contribute considerably to tissue hypoxia. Furthermore, the circulatory adaptations that follow when arterial P_{O_2} is low do not occur because P_{O_2} is normal (see also Chap. 10, p. 246).

Acute Changes of the Hb Dissociation Curve

The Hb dissociation curve changes as a function of blood loss, CO poisoning (see above), and physiological factors such as pH, P_{CO_2}, temperature (Fig. 6-5), and DPG metabolism. The position of the curve can be evaluated roughly if one knows (1) the O_2 capacity and (2) P50, the O_2 tension required to oxygenate 50% of the available O_2 capacity. A low value of P50 indicates high O_2 affinity of Hb and may signify decreased O_2 availability to the tissues. This measurement is particularly useful in conditions in which short-term changes in the dissociation curve's position are suspected. On the longer term, when compensatory changes in O_2 capacity may have occurred, P50 as well as O_2 capacity must be measured. The examples given for Hb variants (Fig. 6-8*B*) show that in that case O_2 transport may occur over a normal range of arterial and venous O_2 tensions, although the P50 varies from 12 mm Hg for Hb Rainier to 40.5 mm Hg for Hb Seattle.[76]

Acidosis and alkalosis. Blood pH variations can cause rapid changes in the position of the Hb dissociation curve. For instance, during treatment of diabetic acidosis, transient alkalosis may impair O_2 availability to the tissues.[8] When pH increases from 7.1 to 7.6, mixed venous P_{O_2} may decrease even though O_2 saturation at an arterial P_{O_2} of 100 mm Hg is slightly higher (Fig. 6-10). The acidotic patient can unload O_2 in the tissues at higher venous P_{O_2}'s. He can transport more oxygen for the same mixed venous P_{O_2} (cf. points at P_{O_2} = 40 mm Hg in Fig. 6-10) and therefore requires a smaller cardiac output for the same O_2 uptake. In patients with heart disease, whose cardiac output can increase only within a small reserve, alkalosis can be especially dangerous while minor degrees of acidosis may be of some advantage in helping to oxygenate tissues (see also pp. 137–142).

DPG metabolism. Red cell DPG levels are altered in several clinical conditions, including lung disease with hypoxemia.[17, 65] During storage of blood 2,3-DPG disappears, and massive transfusions with stored blood can cause significant shifts to the left of the dissociation curve.[14] Patients who require large transfusions (after massive hemorrhage or surgical shock) usually have a decreased O_2 capacity. Therefore, to assess their O_2 transport, one needs to know the O_2 capacity and the P50, as well as the arterial P_{O_2}.

Treatment of Hypoxia

Although administration of supplementary oxygen is an obvious and seemingly simple mode of treating hypoxia, administration of gas with adequately monitored inspired O_2 concentrations requires accurate equipment and constant patient supervision. Monitoring of arterial P_{CO_2} tensions is also required, since patients with ventilatory insufficiency may retain CO_2 during oxygen treatment. Application of

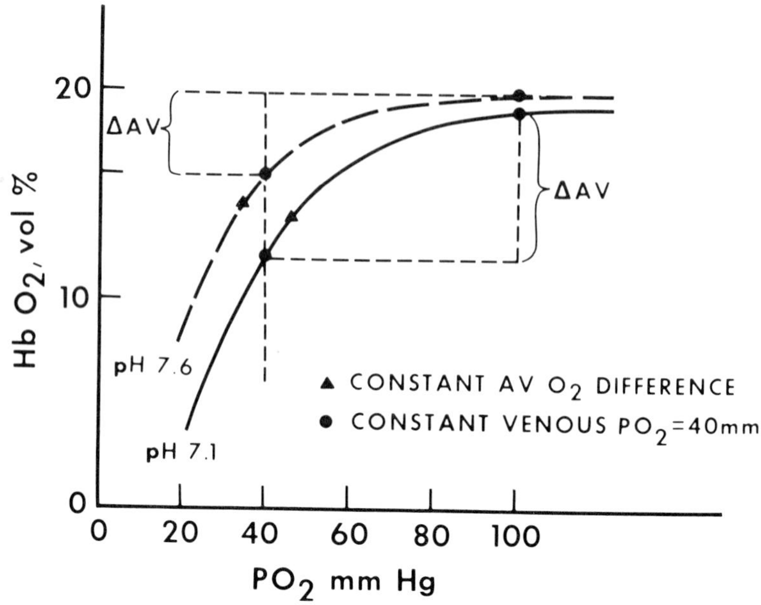

Fig. 6-10. Dissociation curves for alkalotic (pH = 7.6) and acidotic (pH = 7.1) blood. At the same mixed venous P_{O_2} (40 mm Hg; *black circles*), the person with acidosis transports more O_2 per 100 ml blood (i.e., has a larger arteriovenous O_2-content difference, ΔAV) than the person with alkalosis. At a constant ΔAV, the alkalotic person has a lower mixed venous P_{O_2} than the person with acidosis (compare *black triangles*).

the principles of O_2 transport to medicine should include measuring parameters of the dissociation curve, in particular O_2 capacity and P50. Several methods to determine the dissociation curve [27, 100] are now available which could improve evaluation and rational application of oxygen therapy.

As small computers and supporting software become more prevalent, computer-produced diagrams—based on quantitative relationships—will simplify the interpretation of blood gas data. The use of computer-produced tables and nomograms is a first step in this direction.[55, 75] Reliable hardware for measuring the primary data is already available (blood gas electrodes, mass spectrometer). Additional software and quality-controlled features must be developed to incorporate these techniques into user-oriented blood gas analysis systems that take blood samples as input and provide suitable diagrams and time charts as output. With the increasing need for intensive respiratory care in medical and surgical patients, such developments can lead to more effective, as well as more efficient, treatment of patients with ventilatory insufficiency and other conditions leading to tissue hypoxia.

CARBON DIOXIDE TRANSPORT

Carbon dioxide, formed in the tissues, is transported via the bloodstream to its principal site of excretion in the lung capillaries. In blood, CO_2 is physically dissolved as well as chemically bound. Complex physicochemical events in blood allow the transport of large amounts of CO_2, with partial pressure differences between venous and arterial blood much smaller than those that accompany oxygen transport in blood (Fig. 6-1, p. 100). For CO_2, the only large partial pressure drop is that between alveolar and inspired air. Hence, the rate of alveolar ventilation is a crucial factor in CO_2 excretion (see Chap. 5 for relations between PA_{CO_2} and $\dot{V}_A$).

The transport of CO_2 by blood involves major pH-buffering systems of the blood. CO_2 transport is therefore closely linked with the processes that maintain the body's acid-base balance. This chapter focuses on the mechanisms of CO_2 transport, with some reference to other processes (such as bicarbonate excretion or retention in the kidney) which influence the acid-base balance, and which often help compensate for blood pH changes induced by excessive or insufficient excretion of CO_2. The use of blood CO_2 tension, CO_2 content, and pH measurements in assessing acid-base balance is discussed in some detail because of its importance in physiology as well as in clinical medicine.

The broad outlines of CO_2 transport were clearly understood in the early 1930s,[90] but many details at the molecular level have been studied only recently. The importance of reaction rates, of direct binding of CO_2 to hemoglobin, and of carbonic anhydrase was known 40 years ago. However, the factors limiting the rate of equilibration of blood with CO_2, the molecular basis of carbamino-binding of CO_2 to hemoglobin, and the characteristics of different types of carbonic anhydrase have been clarified only in recent years. Also, acid-base disturbances were a topic of intensive research in the 1920s, culminating in the classic manual of Peters and Van Slyke.[84] But only in the past 10 years or so have the concepts based on this early work become fully accepted in clinical practice, largely through technological advances that enabled clinicians to obtain data on arterial blood pH and P_{CO_2} rapidly and accurately.

CO_2 TRANSPORT IN BLOOD

In this section the various modes of CO_2 transport [91] in plasma and in red blood cells are discussed on the basis of the diagrams of Figures 6-11 through 6-15. This is followed by a description of the relations between P_{CO_2} and CO_2 content (the CO_2 dissociation curve) and of the Henderson-Hasselbalch equation. Finally, the reaction velocities involved and the role of carbonic anhydrase are discussed.

Solution and Binding of CO_2 in Blood

Carbon dioxide is formed at the mitochondrial cristae in tissue cells. It diffuses rapidly out of the cells and into the blood (Fig. 6-11). In blood plasma, CO_2 is hydrated to form carbonic acid, H_2CO_3. This reaction proceeds very slowly, as indicated by the dashed arrow in Figure 6-11. The subsequent step—dissociation of H_2CO_3 into HCO_3^- and H^+ ions—is exceedingly fast (like all reactions involving ionic combinations and dissociations). But since the CO_2 hydration step is rate limiting, few bicarbonate ions (HCO_3^-) are formed.

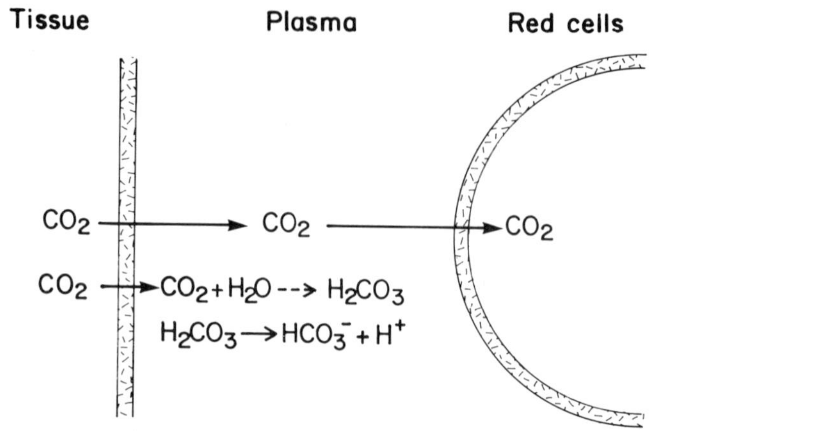

Fig. 6-11. Transport of CO_2 by diffusion from tissues to plasma and red cells. Hydration of CO_2 in plasma (slow reaction—*dashed arrow*). Dissociation of H_2CO_3 into bicarbonate and hydrogen ions.

CO_2 passes readily into the red blood cells. There are no demonstrable diffusion barriers for CO_2 between tissues, plasma, and red cells. Hence, the P_{CO_2} in blood plasma is equal to the P_{CO_2} in the erythrocytes. This diffusion equilibrium is indicated by the double arrow in Figure 6-12. The flux of CO_2 into the red cells is greater than that in the reverse direction because, in the cells, the hydration of CO_2 to H_2CO_3 is catalyzed by an enzyme, carbonic anhydrase. Hence, the rate of H_2CO_3 formation in the cells is several orders of magnitude greater than in

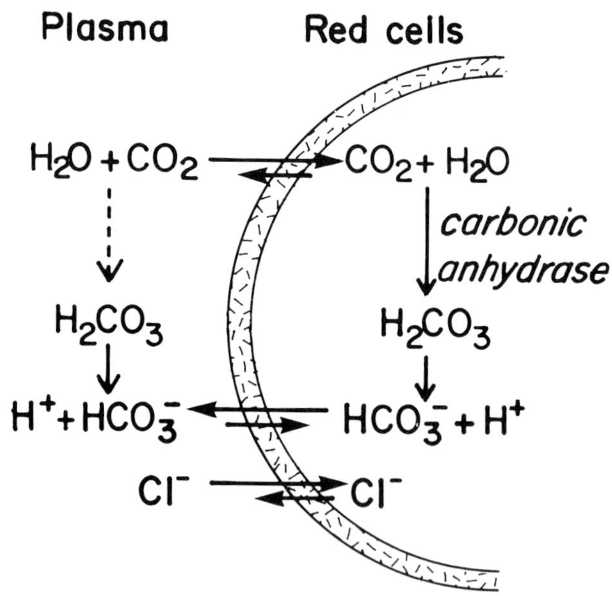

Fig. 6-12. Hydration of CO_2 is accelerated by carbonic anhydrase in red cells (rapid reaction—*drawn arrow*). Net displacement of HCO_3^- from red cells to plasma; replacement by other small anions, mainly chloride, which can pass the red cell membrane (chloride shift).

plasma. In turn, large amounts of bicarbonate and H^+ ions are rapidly formed by dissociation of H_2CO_3 in the red cells.

CHLORIDE SHIFT

The newly formed bicarbonate ions in the red cells diffuse to the plasma. Since cations cannot readily diffuse through the red cell membrane, the loss of bicarbonate ions from the red cells must be offset by an influx of other anions—mainly chloride—from plasma into the red cells, in order to maintain electrical equilibrium within the cells (Fig. 6-12).

These movements of anions—HCO_3^- and Cl^-—are governed by the Gibbs-Donnan principle. The ions that are able to penetrate the red cell wall (e.g., HCO_3^-, Cl^-) adjust their concentrations in plasma and in red cells according to the charges on other ions that do not penetrate the red cell wall (mainly proteinate ions in plasma and Hb^- ions in red cells). In this way, electrical charges on both sides of the red cell membrane are balanced.

The chloride shift is crucial for rapid exchange of CO_2 and allows considerable amounts of HCO_3^-, formed in red cells, to be carried in plasma. Without the chloride shift, the rapid formation of HCO_3^- promoted by carbonic anhydrase in the red cell would be useless because HCO_3^- can move out of the red cells only if other anions move in. Among the small anions in plasma, chloride is the most plentiful; hence it accounts for most of the anions that move into the red cell to replace HCO_3^-.

BUFFERS

The dissociation of H_2CO_3 into HCO_3^- and H^+ is promoted by the presence of anions of weak acids which bind H^+ ions to form un-ionized acid. The presence of these buffer ions (see also p. 126) considerably increases the capacity of blood to carry CO_2. The buffers remove an end product—H^+ ions—of the overall reaction: $CO_2 + H_2O \rightleftarrows HCO_3^- + H^+$. Hence, this reaction is carried to the right; the capacity of the buffers to remove H^+ ions determines to a large extent how much additional CO_2 can be bound as bicarbonate.

The most important buffer is hemoglobin (Fig. 6-13). Plasma proteins too are buffers, but their role in promoting binding of CO_2 as bicarbonate in plasma is less important than that of hemoglobin. Phosphate buffers ($HPO_4^{--}/H_2PO_4^-$)

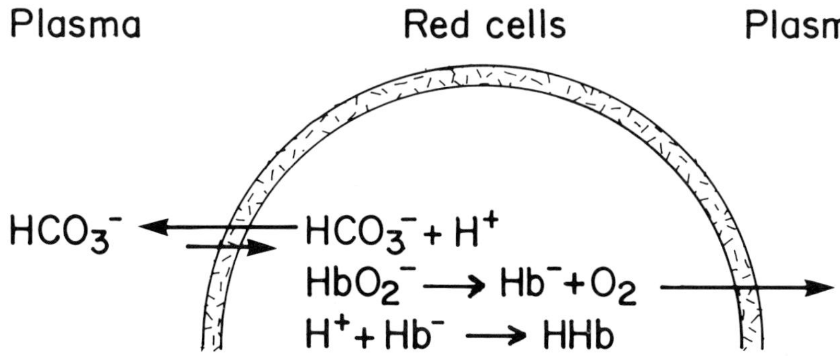

Fig. 6-13. Buffering of H^+ ions formed by dissociation of H_2CO_3 in red cells (see Fig. 6-12). The buffering capacity of Hb is increased by deoxygenation.

also play a relatively minor role. Reduced hemoglobin is more active in binding H^+ ions than oxyhemoglobin. HbO_2 is a relatively strong acid, i.e., many HbO_2 molecules are dissociated in HbO_2^- and H^+ ions. When the HbO_2^- ion is deoxygenated in the tissue capillaries, it yields O_2 and Hb^- ions. Since HHb is a relatively weak acid (i.e., not prone to dissociation into an anion and a cation), many of the Hb^- ions combine with H^+ ions to form HHb (Fig. 6-13). As a result of the increased buffering of H^+ ions, blood with deoxygenated Hb can bind about 60 ml more CO_2 per liter than fully oxygenated blood at the same P_{CO_2} (40 mm Hg) (see Fig. 6-16).

CARBAMINO REACTION

Most CO_2 is carried as HCO_3^- in blood, but an additional amount of CO_2 is bound directly to NH_2 groups of hemoglobin as a carbamino compound (Fig. 6-14). Like bicarbonate formation, this reaction depends on the state of oxygenation of Hb. Reduced Hb can bind more CO_2 as carbamate than HbO_2. In turn, carbamino Hb has a lower oxygen affinity than Hb without bound CO_2. Carbamate binding is also influenced by pH. An increase in pH increases the number of NH_2 groups available for CO_2 binding by shifting the reaction $R - NH_3^+ \rightleftharpoons R - NH_2 + H^+$ (where R = rest of the Hb molecule) to the right.

How CO_2 binding in the carbamate reaction is coupled to oxygenation of Hb is less clear. Early estimates suggested that Hb might bind about three times more CO_2 than HbO_2 at CO_2 partial pressures more than about 25 mm Hg.[31] At that time, the role of organic phosphates in modulating the function of Hb (see p. 111) was not known. We now know that CO_2 and 2,3-diphosphoglycerate (2,3-DPG) compete, at least in part, for the same binding sites on the Hb molecule. The early work [31] on carbamate binding by Hb was very likely done with 2,3-DPG-poor solutions.[70] When 2,3-DPG is added to Hb solutions, carbamate binding decreases; much less CO_2 is then bound when HbO_2 is deoxygenated (at constant pH and P_{CO_2}). Hence, carbamino binding of CO_2 contributes less to the total transport of CO_2 than used to be thought, at least in adult man,[70] i.e., about 10 percent rather than 20 to 30 percent.

The carbamino reaction occurs mainly, perhaps only, at the α-amino groups

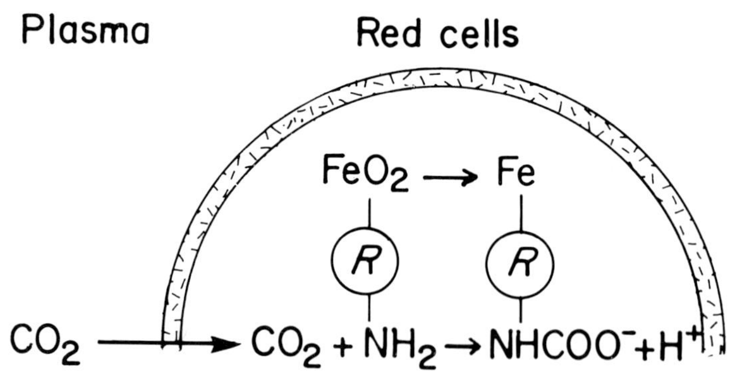

Fig. 6-14. Carbamino binding of CO_2 to Hb. *R* = rest of Hb molecule. Deoxygenation of Hb ($FeO_2 \rightarrow Fe$) promotes carbamino binding by increasing the number of available terminal amino groups.

at the end of the four polypeptide chains of hemoglobin.[2, 79] When the Hb molecule is modified by binding cyanate to these terminal α-amino groups, it binds only minimal amounts of CO_2.[79] Two of these four terminal α-amino groups (those on the β chains) also react with 2,3-DPG. These two α-amino groups are the ones with the highest affinity for CO_2.[70] The effect of binding either CO_2 or 2,3-DPG on the β chain α-amino groups is to decrease the O_2 affinity of Hb. The molecular basis for this change in O_2 affinity is not yet clear.[7] A detailed review of the interactions between Hb, H^+ ions, CO_2, and organic phosphates[56] concludes that only the sum of the effects of CO_2 and DPG can account for the behavior of Hb in blood. Neither DPG nor CO_2 alone is able to lower the oxygen affinity of pure ("stripped"—see p. 111) Hb to that of Hb in blood; together they can.

AMOUNTS OF CO_2 TRANSPORTED

The amounts of CO_2 carried in arterial blood are shown by the white bars in Figure 6-15. Gas exchange in the tissues adds to these amounts. The arteriovenous differences shown in Figure 6-15 indicate how much each transport mode contributes to the transport of CO_2 from the tissue to the lungs, i.e., to the total exchange of CO_2. The bulk of CO_2 ($57 + 24 = 81$ percent) is transported as bicarbonate—70 percent of it in plasma and the rest in red cells. The amount of dissolved CO_2 in plasma and in red cells is proportional to the P_{CO_2}. The constant of proportionality is the solubility coefficient of CO_2 (0.0301 and 0.025 mmol CO_2 per mm Hg per liter for plasma and red cells, respectively). Since the arteriovenous P_{CO_2} difference is small, dissolved CO_2 accounts for only 8 percent of the total amount transported. H_2CO_3 is present in negligible quantities both in plasma and in red cells. Carbamino CO_2 is also a relatively small contributor to CO_2 transport—much less than used to be thought (see previous paragraph).

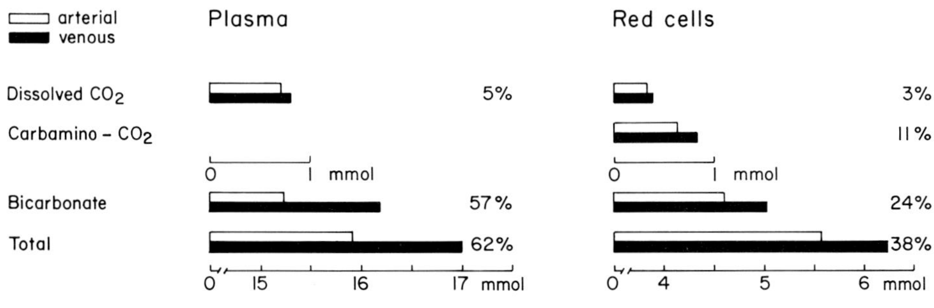

Fig. 6-15. Quantities of CO_2 transported in arterial and venous blood plasma and red cells, in mmol per liter whole blood. The arteriovenous difference for each transport mode represents the amount of CO_2 transported from the tissues to the lungs. The contribution of each transport mode to total CO_2 transport is indicated by the percentage behind each set of bars. The lesser contribution of red cells to total transport is, in part, caused by their smaller relative volume (40% of total blood). However, the amount of bicarbonate carried by 1 liter of plasma is also 60% larger than the amount carried by 1 liter of red cells. Drawn from data in Table 1 of Davenport.[23] Used with permission of University of Chicago Press (copyright 1974).

CO_2 DISSOCIATION CURVE

Blood with deoxygenated Hb binds more CO_2 at the same P_{CO_2} than blood fully saturated with oxygen (Fig. 6-16). The dependence of the CO_2 content on the state of Hb oxygenation is called the Haldane effect (see also p. 110). When HbO_2 is deoxygenated, more H^+ ions can be bound in the salt bridges between the heme groups in the tetramer molecule. This is the molecular basis for the long-known fact that reduced Hb is a weaker acid (i.e., it gives off fewer H^+ ions) than HbO_2. Using the Brønsted definition of a base as a H^+ acceptor, one might also say that reduced Hb is a stronger base (i.e., it accepts more H^+ ions) than HbO_2. By binding more H^+ ions, reduced Hb promotes CO_2 binding, since the reactions $CO_2 + H_2O \rightleftharpoons H_2CO_3^- + H^+$ are carried further to the right by the removal of the H^+ ions.

The changes in the Hb molecule during oxygenation and deoxygenation account for the Bohr effect (see p. 110 and Fig. 6-5) as well as the Haldane effect. Entry of CO_2 into blood, a decrease of pH, or both promotes deoxygenation of Hb by strengthening the salt bridges between the four subunits of the tetramer Hb molecule. There is evidence that CO_2 exerts a specific action in the Bohr effect. At a given pH, the P50 (see p. 117) is greater with CO_2 than without. The specific effect of CO_2 may be related to interaction between carbamate formation and binding of 2,3-DPG to hemoglobin.[6, 7]

The slope of the CO_2 dissociation curve depends on yet other factors than Hb oxygenation.[70] Other conditions being equal, acids (e.g., lactic and pyruvic acids formed by anaerobic glycolysis in working muscles) depress the curve. These relatively strong acids yield many H^+ ions, which compete with H^+ ions contributed by dissociation of H_2CO_3 for buffering by Hb and other buffers.

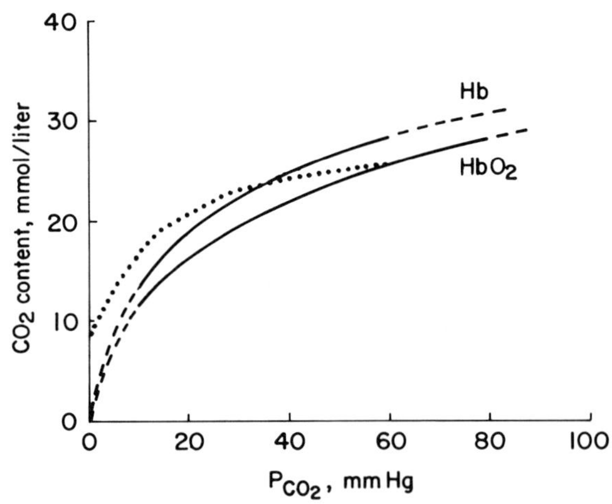

Fig. 6-16. CO_2 dissociation curves for fully oxygenated (HbO_2) and deoxygenated (Hb) blood, from Dill's nomogram (see Chart V in Rahn and Fenn[86]). The dashed portions of the curves are extrapolated beyond the range of the nomogram. The ordinate scale can be converted to volume percent (ml per 100 ml) by multiplying by 2.226. The dotted line is the dissociation curve of separated plasma (see text); after Fig. 3.6 of Michel.[70] Used with permission of Butterworths and the Medical & Technical Publ. Co. (copyright 1974).

Hence, Hb can bind fewer of the latter H^+ ions, and CO_2 binding must therefore decrease. Temperature affects the curve mainly through its influence on the solubility of CO_2, which increases with decreasing temperature. Hence, lowering the temperature displaces the CO_2 dissociation curve slightly upward and to the left; at the same P_{CO_2}, the CO_2 content increases.

More important is the effect of the total Hb concentration. In the physiological range of P_{CO_2}, the CO_2 dissociation curve of blood plasma equilibrated in vitro ("separated plasma") is flat (Fig. 6-16, *dotted line*). Plasma alone cannot transport enough CO_2, even though it can bind a considerable amount of it. At low CO_2 tensions, plasma retains CO_2 in the form of CO_3^{--} ions; lowering the CO_2 tension does not release CO_2 from these ions.[70] At physiological CO_2 tensions, the increase in plasma CO_2 is brought about only by solution of CO_2 and the formation of minimal amounts of H_2CO_3 and HCO_3^- ions, through the uncatalyzed CO_2 hydration reaction (see Fig. 6-11). In contrast, plasma in blood transports about two-thirds of all CO_2 carried from the tissues to the lungs (see Fig. 6-15). Most of this is bicarbonate formed in the red cells through the reactions shown in Figure 6-12. The presence of Hb is crucial in promoting this reaction by buffering of H^+ ions (see Fig. 6-13). Hence, much more CO_2 can be bound in plasma ("true plasma") equilibrated in the presence of red cells at increasing CO_2 tensions (in the range of 20 mm Hg and more) than in "separated plasma." This is reflected in the steepness of the CO_2 dissociation curve of blood, compared to that of the curve of separated plasma, in the physiological range of CO_2 tensions. Unlike the O_2 dissociation curve, the CO_2 dissociation curve does not reach a plateau; the blood CO_2 content continues to increase with further increases in P_{CO_2}.[70] Additional CO_2 is dissolved in proportion to the P_{CO_2}. Hence there is no "fully saturated" point on the curve. One cannot express the CO_2 content of blood as a percentage of full saturation, as is customary for the O_2 content of blood.

THE HENDERSON-HASSELBALCH EQUATION

The reaction

$$HA \rightleftharpoons H^+ + A^-$$

describes the dissociation of an acid (HA) in solution into its component ions, and also the reverse reaction: combination of the two ions to form the un-ionized acid. According to the law of mass action:

$$K[HA] = [H^+][A^-] \quad (1)$$

or:

$$[H^+] = K\frac{[HA]}{[A^-]} \quad (2)$$

where [HA], [H^+], and [A^-] are the concentrations of these three reactants.* If the acid is a strong one, [HA] is small; in solution, most HA is dissociated into ions. Eq. (1) shows that if [HA] is small, K must be large. For less completely ionized (weak) acids, [HA] is large, hence K is small. K is the ionization

* [ ] are used throughout this chapter to indicate concentrations.

constant: the larger K, the stronger the acid. K equals the H^+ concentration in the case that [HA] = [A^-] [Eq. (2)].

HA might, for instance, be acetic acid, a weak acid. If one adds sodium acetate—an almost fully ionized salt ($Na^+ + A^-$)—to a solution of acetic acid, the increase in [A^-] will decrease [H^+], by carrying the reaction $HA \rightleftharpoons H^+ + A^-$ to the left. Hence, addition of the salt suppresses the ionization of the acid. The mixture of a weak acid and one of its salts is a buffer solution. When another acid is added to this mixture, increasing [H^+], the reaction is carried further to the left, further decreasing [H^+] and [A^-]. In other words, the available A^- ions bind some of the excess H^+ ions. The increase of [H^+] is thus less than it would be if the same amount of the other acid were added to a solution without a buffer mixture. It turns out that the buffering action of the weak acid-salt mixture is strongest when HA and A^- are present in equal concentration, i.e., when [H^+] = K in Eq. (2). Weak bases and their salts are also buffer mixtures; here, OH^- ions bind with H^+ ions to form water, and similar considerations apply. Proteins have basic (H^+-accepting, e.g., —NH_2) as well as acidic (H^+-donor, e.g., —COOH) groups, so they can buffer [H^+] changes induced by acids as well as by bases. Especially important is the imidazole group of histidine, since its maximum buffering capacity is in the physiological range of [H^+] in blood (pK, see below, 5.7 to 7.7). Histidine is a component of many proteins, in particular of hemoglobin (about 35 residues per Hb molecule). Hb is a particularly important buffer in blood because of the Bohr and Haldane effects (p. 110). It provides extra buffer capacity in venous blood where it is needed to transport CO_2 and other acids (e.g., lactic acid) formed in the tissues with minimal change of [H^+].

The buffer system HCO_3^-/H_2CO_3 is important in the transport of CO_2 and in buffering other acids. The H^+ ions formed by dissociation of H_2CO_3 must be buffered by other systems, in particular Hb. To apply Eq. (2) to the HCO_3^-/H_2CO_3 system, HA = H_2CO_3 and A^- = HCO_3^-. However, instead of H_2CO_3 one uses αP_{CO_2}. This is warranted because the actual concentrations of H_2CO_3 in blood are minimal. In the presence of carbonic anhydrase (p. 129), the reaction proceeds as if: $H_2O + CO_2 \rightleftharpoons HCO_3^- + H^+$. Here [$CO_2$] = αP_{CO_2}, where α = the solubility coefficient for CO_2. Hence, Eq. (2) is transformed to:

$$[H^+] = K \frac{\alpha P_{CO_2}}{[HCO_3^-]} \tag{3}$$

Taking logarithms and changing signs:

$$-\log [H^+] = -\log K + \log \frac{[HCO_3^-]}{\alpha P_{CO_2}} \tag{4}$$

or:

$$pH = pK + \log \frac{[HCO_3^-]}{\alpha P_{CO_2}} \tag{5}$$

where pK is the negative logarithm of K. This is one of several forms of the Henderson-Hasselbalch equation; for a more detailed treatment of its different forms, see Davenport.[23]

In plasma, dissolved CO_2 and bicarbonate are the only forms in which CO_2 is present (Fig. 6-15). The minimal amount of H_2CO_3 can be neglected without significant error. Hence, for plasma:

$$[\text{Total } CO_2] = [CO_2] + [HCO_3^-] \quad (6)$$

and, since $[CO_2] = \alpha P_{CO_2}$ (see above):

$$[\text{Total } CO_2] = \alpha P_{CO_2} + [HCO_3^-] \quad (7)$$

Substituting Eq. (7) into Eq. (5) and using the value pK = 6.10 (at 38° C†), one has an equation which contains measurable quantities only:

$$pH = 6.10 + \log \frac{[\text{Total } CO_2] - \alpha P_{CO_2}}{\alpha P_{CO_2}} \quad (8)$$

Since α is known (0.0301 mmol/mm Hg/liter plasma at 38° C), Eq. (8) can be used to calculate either pH, [Total CO_2], or P_{CO_2} when the other two of these variables have been measured. Formerly, Eq. (8) was often used to calculate the P_{CO_2} when pH had been measured with a glass electrode,[95] and [Total CO_2] with Van Slyke's manometric or volumetric methods. The latter have been abandoned for routine purposes in most laboratories. Rapid and reliable methods are now available to measure P_{CO_2} with a membrane-covered glass electrode. Therefore, the Henderson-Hasselbalch equations are now mostly used to calculate the CO_2 concentration [using Eq. (8)] or [HCO_3^-] [using Eq. (5)] of blood samples in which pH and P_{CO_2} have been measured. The electrodes measure the H^+ ion concentration in the plasma adjacent to the glass membrane (permeable to H^+ ions) and not that in the red blood cells (the pH in red cells is about 0.2 pH units lower than that in plasma). Therefore, the electrodes provide data that may be inserted in the Henderson-Hasselbalch equation. Since there is an additional form of CO_2 transport (carbamate) in red blood cells, the equation cannot be applied to red blood cells.

Reaction Velocities[41]

Blood spends only brief moments in vessels where exchange of CO_2 can occur. In the lungs, the time during which exchange can take place ("pulmonary contact time") is probably about 0.7 to 1.6 sec at rest and less than 0.5 sec during exercise.[85] In the absence of carbonic anhydrase (p. 129), the dehydration of H_2CO_3 in the lungs would proceed far too slowly for effective excretion of CO_2 in the time available. However, the red cells contain more than sufficient carbonic anhydrase to accelerate H_2CO_3 dehydration, enough so that this process does not limit the rate of CO_2 excretion. Since the ionic reactions as well as the carbamino reactions are inherently quite rapid, it used to be thought that under physiological conditions transcapillary CO_2 exchange occurs rapidly enough for complete equilibrium during the passage of blood through the exchange vessels. However, this is probably not true (Fig. 6-17). Forster and Crandall[40] have described why there may be a considerable delay in final equilibration.

In the red cells, CO_2 entering from the tissues is rapidly hydrated; the P_{CO_2} which is in equilibrium with the intracellular [H_2CO_3] rises to close to the tissue

† The exact value depends on α and hence on temperature. Deviations from the value pK = 6.10 become quantitatively important at temperatures below 30° C.

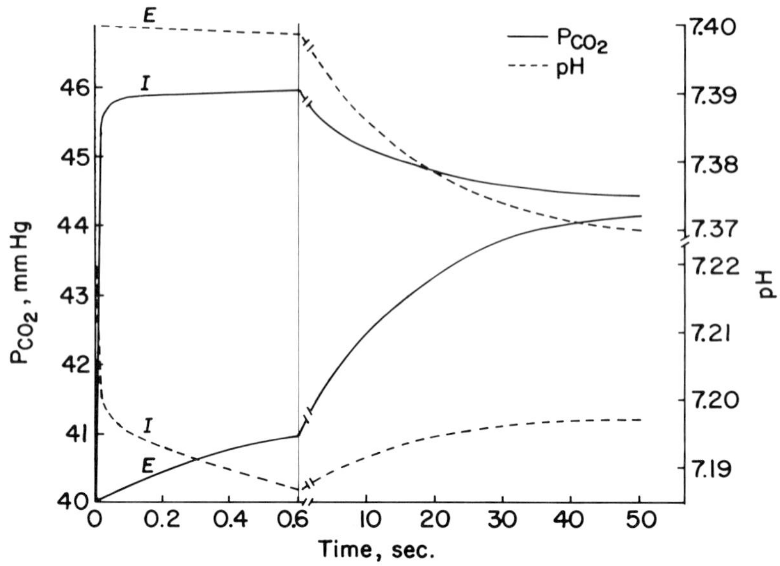

Fig. 6-17. Computed changes of intracellular (*I*) and equilibrated extracellular (*E*) changes in pH and P_{CO_2} in blood. The model assumes that normal whole blood (red cell volume, 40% of total) with a P_{CO_2} of 40 mm Hg enters a tissue capillary at time = 0 and exchanges CO_2 with a tissue of constant P_{CO_2} = 46 mm Hg during a period of 0.6 sec. At t = 0.6 sec, the blood leaves the tissue capillary (*vertical dashed line*). Further equilibration occurs between plasma and red cells after t = 0.6 sec and continues for more than 30 sec. See text for discussion. Redrawn from Forster and Crandall.[40]

P_{CO_2} within 0.2 sec (Fig. 6-17, *drawn line* marked *I*). HCO_3^- is equally rapidly formed and leaves the red cells by exchanging with chloride anions (see Fig. 6-12). This rapid formation of HCO_3^- decreases the intracellular pH to below its final value. The intracellular pH reaches a minimum about 0.6 sec after CO_2 exchange in the tissues begins (Fig. 6-17, *dashed line* marked *I*). Hence, intracellular $[H^+]$ is too high, but H^+ ions cannot leave the cells. They recombine with HCO_3^- ions, to H_2CO_3, which in turn dehydrates to CO_2 and H_2O. The CO_2 diffuses back from the cells to the plasma. In plasma, the initial "equilibrated" P_{CO_2} (the P_{CO_2} which is in equilibrium with the H_2CO_3 concentration) first remains low, since hydration of CO_2 is a slow process in plasma (no carbonic anhydrase present). This is shown by the drawn line marked *E* in Figure 6-17. Gradually, the equilibrated extracellular P_{CO_2} increases, and HCO_3^- is formed in plasma through the reactions of Figure 6-11. When the extracellular HCO_3^- concentration has increased sufficiently, HCO_3^- moves back to the cell; Cl^- moves out simultaneously (reverse chloride shift). In the cells, HCO_3^- recombines with H^+, thus increasing the intracellular pH. At the same time, extracellular pH decreases (*dashed line* marked *E* in Fig. 6-17), since H^+ accumulates in plasma. In effect, H^+ ions are in this way transferred from red cells to plasma, although they do not cross the red cell membrane. Because of the slowness of the hydration of CO_2 in plasma, this final equilibration process occurs largely after the blood has left the gas exchange vessels (i.e., after 0.6 sec has elapsed in Fig. 6-17). Gradually, intracellular and extracellular P_{CO_2} and pH reach their final equilibrium values after more than 30 sec.

Forster and Crandall's analysis[40] is based on a computer simulation of in vivo conditions which ignores the increase in buffering capacity of Hb as it is deoxygenated during gas exchange in the tissues (see Fig. 6-13). However, another analysis that does take O_2 exchange into account also shows a considerable delay in final equilibration of P_{CO_2} and pH.[48] Experimentally, rapid recordings of extracellular pH, during equilibration of diluted human blood with a high-CO_2, low-pH, bicarbonate buffer solution, show that pH equilibrium requires about 10 sec. When carbonic anhydrase was added to the extracellular fluid, less than 20 msec was required.[40] Hence, it seems well established that the rate of the uncatalyzed reaction $CO_2 + H_2O \rightleftharpoons H_2CO_3$ limits the rate at which pH is equilibrated in red cell suspensions. The computer simulations support the idea that this is also true for blood under physiological conditions of gas exchange.

CARBONIC ANHYDRASE[68]

It has long been known that dehydration of H_2CO_3, to CO_2 and H_2O, is too slow, in vitro, to explain the rate of CO_2 excretion in the lungs. The discovery of carbonic anhydrase in red blood cells provided an explanation why the in vivo processes—dehydration of H_2CO_3 and hydration of CO_2—take so much less time. Carbonic anhydrase is a protein with a molecular weight of about 30,000. In man, two forms of the enzyme exist (forms B and C); x-ray diffraction studies have provided details about their structure.[54, 67] However, the mechanism of the catalytic action of carbonic anhydrase is not yet fully understood.[104] Essential to this action, which speeds up the hydration of CO_2 by a factor of 10^9, is the presence of zinc, one atom per molecule. Cobalt (Co^{++}) can replace zinc, but the enzyme is then less active. With other metals or without any, carbonic anhydrase is almost inactive in hydrating CO_2. Although human red cells contain mostly carbonic anhydrase B (85 percent of the total), this form of the enzyme is probably not active in CO_2 hydration. Carbonic anhydrase C is about 20 times more active than B; the small amount of C present in red cells is sufficient to provide excess enzyme activity for dehydration and hydration of CO_2—even during maximum exercise.[69]

The action of carbonic anhydrase, especially C,[69] is inhibited by several drugs, including sulfanilamide and acetazolamide (Diamox®). Because of the excess capacity of carbonic anhydrase C, therapeutic doses of drugs which inhibit the enzyme do not impede CO_2 transport and excretion (although they may affect CO_2 hydration elsewhere in the body, e.g., in the kidneys), at least not in healthy man at rest. However, large doses of acetazolamide (50 or 100 mg/kg) decrease the rate of CO_2 excretion by the lungs in dogs.[17a, 49] Hyde calculated that, under these conditions, the P_{CO_2} in blood at the end of a pulmonary capillary should be considerably higher than the alveolar P_{CO_2}. These results suggest that inhibition of carbonic anhydrase might limit the rate of CO_2 excretion during heavy exercise or in patients with severe reductions of the gas-exchanging surface area of the lung alveoli.

CO_2 TRANSPORT IN VIVO

During transport of CO_2 in the intact organism, additional events take place which do not occur when blood is equilibrated with CO_2 in vitro. These events include: (1) exchange of ions between blood plasma and extracellular tissue fluid; and (2) exchange of CO_2 with tissues where it can be stored.

This section briefly describes these aspects of CO_2 transport in vivo and also some consequences of the delayed equilibrium in blood after passage through the tissues or lungs (p. 127). The importance of the ventilation-perfusion relations in the lungs for adequate removal of CO_2 will also be discussed.

CO_2 Dissociation Curve in Vivo

When blood is equilibrated at a given P_{CO_2} in vitro, all bicarbonate formed remains in the red cells and the blood plasma. When a person inhales a CO_2-air mixture which yields the same P_{CO_2} in arterial blood as existed during the in vitro equilibration, a large fraction of the bicarbonate enters extracellular tissue fluid. Hence, for the same P_{CO_2} change, the changes in plasma bicarbonate (and total CO_2) concentrations are less in vivo than in vitro. Also, some buffering occurs in vivo in cells other than red cells. The binding of H^+ by intracellular protein buffers leaves additional bicarbonate in the extracellular fluid. Intracellular buffering in tissues other than the kidneys may account for more than 50 percent of total buffering in vivo.[99] Thus, in vivo plasma bicarbonate levels are influenced by two opposing mechanisms: (1) dilution of bicarbonate in extracellular fluid; and (2) additional accumulation of bicarbonate in extracellular fluid due to intracellular buffering of H^+ ions.[23] If these opposing effects were equal they would cancel one another. However, they often differ in magnitude; this means that for the same P_{CO_2}, the bicarbonate content of plasma from blood equilibrated in vitro differs from the bicarbonate content of blood plasma equilibrated in vivo. In vivo CO_2 dissociation curves have been determined in man and in animals during acute as well as longer term CO_2-exposure experiments in an environmental chamber. The differences between the in vivo and in vitro dissociation curves are well illustrated in Davenport's book.[23] In principle, it is clearly not correct to use in vitro dissociation curves to calculate changes in CO_2 contents of blood plasma in vivo. But in practice, the application of in vivo curves poses many problems. The scatter of in vivo data is considerable (see, e.g., Fig. 18 in ref. 23 and Table 6 in ref. 19). Moreover, at a given P_{CO_2} the total amount of CO_2 stored in the body increases with time (see next section). Hence, in assessing the acid-base balance of patients with, e.g., chronic respiratory acidosis (p. 137), one would need to know how this condition has developed in time in order to apply appropriate in vivo dissociation curves. In the range of pH 7.2 to 7.6, the difference between in vivo and in vitro dissociation curves is small. In most applications, in vitro CO_2 dissociation curves may be used as long as it is understood that no quantitative estimates of base excess or base deficit (see p. 142) can be made on the basis of in vitro data.[94] The in vitro curves are straight lines on a log $[CO_2]$-log P_{CO_2} diagram (see Figs. 6-19 to 6-22), which facilitates the qualitative assessment of acid-base changes.

In vivo CO_2 equilibration studies have clearly demonstrated that CO_2 buffering differs considerably in states of acute and chronic hypercapnia (Fig. 6-18). In dogs previously made chronically hypercapnic by several days' exposure to CO_2-enriched air, $[H^+]$ ion changes during superimposed acute changes in inspired P_{CO_2} were much smaller than the $[H^+]$ ion changes in control animals that previ-

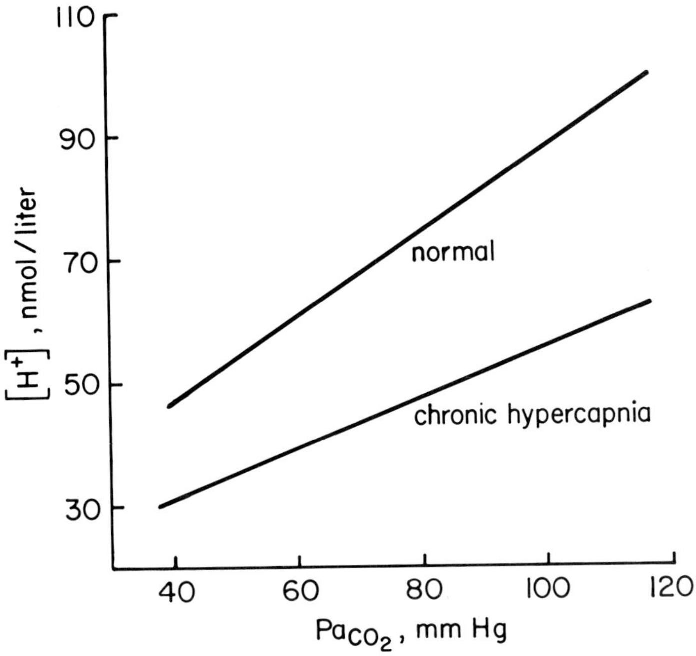

Fig. 6-18. Hydrogen concentration of blood plasma as a function of arterial P_{CO_2} in a normal dog (baseline Pa_{CO_2} approx. 40 mm Hg) and in a dog with induced chronic hypercapnia (6 days at Pa_{CO_2} of approx. 110 mm Hg). From Goldstein et al.[43]

ously had breathed air.[43] The principal reason why the chronically hypercapnic animal is better able to buffer H^+ ions during acute changes in P_{CO_2} is its increased bicarbonate level. The change in $[H^+]$ depends on the ratio

$$\frac{P_{CO_2}}{[HCO_3^-]}$$

as is obvious from Eq. (3) (p.126). Hence, for the same absolute change of P_{CO_2} (in mm Hg), $[H^+]$ will change less, the larger $[HCO_3^-]$. The difference between the control and hypercapnic animals is clear only when absolute H^+ concentration, not the logarithmic pH scale, is used, as in Figure 6-18. In that figure the interval from 30–50 nmol/1 H^+ corresponds to 0.22 pH units; the interval from 70–90 nmol/1 H^+ corresponds to only 0.10 pH units. When using the pH scale, it is important to keep in mind that pH is not linearly related to $[H^+]$: small changes in $[H^+]$ influence pH more, the more alkaline the blood. The reader should also be aware that pH units should be converted to $[H^+]$ whenever one wants to calculate averages from a series of data and for other statistical calculations.

CO_2 Stores

The human body contains more than 100 liters CO_2, all but 3 liters of it stored in the tissues.[19] The lungs contain about 0.2 liters CO_2, most of it in alveolar gas; blood contains about 2.5 liters (5 liters blood at about 500 ml

CO_2/liter at normal P_{CO_2}). The tissues contain CO_2 in solution as bicarbonate and perhaps in carbamino compounds. But more than 90% of the tissue CO_2 is stored as carbonate (CO_3^{--}) in bone. Some tissues (those with high rates of blood perfusion) reach a steady state of CO_2 storage within minutes after a change in arterial P_{CO_2}; tissues with lesser perfusion rates may take an hour or more to equilibrate. And in animal experiments bone continues to accumulate CO_2 even 6 to 8 weeks after exposure to CO_2-enriched air begins.[87] So far, no definite saturation of the body CO_2 stores has been described.

Not only the time course of equilibration, but also the CO_2 binding capacity of different body tissues varies considerably. Data from different sources [99] show that (at $P_{CO_2} = 50$ mm Hg) muscle may have a [CO_2] of about 13 mmol/kg wet tissue, heart and brain of about 16 mmol/kg, and bone 450 mmol/kg. Bones and tendons are high-capacity buffers, but their exchange rates with extracellular fluid and plasma are so slow that their role as CO_2 stores becomes clear only in long-term experiments.[87] As a source of tissue buffering, however, bone is important on the shorter term—mainly because it releases sodium ions in exchange for H^+ ions. In 5-hour experiments with rats and dogs, sodium release from bone accounted for a major share of the tissue buffering of hydrochloric acid infused into the bloodstream.[11]

CO_2 Exchange in the Lungs

ALVEOLAR-ARTERIAL P_{CO_2} DIFFERENCE

When human subjects rebreathe in a bag, CO_2 exchange between blood and alveolar gas can be abolished. If this is done during exercise—thus increasing the amounts of CO_2 to be excreted via the lungs—alveolar P_{CO_2} is often higher than the arterial or the mixed venous P_{CO_2}.[45, 53] Similar findings in dogs who inhaled 5 to 10 percent CO_2 have led to the suggestion that passive diffusion may not suffice to account for CO_2 exchange in the lungs.[50] However, Forster and Crandall [40] have provided an explanation that requires no sweeping revisions of the view that CO_2 exchange in the lungs is by passive diffusion alone. They point out that blood may return to the lungs with a P_{CO_2} higher than the equilibrated P_{CO_2} (46 mm Hg versus about 44 mm Hg in their example, Fig. 6-17). Alveolar P_{CO_2} is in equilibrium with the higher value; arterial P_{CO_2} is closer to the lower, equilibrated value. In some rebreathing + exercise, as well as CO_2 exposure experiments, larger alveolar-arterial P_{CO_2} differences than those suggested by Figure 6-17 have been found. But this does not invalidate Forster and Crandall's argument since these experimental conditions would enlarge the difference between mixed venous and equilibrated P_{CO_2} in their analysis.

VENTILATION-PERFUSION DISTRIBUTION

An arterial-alveolar P_{CO_2} difference (i.e., $PA_{CO_2} < Pa_{CO_2}$) indicates the presence of hyperventilated lung zones (Chap. 5). Nonuniformity of $\dot{V}_A/\dot{Q}$ ratios in the lungs can also explain why arterial P_{CO_2} is often high in patients with chronic airway obstruction. Computer simulations show that, all other conditions being equal, increased variability of $\dot{V}_A/\dot{Q}$ ratios throughout the lungs leads to increased arterial and venous P_{CO_2} when CO_2 production is constant.[29, 103] In such nonuniform lungs, hyperventilation of some areas is not sufficient to compensate for the rise in blood P_{CO_2} that results from underventilation in other areas. The effect of $\dot{V}_A/\dot{Q}$ nonuniformity in causing CO_2 retention is especially marked in lung models with series ventilation (see Chap. 4). Therefore, clinical conditions associated with series ventilation (e.g., lower airway obstruction with collateral ventilation of lung areas behind the obstructions) are likely to lead to CO_2 retention. Although an increase in total ventilation (for instance, by a respirator) may help to increase CO_2 output and to decrease arterial P_{CO_2}, treatment of the conditions underlying the nonuniform $\dot{V}_A/\dot{Q}$ distribution (e.g., removal of secretions from obstructed airways) is fundamental in removing a principal cause of CO_2 retention.[103]

ACID-BASE DIAGRAMS

The relations between pH, P_{CO_2}, and total CO_2 content determined by the Henderson-Hasselbalch equation (p. 126) can be summarized in nomograms that enable one to read the unknown value when the two others are known. Examples of such nomograms, first worked out by L. J. Henderson,[47] are given in references 25, 26, and 86. For clinical purposes, the same relations are visualized more easily in diagrams that contain two of the three variables on the ordinate and the abscissa, with the third as a parameter. Well-known examples are the pH-$[HCO_3^-]$ diagram of Davenport [23] and the pH-log P_{CO_2} diagram of Astrup and Siggaard-Andersen.[96] This chapter uses one of the earliest of these diagrams, first introduced by Peters in 1923 [83] and later used in an extensive clinical study by Møller.[73] Figure 6-19 shows that in the Peters diagram log $[CO_2]$ is plotted against log P_{CO_2}, with pH as the parameter. Since log scales are used for both $[CO_2]$ and P_{CO_2}, the relation between $[CO_2]$ and P_{CO_2} at a constant pH is a straight line [see Eq. (8)]. The relation between $[CO_2]$ and P_{CO_2} (the CO_2 dissociation curve, see Fig. 6-16) is also a straight line.[83] Its position depends on the factors discussed on p. 124 (Fig. 6-16). Because the diagram uses logarithmic scales, some aspects of acid-base balance are not well expressed in it. For instance, the difference in H^+ buffering between hypercapnic and control animals (see p. 130) causes only a minor difference in the slope of log $[CO_2]$ — log P_{CO_2} lines; the difference is better seen when plotted as $[H^+]$ versus P_{CO_2} (Fig. 6-18). For qualitative purposes, however, the logarithmic scales of the Peters diagram allow easy distinction between respiratory and nonrespiratory disturbances of acid-base balance.

Figure 6-19 includes normal values for pH, P_{CO_2}, and $[CO_2]$ from different sources.[16, 95] Only the portion of the diagram between the lines for pH = 7.70 and pH = 6.80 concerns conditions likely to be encountered in healthy or diseased persons. pH values higher than 7.70 or lower than 6.80 have rarely, if at all, been observed and are probably incompatible with life. This range of pH values corresponds to a sevenfold change in H^+ concentrations (150 nmol/liter at pH 6.80; 20 nmol/liter at pH = 7.70). Figures 6-19 through 6-22 use $[CO_2]$, which is less than 2 mmol/liter higher than $[HCO_3^-]$ at $P_{CO_2} < 65$ mm Hg. For most qualitative purposes, the difference may be ignored. Equation (7) (p. 127) allows conversion of $[CO_2]$ to $[HCO_3^-]$ and vice versa if P_{CO_2} is known.

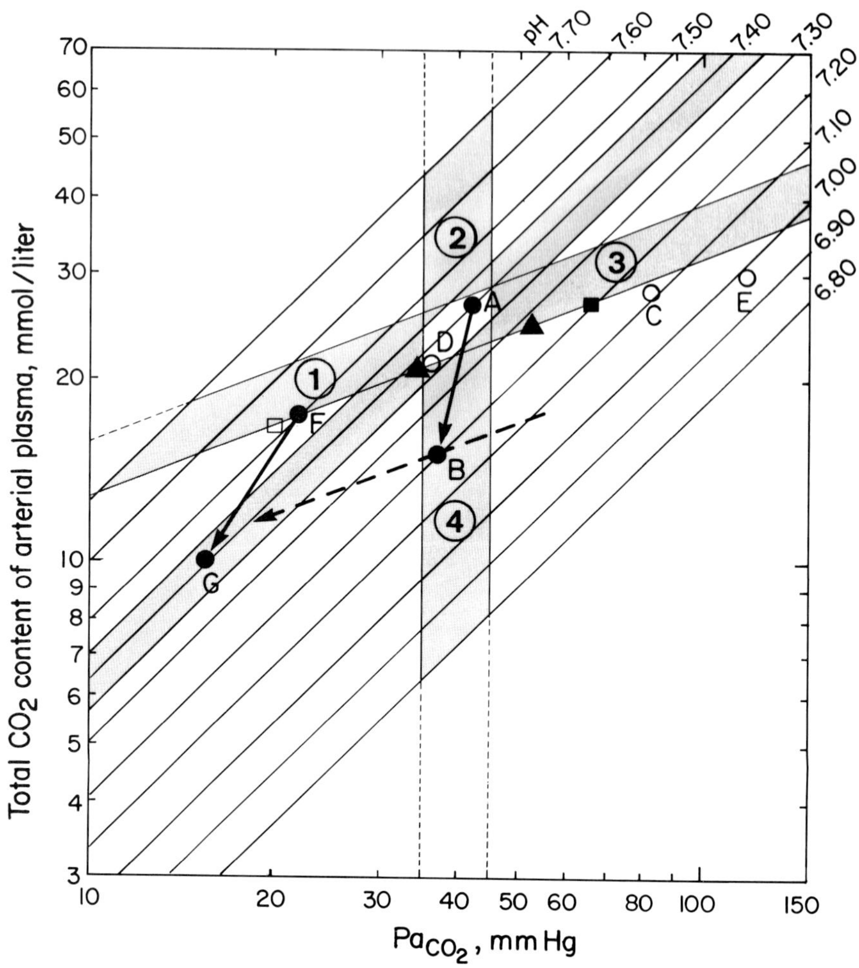

Fig. 6-19. This and the following figures use the Peters diagram [83] for a graphical assessment of changes in acid-base status. Pa_{CO_2} (abscissa) and $[CO_2]$ of arterial plasma are plotted on log scales. Hence, lines for equal pH run at a 45° angle in the diagram (see Eq. 5, p. 126). Range of normal pH values is indicated by shading between the pH lines for pH = 7.35 and for pH = 7.45. Range of normal Pa_{CO_2} values (35–45 mm Hg) is indicated by the vertical gray area. Two upward sloping lines enclosing another gray area are CO_2 dissociation curves. Lower one of these is the same as the curve for fully oxygenated blood in Fig. 6-16. Upper CO_2 dissociation curve is parallel to the lower one; in the range of normal P_{CO_2} and pH, it indicates the upper limits of normal $[CO_2]$ (approx. 28 mmol/liter).

Areas designated by circled numbers *1* to *4* represent respiratory alkalosis (*1*), nonrespiratory alkalosis (*2*), respiratory acidosis (*3*), and nonrespiratory acidosis (*4*). Specific data points are as follows: ▲: points A_2 and A_3 in Fig. 5-4, p. 85; □: acute hyperventilation; ■: breath holding after O_2 inspiration.[86] Arrow *AB*: average control (*A*) and postexercise data points in healthy athletes.[16] Arrow *FG*: acute respiratory alkalosis on first exposure to high altitude (*F*), followed by compensation during altitude acclimatization (to *G*). Data from Rahn and Fenn.[86] ○: (*C, D, E*): three data points obtained over a 15-hour period in a patient with intermittent acute respiratory acidosis (p. 138 in ref. 73). Dashed arrow through *B*—see text for explanation.

Acid-Base Changes under Physiological Conditions

Figure 6-19 illustrates the changes in acid-base status that occur during hypoventilation, hyperventilation, breath holding, and exercise in healthy persons.

HYPO- AND HYPERVENTILATION

The changes in alveolar gas tensions, as a function of changes in alveolar ventilation, are discussed in Chapter 5. Using the graphical methods of Rahn and Fenn,[86] one can obtain the values for CO_2 content which correspond to points A_2 and A_3 in Figure 5-4 (p. 85). Rahn and Fenn's diagrams use the classic data for the CO_2 dissociation curve also used in Figures 6-16 and 6-19, i.e., the nomogram of Dill et al.[25] based on in vitro studies of A. V. Bock's blood. The resulting $[CO_2] - P_{CO_2}$ points are plotted in Figure 6-19 (▲). They lie on the CO_2 dissociation curve from which they are derived. The changes between these points, in time, occur along a curve that closely follows the CO_2 dissociation curve. During strenuous hyperventilation, alveolar and arterial P_{CO_2} may decline to 20 mm Hg or even lower (□ in Fig. 6-19). Such values can be obtained, for instance, in relaxed healthy subjects who are hyperventilated in an iron lung.

BREATH HOLDING

The breaking point of breath holding (see also p. 249) after breathing air at sea level commonly occurs when the alveolar P_{CO_2} is about 50 mm Hg. After breathing of oxygen-enriched air, P_{CO_2} may rise to about 65 mm Hg before the breaking point occurs.[86] The corresponding $[CO_2] - P_{CO_2}$ point is shown in Figure 6-19 (■).

EXERCISE

During strenuous exercise, lactic and pyruvic acids are formed in the working muscles as end products of anaerobic glycolysis. These acids are transported by the blood to the liver, where resynthesis of glucose takes place. The bicarbonate system in blood buffers these acids, thus limiting the extent to which pH decreases during heavy exercise. As a result, the CO_2 content of plasma decreases considerably. In principle, P_{CO_2} should not change—if alveolar ventilation increases in proportion to CO_2 production by the tissues (see Fig. 5-4 and its discussion, p. 85). Actually, alveolar ventilation usually increases slightly more than is needed to maintain a constant P_{CO_2} (see p. 250), and hence alveolar and arterial P_{CO_2} often decline a few mm Hg during heavy exercise. Average results of acid-base studies in 11 healthy young men[16] are included in Figure 6-19 ($A \rightarrow B$). During exercise, $[CO_2]$ and pH decrease considerably; P_{CO_2} decreases only 5 mm Hg. In this example of exercise acidosis, $[CO_2]$ decreases 11.5 mmol/liter. A small part of this decrease is due to the decrease of P_{CO_2}; this part can be estimated by drawing a straight line through point B parallel to the CO_2 dissociation curve (*dashed line* in Fig. 6-19). The vertical distance between point A and the dashed line is the amount by which $[CO_2]$ would have decreased if P_{CO_2} had been kept constant, i.e., 10.5 mmol/liter, or 1 mmol/liter less than the actual $[CO_2]$ decrease.

The decrease of $[CO_2]$ at a constant P_{CO_2} is related to the amount of acids other than CO_2 added to the blood. However, since the bicarbonate system is not the only blood buffer system, the decrease of $[CO_2]$ underestimates the actual amount of acids added. In the exercise experiments shown by line AB in Figure

6-19, blood lactic and pyruvic acid concentrations together increased by about 12 mmol/liter, i.e., 1.5 mmol/liter more than the decrease of [CO_2] at constant P_{CO_2}.[16]

HIGH ALTITUDE

When a healthy person is acutely transported from sea level to an altitude of about 20,000 ft (6130 meters), hyperventilation brings his alveolar P_{CO_2} down to about 22 mm Hg (data from Rahn and Fenn;[86] compare also Fig. 10-10, p. 251). Blood [CO_2] decreases according to the CO_2 dissociation curve, and pH increases to 7.50 (point F in Fig. 6-19). Acclimatization to altitude is accompanied by increased hyperventilation (p. 252) and by a considerable decrease in [CO_2], the latter largely through excretion of bicarbonate by the kidneys. An extreme case, based on an observation in an acclimatized man at 23,000 ft (7050 meters) [86] is shown as point G in Fig. 6-19. Acclimatization returns blood pH to a normal value, 7.40; plasma [CO_2] (derived from Dill et al.'s data for high-altitude residents [26]) must have been as low as about 10 mmol/liter.

ACIDOSIS AND ALKALOSIS

The examples discussed in the preceding section show that the acid-base status of healthy persons can vary considerably. Hyperventilation, voluntary or induced by exposure to high altitude, may increase pH to 7.50 or more. All conditions associated with an increase of blood pH beyond the normal range are called alkalosis. Hyperventilation leads to respiratory alkalosis. All points in gray area 1 in Figure 6-19 are associated with respiratory alkalosis (pH $>$ 7.45; $P_{CO_2} < 35$ mm Hg; [CO_2] at values between the two CO_2 dissociation curves). Apart from voluntary hyperventilation and exposure to high altitude, respiratory alkalosis also occurs in anxiety states (hyperventilation syndrome), in pregnancy, perhaps through a stimulating effect of progesterone on ventilatory drive, and in hyperthyroidism.

The points in gray area 2 (Fig. 6-19) are associated with alkalosis (pH $>$ 7.45), normal P_{CO_2} (between 35 and 45 mm Hg), and increased [CO_2]. The increased [CO_2] cannot be explained by a decrease of alveolar ventilation (which would increase P_{CO_2}). It must be due to nonrespiratory causes, e.g., loss of acid by repeated vomiting, or ingestion of large amounts of alkaline salts (e.g., sodium bicarbonate). The commonly used name for this condition is "metabolic alkalosis." However, Comroe's term "nonrespiratory" is preferable;[20] alkalosis induced by vomiting or salt ingestion has little to do with metabolic processes in the tissues.

Conditions associated with a low pH ($<$7.35) are called acidosis. Again, two types exist. Respiratory acidosis (gray area 3 in Fig. 6-19) is caused by insufficient excretion of CO_2 due to a decrease in overall alveolar ventilation (including breath holding) or to pronounced nonuniform distribution of $\dot{V}_A/\dot{Q}$ ratios (p. 87). P_{CO_2} is more than 45 mm Hg; [CO_2] is increased according to the CO_2 dissociation curve of the subject, which lies between the two [CO_2]-P_{CO_2} lines of Figure 6-19. Nonrespiratory acidosis, as during exercise, on the other hand, is a condition of low pH and normal P_{CO_2} (gray area 4 in Fig. 6-19).

Exercise, hyperventilation and breath holding are conditions in which acid-base changes occur in, at most, a few minutes. Respiratory acidosis and alkalosis, and also nonrespiratory acidosis, are seen in their pure form when they develop rapidly. Metabolic alkalosis is rarely, if ever, seen in its pure, uncompensated form—it develops too slowly (e.g., after several days of intensive vomiting).

PROLONGED ACIDOSIS AND ALKALOSIS; COMPENSATION

The acid-base changes during acclimatization to high altitude are a perfect example of what happens when respiratory alkalosis persists and even becomes more severe with time. Bicarbonate excretion via the kidney reduces [CO_2]; the ratio HCO_3^-/P_{CO_2} [see Eq. (5); p. 126] decreases and pH returns toward normal. The HCO_3^- changes compensate for the primary P_{CO_2} change. Line FG (Fig. 6-19) is a compensatory pathway. The condition at point G is a fully compensated respiratory alkalosis (pH = 7.40). Points between F and G represent conditions of partially compensated respiratory alkalosis. However, much confusion can arise because the same point on the diagram can be reached via different pathways and by different mechanisms. For instance, points very close to G might be reached by healthy persons who voluntarily hyperventilate shortly after heavy exercise. Point B indicates their condition immediately (1 to 3 min) after exercise. Voluntary hyperventilation would move the acid-base point to the left, along a CO_2 dissociation curve that corresponds to their lower buffering capacity (*dashed line* through B). Their P_{CO_2} decreases and their pH rapidly returns toward normal values. Hence, when they reach a point near G, they have a combination of acute nonrespiratory acidosis and acute respiratory alkalosis. The same combination could also occur when a healthy person who hyperventilates at altitude develops an added nonrespiratory acidosis by exercise; this person might move his acid-base point within a few minutes along a course similar to that of line FG. Thus, to interpret the conditions and mechanisms that lead to changes in a person's acid-base status, one must know the conditions under which the changes developed, as well as the time course involved. Similar points can be reached (1) rapidly by a combination of respiratory alkalosis and nonrespiratory acidosis, or (2) slowly during development of a compensated respiratory alkalosis. The reason for the similarity is, of course, that the diagram does not tell us whether [CO_2] decreased rapidly due to addition of other acids to blood (exercise) or slowly due to compensatory renal bicarbonate excretion. Confusion about the interpretation of acid-base changes in clinical conditions is often based on failure to understand this basic limitation of any acid-base diagram (see next section).

ACIDOSIS AND ALKALOSIS IN DISEASE

In order for us to explore changes in the relations between [CO_2], P_{CO_2}, and pH in areas of the diagram that have not yet been discussed, some examples of acidosis and alkalosis in disease are illustrated in Figures 6-19 through 6-21.

The first example concerns *acute respiratory acidosis* (points C, D, and E in Fig. 6-19). As other clinical data in this section, these are from Møller's work [73] based on arterial blood sampling, electrometric pH determination, determination of plasma [CO_2] with Van Slyke's manometric method, and calculation of P_{CO_2} from pH and [CO_2] [Eq. (8)]. Point C represents respiratory acidosis in an unconscious man (barbiturate intoxication). During various treatments over a 15-hour period, his condition varied from normal (D) to severe acute respiratory acidosis (E). Since 15 hours is too short for an important contribution of compensatory changes, a line through points C, D, and E is nearly parallel to the CO_2 dissociation curve. The slight deviation may be due to the difference between in vivo and in vitro CO_2 dissociation curves.

Acute respiratory acidosis often accompanies exacerbations of ventilatory insufficiency in patients with chronic airway obstruction (Chap. 12, p. 296). Other conditions that may lead to respiratory acidosis are chest injuries, neurological disease (see Chap. 10), paralysis of respiratory muscles, and intoxication with drugs that depress ventilatory drive (p. 256). Nonrespiratory alkalosis also leads to increases in Pa_{CO_2} (see below). Partial compensation of the acute acidosis is the rule when ventilatory insufficiency develops slowly. Examples of data obtained in patients with chronic airway obstruction are shown in Figure 6-20 (●). When P_{CO_2} is more than 60 mm Hg, the CO_2 content is usually increased too, so that pH is closer to its normal value than in acute respiratory acidosis with the same P_{CO_2}. The course of events in a patient who developed ventilatory insufficiency after surgical removal of one lung[73] is particularly illustrative (Fig. 6-20). After surgery, complications resulted in ventilatory insufficiency (*1*). Oxygen treatment was accompanied by acute retention of CO_2 (arrow to *2*): 100% O_2 often decreases ventilatory drive in patients with lung disease (Chap. 10, p. 257). Five days later (*3*), compensatory bicarbonate retention has increased pH to the normal limit. Respirator treatment leads to short-term removal of CO_2 (*4*), but this did not last long enough to allow a return of [CO_2] toward normal levels. The patient's condition worsened, with alternating CO_2 retention (*4* → *5*) and removal by respirator treatment (*5* → *6*), and with gradually increasing [CO_2] with the final point (*9*) representing severe, partially compensated respiratory acidosis. At that point, pH was 7.29, i.e., $[H^+] = 51$ nmol/liter. Without compensatory bicarbonate retention, $[H^+]$ at the same P_{CO_2} would have been about double (pH = 7.00; $[H^+] = 100$ nmol/liter).

Examples of *nonrespiratory acidosis* and *alkalosis* are shown in Figure 6-21. Since these conditions, in contrast to respiratory acidosis and alkalosis, usually develop in the course of days rather than hours (with the exception of exercise acidosis, Fig. 6-19), some degree of compensation is the rule when the first clinical observations are made. In the case of diabetes (○ in Fig. 6-21), the acidosis is due to accumulation of acetoacetic and β-hydroxybutyric acids in blood. The acidemia is buffered by HCO_3^- ions (see discussion on exercise acidosis, p. 135) and, as a result, [CO_2] declines. Without this buffering process, pH would rapidly decrease to values incompatible with life. In spite of buffering, blood pH decreases to levels sufficient to stimulate the ventilatory drive (Chap. 10, p. 244), so P_{CO_2} decreases. Alveolar hyperventilation is a compensatory process since the decline of P_{CO_2} returns the ratio $[HCO_3^-]/P_{CO_2}$ [see Eq. (5)] in the direction of normal. Hence, pH increases toward normal. The patient whose data[73] are shown in Figure 6-21 (○) was initially in diabetic precoma with severe acidosis. If her P_{CO_2} had remained within normal limits while the acidosis developed, her pH would have decreased along a vertical line to 6.80 at a [CO_2] of about 7 mmol/liter (□ in Fig. 6-21). Further decrease of pH is probably fatal. Compensatory hyperventilation (displacing the acid-base changes in the direction of the lower arrow in Fig. 6-21) helped maintain pH at higher levels, compatible with survival, and allowed [CO_2] to decrease to very low levels. Thus, the compensatory process allows maximum usage of the buffering capacity of the bicarbonate system. During insulin treatment, the acidemia decreased and the com-

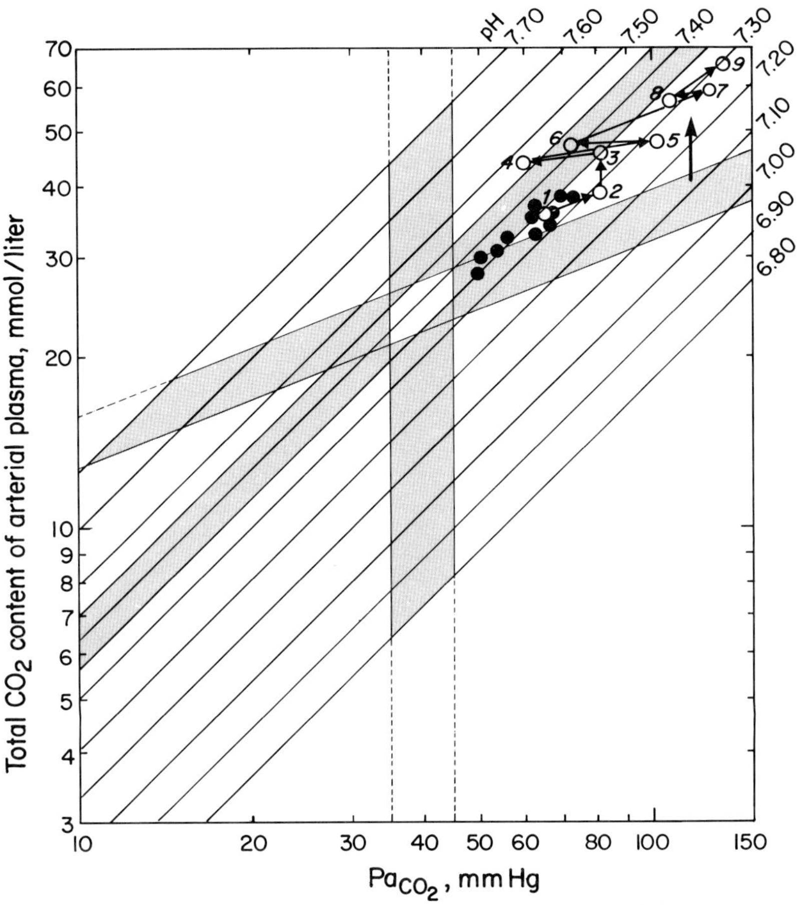

Fig. 6-20. (See legend to Fig. 6-19.) ●: data points for individual patients with various degrees of ventilatory insufficiency owing to chronic lung disease including emphysema (data from Fig. 47 in ref. 73). ○: *1* to *9*, consecutive data points in a patient with increasing ventilatory insufficiency (see text; data from Fig. 42 in ref. 73). Vertical arrow to right of data: direction of compensatory changes in CO_2 content in respiratory acidosis.

pensatory hyperventilation subsided concomitantly. After 7 hours' treatment, a moderate, partially compensated acidosis remained (*4* in Fig. 6-21). Subsequently, all values returned to normal.

The opposite course of events occurs during treatment of metabolic alkalosis (● in Fig. 6-21). The initial status of the patient whose data are shown resulted from severe and frequent vomiting.[73] The loss of H^+ ions through vomiting of the acid contents of the stomach is first buffered by the bicarbonate system, leading to an increased [HCO_3^-] and hence an increased [CO_2] according to Eq. (7) (p. 127). The increased pH results in a decrease of ventilatory drive (Chap. 10, p. 244) and thus in an increase of P_{CO_2}. Without this compensatory change of P_{CO_2} (in the direction of the upper arrow in Fig. 6-21), pH would have increased to 7.70, a dangerously high value; as a result of the partial compensation, pH increased only to 7.55. The compensatory hypoventilation may be severe enough to decrease the arterial P_{O_2}. During treatment

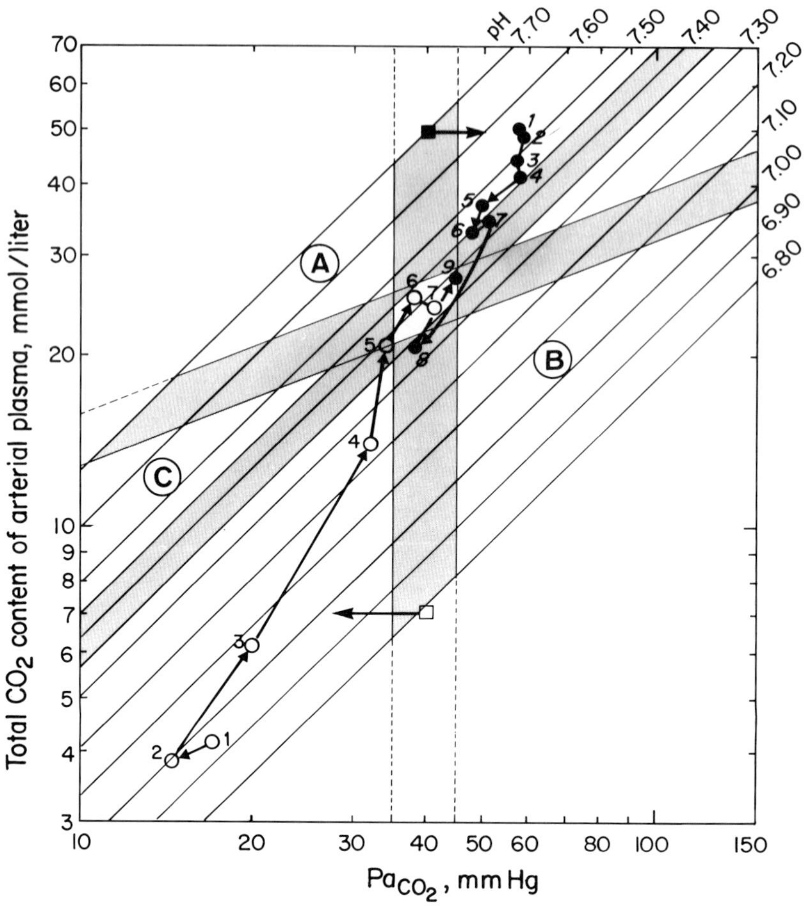

Fig. 6-21. Consecutive data points from a patient with severe diabetic acidosis (○ *1* to *7*) and from a patient with nonrespiratory alkalosis (● *1* to *9*). See text for discussion. Data from Figs. 21 and 63 in ref. 73. Horizontal arrows: direction of compensatory changes in P_{CO_2} in nonrespiratory acidosis (*lower arrow*) and in nonrespiratory alkalosis (*upper arrow*). Areas *A* (combined respiratory and nonrespiratory alkalosis), *B* (combined respiratory and nonrespiratory acidosis), and *C* (respiratory alkalosis with nonrespiratory loss of buffering capacity) are discussed in the text.

all changes reverted to normal. Initially, both $[CO_2]$ and pH decreased toward normal, leading to a state of slight but fully compensated nonrespiratory alkalosis (data point *7* in Fig. 6-21). Next, P_{CO_2} as well as $[CO_2]$ and pH returned to normal.

Three additional areas in the CO_2 — P_{CO_2} diagram are indicated by *A, B,* and *C* in Figure 6-21. Points in *A* represent combinations of respiratory (since P_{CO_2} is low) and nonrespiratory (since $[CO_2]$ is high) alkalosis. Points in *B* represent combinations of respiratory (since P_{CO_2} is high) and nonrespiratory (since $[CO_2]$ is low) acidosis. Experimentally, this condition develops in healthy men who inhale 4 percent CO_2 in air while exercising.[89] Points in *C* may represent (1) partially compensated respiratory alkalosis (see discussion of pathway *FG* in Fig. 6-19, p. 134), or (2) combinations of acute respiratory alkalosis and a degree of nonrespiratory bicarbonate loss (as in nonrespiratory acidosis) insufficient to decrease pH to normal.

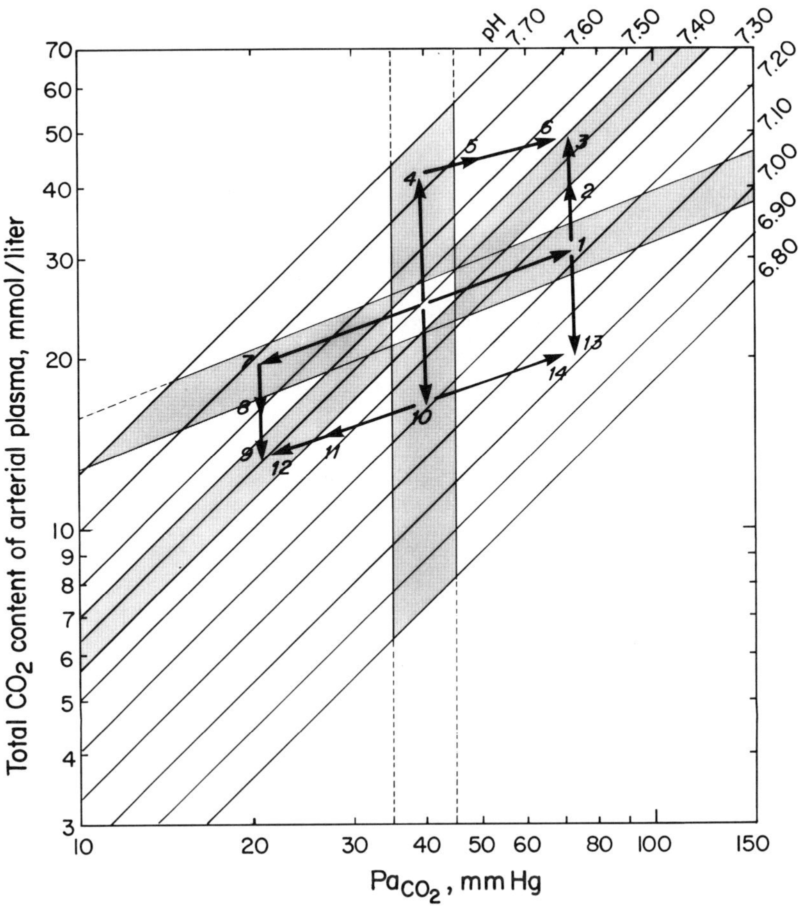

Fig 6-22. Schematic representation of different pathways in acid-base disorders that may lead to similar end results. See text for discussion.

To emphasize again that points plotted on an acid-base diagram need to be interpreted on the basis of knowledge of the sequence of physiological or pathological events that lead to an acid-base disturbance, Figure 6-22 summarizes several possible pathways. Pathway *1-2-3* represents acute respiratory acidosis (*1*) followed by partial (*2*) and full (*3*) compensation. Pathway *4-5-6* represents acute nonrespiratory alkalosis (*4*) followed by partial (*5*) and full (*6*) compensation. Note that both pathways may eventually lead to very similar points (*3* and *6*) on the diagram. However, full compensation of either respiratory or nonrespiratory alkalosis is the exception rather than the rule. But the clinician needs to keep in mind that any point in the upper right quadrant of the diagram might, in principle, result from combinations of respiratory acidosis and nonrespiratory alkalosis. Usually, but not always, the clinical history clarifies which is the primary event. Along the same lines, pathway *7-8-9* indicates acute, partially and fully compensated respiratory alkalosis, and pathway *10-11-12* acute, partially and fully compensated nonrespiratory acidosis. Again, the end results (*9* or *12*) may be similar, but the pathophysiological events different. Combinations of respiratory and nonrespiratory acidosis (in area *B* of the diagram,

Fig. 6-21) may result from either one of these as the primary and the other as a secondary event (pathways *1–13* or *10–14* in Fig. 6-22).

Among acid-base diagrams, the Peters diagram has the advantage of clearly contrasting the direction of changes owing to the most important primary events: excessive excretion or retention of CO_2 in the lungs, and changes in CO_2 content caused by addition of acids other than CO_2 to blood (or their loss). The examples of combined respiratory and nonrespiratory disorders discussed by Schwartz and Relman[94] are easily understood when plotted in the Peters diagram. When the usefulness as well as the limitations of the diagram are understood, there is little need for the additional use of derived values such as standard bicarbonate and base excess (see refs. 23, 94, 96). Standard bicarbonate is the $[HCO_3^-]$ in a sample of blood equilibrated in vitro at $P_{CO_2} = 40$ mm Hg and a high P_{O_2}, so that Hb is saturated. The equilibration moves the acid-base point of the sample, if its original $P_{CO_2} \neq 40$ mm Hg, along a CO_2 dissociation curve (e.g., from *12* to *10* or from *14* to *10* in Fig. 6-22). Thus, a decrease of standard bicarbonate reflects addition of acids other than CO_2 to blood *or* bicarbonate excretion through the kidney. Base excess and deficit express changes in total buffer anion concentrations in blood (including protein and phosphate buffer anions). Base excess or deficit can be calculated from nomograms.[23, 96] A base excess occurs when total base anions increase (through ingestion of base or retention of bicarbonate by the kidney); a base deficit occurs under the conditions just described for a decrease in standard bicarbonate.

Neither standard bicarbonate (SB) nor base excess (+BE) or deficit (−BE) values offer much additional help to the clinician who needs to find out how an abnormal acid-base status in a patient has developed. Understanding the various pathways in the Peters diagram can help to indicate which mechanisms may be involved. As quantitative guidelines, neither SB and BE nor the Peters diagram (nor other acid-base diagrams) are accurate enough, largely because they ignore the complexities of in vivo buffering processes (p. 130). Neither SB nor BE gives an accurate indication of the amounts of acid or base added to or lost from blood in vivo. For both lactic acidemia of exercise [16] and other forms of organic-acid acidemia [12] there is evidence that SB and BE values are inaccurate as quantitative indices of acidemia.

In diagnosis and treatment of acid-base disorders, the physician should avoid using any single set of measured or derived values on acid-base status as magic numbers. Plotting a sequence of observations in a Peters diagram may be of help. Together with all relevant clinical information, one may then be able to find out which is the most likely train of pathophysiological events that led to the patient's condition. This understanding is crucial for rational treatment. In the management of patients with acid-base disorders, who are often critically ill, the implications of acidosis and alkalosis for oxygen transport (see p. 117 and Fig. 6-10, p. 118) should also be taken into account.

SUMMARY

Oxygen diffuses from alveolar air, via the alveolocapillary diffusion barrier, to red cells in lung capillaries. In the red cells, oxygen is bound to hemoglobin and transported to tissues. The overall diffusion characteristics of the alveolo-capillary interface can be assessed by measuring the diffusion capacity (D_L) using a single-breath, rebreathing, or steady-state method with CO in the inspired gas mixture. D_{LCO} depends on $\dot{V}_A/\dot{Q}$ distribution as well as on diffusion through the interface; a low D_{LCO} value often primarily reflects nonuniform ventilation-perfusion relations and is an early sign of certain lung diseases.

The binding of O_2 to hemoglobin involves successive binding of O_2 to Fe atoms in the four heme groups in Hb. Heme-heme interaction and the Bohr effect alter the affinity of Hb for O_2 during the binding process and promote O_2 unloading in the tissues. Organic phosphates in the red cell (primarily 2,3-DPG) also alter the O_2 affinity of Hb and may regulate O_2 binding. Myoglobin, fetal Hb, and Hb variants have O_2 affinities that differ from those of adult Hb (HbA). Through compensatory changes in O_2 capacity, O_2 transport may proceed normally in persons with high or low affinity Hb variants.

Significant tissue hypoxia probably occurs when the capillary P_{O_2} decreases below about 20 mm Hg. Facilitation of diffusion is of minor importance in vivo. In disease, the arterial as well as the venous P_{O_2} need to be taken into account when assessing tissue oxygenation. Moderate arterial hypoxemia can lead to tissue hypoxia when cardiac output is low and the arteriovenous oxygen content difference is large. Arterial hypoxemia in lung disease usually results from overall hypoventilation or nonuniform $\dot{V}_A/\dot{Q}$ ratios, or both. Alteration of O_2 transport in anemia, CO poisoning, alkalosis and acidosis, and following massive blood transfusion results in part from changes in the Hb-O_2 dissociation curve. These changes can be assessed by measuring P50 (the P_{O_2} required for 50 percent oxygenation of Hb) and the blood's O_2 capacity. To evaluate oxygen therapy and other modes of treatment in respiratory failure, one should consider all factors that result in tissue hypoxia rather than arterial P_{O_2} measurements alone.

Carbon dioxide is transported from tissues to the lungs (1) in solution in plasma and red cells, (2) as bicarbonate in plasma and red cells, and (3) bound to hemoglobin in a carbamino compound. Rapid exchange of CO_2 in tissue and lung capillaries is promoted by carbonic anhydrase in red cells and by the chloride shift. Most CO_2 is transported as bicarbonate. H^+ ions released by dissociation of H_2CO_3 are mainly buffered by hemoglobin; in turn, the CO_2—HCO_3^- system is an important buffer for H^+ ions released by acids other than CO_2. The relations among [H^+] or pH, Pa_{CO_2}, total CO_2 content, and bicarbonate content of plasma are given by various forms of the Henderson-Hasselbalch equation. In vivo these relations are affected by dilution of bicarbonate in extracellular fluid and by tissue buffering. Hence, in vivo CO_2 dissociation curves ([CO_2] versus P_{CO_2}) differ from in vitro CO_2 dissociation curves. Since the body contains tissues with varying CO_2 storage capacities and CO_2 exchange rates, the in vivo CO_2 dissociation curve depends on the time allowed for equilibration at any given P_{CO_2}—the longer, the higher the total body CO_2 content. Exchange of CO_2 in the lungs depends on total alveolar ventilation and on the distribution of ventilation-perfusion ratios (see also Chap. 5). Experimental findings of higher alveolar than arterial P_{CO_2} are probably best explained by delayed equilibration between red cells and plasma, leading to a lower arterial P_{CO_2} than occurs at the end of the gas exchanging lung capillaries.

The relations among Pa_{CO_2}, pH, and plasma CO_2 content can be used to assess changes in acid-base status induced by hyper- or hypoventilation (respiratory alkalosis; respiratory acidosis) or by addition to or loss of acid from blood (non-respiratory acidosis or alkalosis), as well as by combinations of these disorders. The interpretation of acid-base status in these diagrams requires knowledge of the type and time course of physiological or pathological events that have led to the acid-base disorder.

REFERENCES

1. Arndt H, King TKC, Briscoe WA: Diffusing capacities and ventilation: perfusion ratios in patients with the clinical syndrome of alveolar capillary block. J. Clin Invest 49:408–422, 1970
2. Arnone A: X-ray studies of the interaction of CO_2 with human deoxyhaemoglobin. Nature 247:143–145, 1974
3. Asakura T, Sato Y, Minakami S, Yoshikawa H: Effect of deoxygenation of intracellular hemoglobin on red cell glycolysis. J Biochem (Tokyo) 59:524–526, 1966
4. Åstrand I, Åstrand P-O, Christensen EH, Hedman R: Myohemoglobin as an oxygen-store in man. Acta Physiol Scand 48:454–460, 1960
5. Barcroft J: The Respiratory Function of the Blood. Part II, Haemoglobin. London, Cambridge University Press, 1928
6. Bauer C: Antagonistic influence of CO_2 and 2,3 diphosphoglycerate on the Bohr effect of human haemoglobin. Life Sci 8(II):1041–1046, 1969
7. Bauer C: On the respiratory function of haemoglobin. Rev Physiol Biochem Pharmacol 70:1–31, 1974
8. Bellingham AJ, Detter JC, Lenfant C: The role of hemoglobin affinity for oxygen and red cell 2,3-diphosphoglycerate in the management of diabetic ketoacidosis. Trans Assoc Am Physicians 83:113–120, 1970
9. Benesch R, Benesch RE: Intracellular organic phosphates as regulators of oxygen release by haemoglobin. Nature 221:618–622, 1969
10. Benesch RE, Benesch R, Renthal R, Gratzer WB: Cofactor binding and oxygen equilibria in haemoglobin. Nature [New Biol] 234:174–176, 1971
11. Bettice JA, Gamble JL Jr: Skeletal buffering of acute metabolic acidosis. Am J Physiol 229:1618–1624, 1975
12. Biervliet JP van, Stekelenburg GJ van, Duran M, Wadman SK: Letter to the editor: Base excess and organic acidaemia. Lancet 2:1518–1519, 1974
13. Bjure, J, Söderholm B: "Pulmonary diffusing capacity"—a critical review of its value as a lung function test. Scand J Clin Lab Invest 22:167–170, 1968
14. Bordiuk JM, McKenna PJ, Giannelli S Jr, Ayres SM: Alterations in 2–3 diphosphoglycerate and O_2 hemoglobin affinity in patients undergoing open heart surgery. Circulation 43 (suppl 1):141–146, 1971
15. Bouhuys A, Georg J, Jönsson R, Lundin G, Lindell S-E: The influence of histamine inhalation on the pulmonary diffusing capacity in man. J Physiol (Lond) 152:176–181, 1960
16. Bouhuys A, Pool J, Binkhorst RA, van Leeuwen P: Metabolic acidosis of exercise in healthy males. J Appl Physiol 21:1040–1046, 1966
17. Brewer GJ, Eaton JW: Erythrocyte metabolism: interaction with oxygen transport. Science 171:1205–1211, 1971

17a. Cain SM, Otis AB: Carbon dioxide transport in anesthetized dogs during inhibition of carbonic anhydrase. J Appl Physiol 16:1023–1028, 1961

18. Cerretelli P, Cruz JC, Farhi LE, Rahn H: Determination of mixed venous O_2 and CO_2 tensions and cardiac output by a rebreathing method. Respir Physiol 1:258–264, 1966
19. Cherniack NS, Longobardo GS: Oxygen and carbon dioxide gas stores of the body. Physiol Rev 50:196–243, 1970
20. Comroe JH Jr: Physiology of Respiration, ed 2. Chicago, Year Book Medical Publishers, 1974
21. Cotes JE: Lung Function; Assessment and Application in Medicine, ed 2. Oxford and Edinburgh, Blackwell Scientific Publications, 1968

22. Cotes JE, Hall AM: The transfer factor for the lung; normal values in adults, in Arcangeli P (ed): Introduction to the Definition on Normal Values for Respiratory Function in Man. Alghero, Panminerva Medica, 1970, pp 327–343
23. Davenport HW: The ABC of Acid-Base Chemistry, ed 6. Chicago, University of Chicago Press, 1974
24. DeGraff AC Jr, Grover RF, Johnson RL Jr, Hammond JW Jr, Miller JM: Diffusing capacity of the lung in Caucasians native to 3,100 m. J Appl Physiol 29:71–76, 1970
25. Dill DB, Edwards HT, Consolazio WV: Blood as a physicochemical system. XI. Man at rest. J. Biol Chem 118: 635–648, 1937
26. Dill DB, Talbott JH, Consolazio WV: Blood as a physicochemical system. XII. Man at high altitudes. J Biol Chem 118:649–666, 1937
27. Duc G, Engel K: A method for determination of oxyhemoglobin dissociation curves at constant temperature, pH and pCO_2. Respir Physiol 8:118–126, 1969
28. Eaton JW, Skelton TD, Berger E: Survival at extreme altitude: protective effect of increased hemoglobin-oxygen affinity. Science 183:743–744, 1974
29. Evans JW, Wagner PD, West JB: Conditions for reduction of pulmonary gas transfer by ventilation-perfusion inequality. J Appl Physiol 36:533–537, 1974
30. Fenn WO: Partial molar volumes of oxygen and carbon monoxide in blood. Respir Physiol 13:129–140, 1971
31. Ferguson JKW: Carbamino compounds of CO_2 with human haemoglobin and their role in the transport of CO_2. J Physiol (Lond) 88:40–55, 1936
32. Filley GF, MacIntosh DJ, Wright GW: CO uptake and pulmonary diffusing capacity in normal subjects at rest and during exercise. J Clin Invest 33: 530–539, 1954
33. Finch CA, Lenfant C: Oxygen transport in man. N Engl J Med 286:407-415, 1972
34. Finley TN, Swenson EW, Comroe JH Jr: The cause of arterial hypoxemia at rest in patients with "alveolar-capillary block syndrome." J Clin Invest 41:618–622, 1962
35. Flenley DC, Miller HC, King AJ, Kirby BJ, Muir AL: Oxygen transport in acute pulmonary oedema and in acute exacerbations of chronic bronchitis. Br Med J 1:78–81, 1973
36. Forster RE: Carbon monoxide and the partial pressure of oxygen in tissue. Ann N Y Acad Sci 174:233–241, 1970
37. Forster RE: Diffusion of gases, in Fenn WO, Rahn H (eds): Handbook of Physiology, Section 3: Respiration, vol I. Washington, D.C., American Physiological Society, 1964, pp 839–872
38. Forster RE: Exchange of gases between alveolar air and pulmonary capillary blood: pulmonary diffusing capacity. Physiol Rev 37:391–452, 1957
39. Forster RE: Interpretation of measurements of pulmonary diffusing capacity, in Fenn WO, Rahn H (eds): Handbook of Physiology, Section 3: Respiration, vol II. Washington, D.C., American Physiological Society, 1965, pp 1453–1468
40. Forster RE, Crandall ED: Time course of exchanges between red cells and extracellular fluid during CO_2 uptake. J Appl Physiol 38:710–718, 1975
41. Forster RE, Edsall JT, Otis AB, Roughton FJW (eds): CO_2: Chemical, Biochemical, and Physiological Aspects. NASA SP-188, Washington, D.C., Office of Technology Utilization, National Aeronautics and Space Administration, 1969
42. Glazier JB, Hughes JMB, Maloney JE, West JB: Measurements of capillary dimensions and blood volume in rapidly frozen lungs. J Appl Physiol 26:65–76, 1969
43. Goldstein MB, Gennari FJ, Schwartz WB: The influence of graded degrees of chronic hypercapnia on the acute carbon dioxide titration curve. J Clin Invest 50:208–216, 1971
44. Gurtner GH, Fowler WS: Interrelationships of factors affecting pulmonary diffusing capacity. J Appl Physiol 30: 619–624, 1971
45. Guyatt AR, Yu CJ, Lutherer B, Otis AB: Studies of alveolar-mixed venous CO_2 and O_2 gradients in the rebreathing dog lung. Respir Physiol 17:178–194, 1973
46. Hatzfeld C, Wiener F, Briscoe WA: Effect of uneven ventilation-diffusion

ratios on pulmonary diffusing capacity in disease. J Appl Physiol 23:1–10, 1967

47. Henderson LJ: Blood: A Study in General Physiology. New Haven, Yale University Press, 1928
48. Hill EP, Power GG, Longo LD: Mathematical simulation of pulmonary O_2 and CO_2 exchange. Am J Physiol 224:904–917, 1973
49. Hyde RW: Influence of carbonic anhydrase activity on the exchange of CO_2 across the alveolar-capillary membrane, in Forster et al. (eds) (see ref. 41), pp 261–265
50. Jennings DB, Chen CC: Negative arterial-mixed expired P_{CO_2} gradient during acute and chronic hypercapnia. J Appl Physiol 38:382–388, 1975
51. Jöbsis FF: Basic processes in cellular respiration, in Fenn WO, Rahn H (eds): Handbook of Physiology, Section 3: Respiration, vol I. Washington, D.C., American Physiological Society, 1964, pp 63–124
52. Johnson RL Jr, Taylor HF, DeGraff AC Jr: Functional significance of a low pulmonary diffusing capacity for carbon monoxide. J Clin Invest 44: 789–800, 1965
53. Jones NL, Campbell EJM, Edwards RHT, Wilkoff WG: Alveolar-to-blood P_{CO_2} difference during rebreathing in exercise. J Appl Physiol 27:356–360, 1969
54. Kannan KK, Notstrand B, Fridborg K, Lövgren S, Ohlsson A, Petef M: Crystal structure of human erythrocyte carbonic anhydrase B: Three-dimensional structure at a nominal 2.2-Å resolution. Proc Natl Acad Sci USA 72:51–55, 1975
55. Kelman GR, Nunn JF: Computer Produced Physiological Tables, for Calculations Involving the Relationship Between Blood Oxygen Tension and Content. New York, Appleton-Century-Crofts, 1968
56. Kilmartin JV, Rossi-Bernardi L: Interaction of hemoglobin with hydrogen ion, carbon dioxide, and organic phosphates. Physiol Rev 53:836–890, 1973
57. Kreuzer F: Facilitated diffusion of oxygen and its possible significance; A review. Respir Physiol 9:1–30, 1970
58. Kreuzer F, van Lookeren Campagne P: Resting pulmonary diffusing capacity for CO and O_2 at high altitude. J Appl Physiol 20:519–524, 1965
59. Kruhøffer P: Studies on the lung diffusion coefficient for carbon monoxide in normal human subjects by means of $C^{14}O$. Acta Physiol Scand 32:106-123, 1954
60. Kutchai H: O_2 uptake by 100 mu layers of hemoglobin solution: theory vs. experiment. Respir Physiol 11: 378–383, 1971
61. Lawson WH Jr: Rebreathing measurements of pulmonary diffusing capacity for CO during exercise. J Appl Physiol 29:896–900, 1970
62. Lawson WH Jr, Johnson RL Jr: Gas chromatography in measuring pulmonary blood flow and diffusing capacity. J Appl Physiol 17:143–147, 1962
63. Lenfant C, Sullivan K: Adaptation to high altitude. N Engl J Med 284: 1298–1309, 1971
64. Lenfant C, Torrance J, English E, Finch CA, Reynafarje C, Ramos J, Faura J: Effect of altitude on oxygen binding by hemoglobin and on organic phosphate levels. J Clin Invest 47:2652–2656, 1968
65. Lenfant C, Ways P, Aucutt C, Cruz J: Effect of chronic hypoxic hypoxia on the O_2-Hb dissociation curve and respiratory gas transport in man. Respir Physiol 7:7–29, 1969
66. Lewis BM, Lin T-H, Noe FE, Hayford-Welsing EJ: The measurement of pulmonary diffusing capacity for carbon monoxide by a rebreathing method. J Clin Invest 38:2073–2086, 1959
67. Liljas A, Kannan KK, Bergstén PC, Fridborg K, Järup L, Lövgren S, Paradies H, Strandberg B, Waara I: X-ray diffraction studies on the structure of carbonic anhydrase, in Forster et al. (eds) (see ref. 41), pp 89–98
68. Maren TH: Carbonic anhydrase: chemistry, physiology, and inhibition. Physiol Rev 47:595–781, 1967
69. Maren TH, Rayburn CS, Liddell NE: Inhibition by anions of human red cell carbonic anhydrase B: physiological and biochemical implications. Science 191:469–472, 1976
70. Michel CC: The transport of oxygen and carbon dioxide by the blood, in Widdicombe JG (ed): Respiratory Physiology (MTP Internat Rev Sci) (Physiology, series 1, vol 2). London,

Butterworths, and Lancaster, Lancs., Medical & Technical Publishing Co., 1974, pp 67–104

71. Miller JM, Johnson RL Jr: Effect of lung inflation on pulmonary diffusing capacity at rest and exercise. J Clin Invest 45:493–500, 1966
72. Moll W: Oxygen supply of the human fetus. Bull Physiopathol Respir (Nancy) 9:1345–1364, 1973
73. Møller B: The Hydrogen Concentration in Arterial Blood. A Clinical Study of Patients with Diabetes Mellitus and Diseases of the Kidneys, Lungs, and Heart. Aarhus, Universitetsforlag, 1959
74. Morimoto H, Lehman H, Perutz MF: Molecular pathology of human haemoglobin: stereochemical interpretation of abnormal oxygen affinities. Nature 232: 408–413, 1971
75. Olszowka AJ, Rahn H, Farhi LE: Blood Gases: Hemoglobin, Base Excess, and Maldistribution. Philadelphia, Lea & Febiger, 1973
76. Parer JT: Oxygen transport in human subjects with hemoglobin variants having altered oxygen affinity. Respir Physiol 9:43–49, 1970
77. Pascual RS, Mosher MB, Sikand RS, DeConti RC, Bouhuys A: Effect of bleomycin on pulmonary function in man. Am Rev Respir Dis 108:211–217, 1973
78. Paton JB, Peterson E, Fisher DE, Behrmann RE: Oxygen dissociation curves of fetal and adult baboons. Respir Physiol 12:283–290, 1971
79. Perrella M, Kilmartin JV, Fogg J, Rossi-Bernardi L: Identification of the high and low affinity CO_2-binding sites of human haemoglobin. Nature 256:759–761, 1975
80. Perutz MF: Haemoglobin: The molecular lung. New Sci and Sci J 50: 676–679, 1971
81. Perutz MF: Haemoglobin: Genetic abnormalities. New Sci and Sci J 50: 762–765, 1971
82. Perutz MF: Stereochemistry of cooperative effects of hemoglobin. Nature 228:726–739, 1970
83. Peters JP: Studies of the carbon dioxide absorption curve of human blood. III. A further discussion of the form of the absorption curve plotted logarithmically, with a convenient type of interpolation chart. J Biol Chem 56:745–750, 1923
84. Peters JP, Van Slyke DD: Quantitative Clinical Chemistry, vol 2: Methods. Baltimore, Williams & Wilkins, 1932
85. Piiper J: Rates of chloride-bicarbonate exchange between red cells and plasma, in Forster et al. (eds) (see ref. 41), pp 267–273
86. Rahn H, Fenn WO: A Graphical Analysis of the Respiratory Gas Exchange; the O_2-CO_2 Diagram. Washington, D.C., American Physiological Society, 1955
87. Reichart E, Claudon F, Sablière S: Le stockage carbonique dans divers organes au cours de l'hypercapnie chronique expérimentale. Bull Eur Physiopathol Respir 12:19–32, 1976
88. Remmers JE, Mithoeffer JC: The carbon monoxide diffusing capacity in permanent residents at high altitudes. Respir Physiol 6:233–244, 1969
89. Rizzo A, Gimenez M, Horsky P, Saunier C: Influence d'une atmosphère de CO_2 à 4% sur le comportement métabolique à l'exercice d'hommes jeunes. Bull Eur Physiopathol Respir 12:209–219, 1976
90. Roughton FJW: Recent work on carbon dioxide transport by the blood. Physiol Rev 15:241–296, 1935
91. Roughton FJW: Transport of oxygen and carbon dioxide, in Fenn WO, Rahn H (eds): Handbook of Physiology, Section 3: Respiration, vol I. Washington, D.C., American Physiological Society, 1964, pp 767–825
92. Roughton FJW, Forster RE: Relative importance of diffusion and chemical reaction rates in determining rate of exchange of gas in the human lung, with special reference to true diffusion capacity of pulmonary membrane and volume of blood in the lung capillaries. J Appl Physiol 11:290–302, 1957
93. St. Helen R, Roughton FJW, Fatt I: Polarographic studies of oxygen-hemoglobin equilibria at very low saturations. J Appl Physiol 30:575–579, 1971
94. Schwartz WB, Relman AS: A critique of the parameters used in the evaluation of acid-base disorders. N Engl J Med 268:1382–1388, 1963
95. Severinghaus JW: Blood gas concentrations, in Fenn WO, Rahn H (eds):

Handbook of Physiology, Section 3: Respiration, vol II. Washington, D.C., American Physiological Society, 1965, pp 1475–1487
96. Siggaard-Andersen O: The acid-base status of the blood. Scand J Clin Lab Invest 15 (suppl 70):1–134, 1963
97. Sirs JA: The kinetics of the reaction of carbon monoxide with fully oxygenated haemoglobin in solution and erythrocytes. J Physiol (Lond) 236:387–401, 1974
98. Stamatoyannopoulos G, Bellingham AJ, Lenfant C, Finch CA: Abnormal hemoglobins with high and low oxygen affinity. Annu Rev Med 22:221–234, 1971
99. Tenney SM, Lamb TW: Physiological consequences of hypoventilation and hyperventilation, in Fenn WO, Rahn H (eds): Handbook of Physiology, Section 3: Respiration, vol II. Washington, D.C., American Physiological Society, 1965, pp 979–1010
100. Torrance JD, Lenfant C: Methods for determination of O_2 dissociation curves, including Bohr effect. Respir Physiol 8:127–136, 1969
101. Tribukait B: Experimentelle Untersuchungen zur Regulation der Erythropoiese unter besonderer Berücksichtigung der Bedeutung des Sauerstoffs. Acta Physiol Scand 58 (suppl 208): 1–47, 1963
102. Weibel ER: Morphological basis of alveolar-capillary gas exchange. Physiol Rev 53:419–495, 1973
103. West JB: Causes of carbon dioxide retention in lung disease. N Engl J Med 284:1232–1236, 1971
104. Woolley P: Models for metal ion function in carbonic anhydrase. Nature 258:671–682, 1975
105. Zierler KL: Diffusion of gases in peripheral tissue, in: Physiology in the Space Environment, vol II, Respiration. Washington, D.C., National Academy of Sciences, National Research Council, 1967, pp 79–86

Chapter 7

Pressure-Volume Relations

During breathing, the lungs inflate and deflate cyclically. The movements of the lungs and chest cage result from the force of respiratory muscles and the elastic properties of the structures themselves. In the chest cage, forces are generated actively by muscle contraction and passively by chest cage elastic recoil. The special properties of the pleural space allow transmission of these forces from the chest cage to the lungs. The forces applied by the chest cage are spent in overcoming opposing forces—chest and lung elastic recoil and airway resistance—in the lungs as well as in the chest cage. The interaction between applied and opposing forces causes pressures within the lungs and pleural space to deviate from atmospheric pressure. To understand lung and chest cage elastic recoil and the generation of pleural and alveolar pressures, pressure-volume diagrams of the lungs and chest are indispensable. The pressure-volume relations are also used to describe the maximum pressures that the respiratory muscles can generate, the work of breathing, and the factors that limit inspiratory and expiratory volume excursions. We shall consider first only conditions where airflow is zero or minimal, and, hence, where resistive and inertial forces are negligible. Airflow is introduced as an additional variable in Chapter 8; this chapter concentrates on the properties of the breathing pump, and Chapter 8 focuses on those of the airways, the complex plumbing system connected to the pump.

MOVEMENTS OF LUNGS AND CHEST

The lungs are enclosed by the rib cage, the soft tissues of the neck, and the diaphragm. These form the chest cage, which is expanded by the action of the diaphragm, the external intercostal muscles, and certain accessory muscles. The abdominal contents and wall are also displaced during breathing. Thus, the term chest wall, commonly used in lung mechanics, is an anatomical and physiological abstraction; the chest wall's properties are determined by all structures outside the lungs that move during breathing.

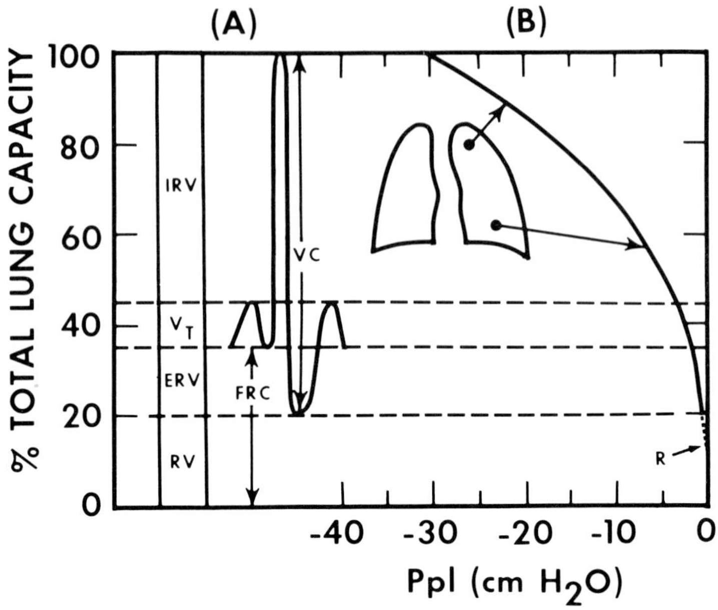

Fig. 7-1. *A.* Subdivisions of the total lung capacity (TLC). *Abscissa.* Time. IRV = inspiratory reserve volume; V_T = tidal volume; ERV = expiratory reserve volume; RV = residual volume; IC = inspiratory capacity; FRC = functional residual capacity; VC = vital capacity. The spirographical curve shows two tidal breaths and a VC maneuver. *B.* Static pressure-volume or static recoil curve. *Abscissa.* Pleural pressure (cm H_2O). R = resting position of the lungs in healthy young persons (zero recoil force). In older persons and in particular in obstructive airway diseases, R increases (see discussion on airway closure, p. 63). Diagram of vertical lungs shows that areas in the lung top operate at higher volume than areas in bottom lung zones; the former have a lower compliance than the latter because of the curvature of the recoil curve (see also Chap. 4).

The lungs and chest always move together in healthy persons (see next section). During quiet breathing, the tidal volume (V_T) is a small fraction of the maximal volume excursion (the vital capacity, VC; Fig. 7-1). At the point of maximum expiration, the lungs still contain air (residual volume, RV), and further collapse can occur only when the chest is opened. The lungs then assume their resting volume (R in Fig. 7-1).

When excised lungs are inflated with air through the trachea, all linear dimensions increase by the same fraction; the lungs behave isotropically.[68] The lungs within the chest cage, however, can assume different shapes at the same volume. Thus, the configuration of lungs in situ depends not only on their volume, but also on the shape of the chest cage.[49] If lung volume is kept constant by closing the glottis, different configurations of chest and abdomen (and thus indirectly of the lungs) can be produced—first by expanding the chest and retracting the abdominal wall, and next by drawing in the chest and expanding the abdomen.

Role of the Pleural Space

The chest cage and the lungs are each covered with a pleural membrane that allows the lungs to move, to some extent, independently from the chest wall. Con-

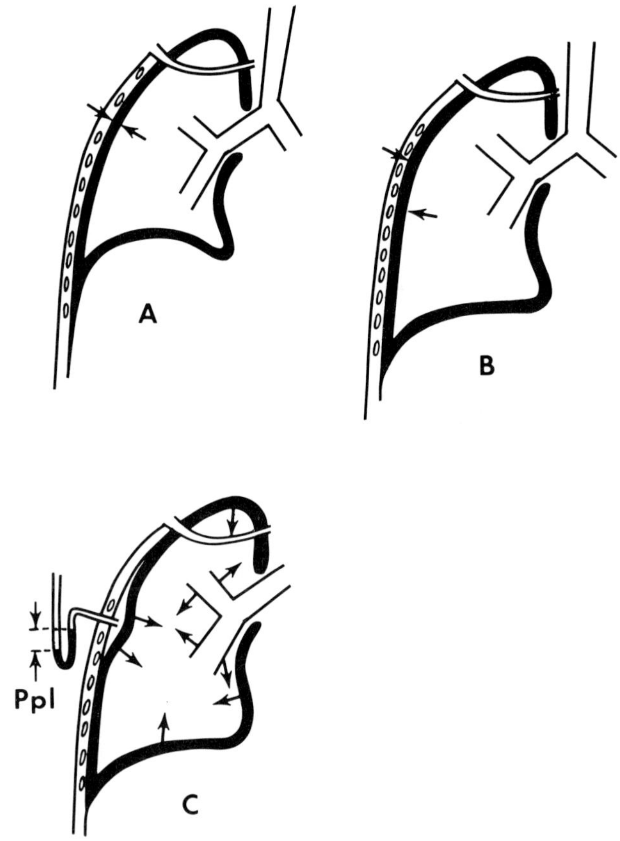

Fig. 7-2. Diagram of airways, lungs, pleural space (*black zone*), and rib cage. Points on the pleural membrane's two layers, which are in apposition (*arrows* in *A*), move apart when the lung expands in *B*. The retractile or recoil force (*arrows* in *C*) results in a distending force exerted on the airways and in subatmospheric (negative) pleural pressure.

sequently, when the lungs increase in volume, points that are in apposition near maximum expiration move apart (Fig. 7-2*A* and *B*). This enables the lungs to enlarge downward in response to contraction of the diaphragm. The pleural space contains no gas and only a minimal amount of liquid (about 2 ml) dispersed over a large surface area. Since the sum of the partial pressures of the gases in venous and even arterial blood is less than atmospheric,[27] any gas in the pleural space is absorbed into the blood. Also, any additional liquid is absorbed because capillary oncotic pressures in the pleura are low.[1] Therefore, the space between the pleural membrane is narrow (5–10 μm in cats[2]), and the lungs remain in close contact with the chest wall. This enables forces to be transmitted from the chest to the lungs and causes the lungs to follow all volume changes of the chest cage.

Viscoelastic Behavior of the Lungs

The lungs are elastic: they expand when stresses are applied and recoil passively when stresses are released. Lung tissue also has viscous properties: it responds to applied stress with some delay in deformation. Thus, the lungs are a viscoelastic, rather than a purely elastic, organ. The physical properties of such bodies are complex;[15, 68] a guide to terminology and definitions is available.[50]

Elastic recoil. The tensile strength of lung tissue is probably provided by strong, collagenic connective tissue fibers.[64] Although the extensibility of lung tissue is often attributed to the presence of elastic fibers, their close association with collagen fibers limits the extent to which the elastic fibers can be stretched. The recoil properties of the lungs as a whole relate less to the properties of the single fibers than to the arrangement of collagen and elastic fibers in a network (Fig. 7-3). When the lung tissue is stretched, the helical fiber network around alveoli and alveolar ducts uncoils.[65] Under the electron microscope, the alveolar surface is smooth and flat, regardless of lung volume.[32] The alveolar wall, therefore, distends and retracts without folding; it appears to have inherent elastic properties.[33, 72] The alveolar surface film (Chap. 1) also contributes considerably to the lung's elastic recoil, at higher lung volumes providing the major portion of the recoil force.[7]

Hysteresis. This term refers to "the failure of a system to follow identical paths of response upon application of and withdrawal of a forcing agent."[50] In air-filled excised lungs, pressure-volume curves during inflation and deflation differ markedly (Fig. 7-4). To a large extent, lung hysteresis is a function of the alveolar

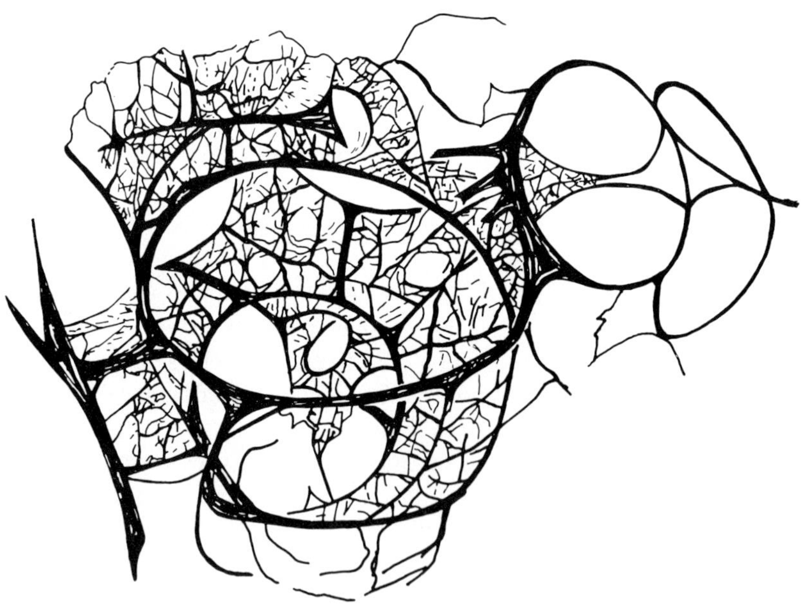

Fig. 7-3. Elastic fiber network arranged in a helical form around an alveolar duct and its alveoli. From reference 65.

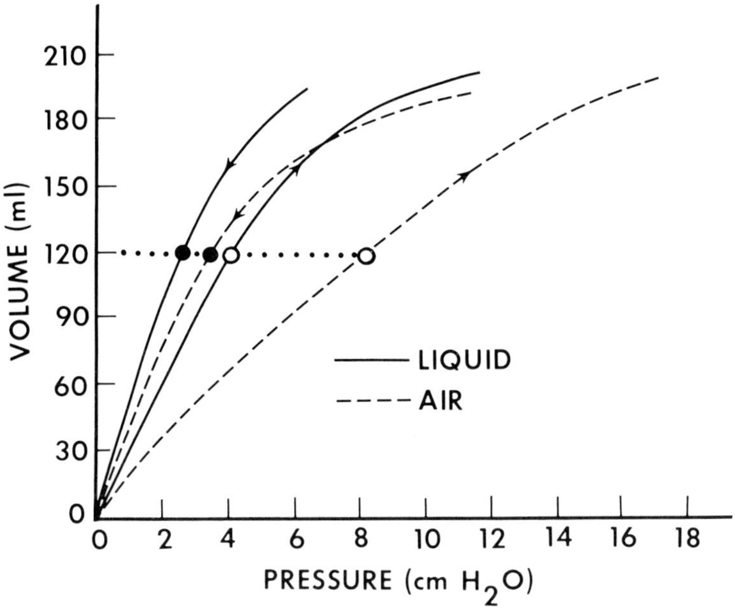

Fig. 7-4. Pressure-volume curves of cat lungs in situ inflated with liquid (Ringer-Locke solution) or air and subsequently deflated. The surface area between the inflation and deflation curves is greater for air than for liquid, reflecting the contribution of the air-liquid interface to hysteresis. Redrawn from reference 31.

surface film—hysteresis decreases when the lungs are filled with saline and the air-liquid interface is abolished. During quiet breathing, this may account for about ⅞ of the hysteresis of excised lungs.[39] How much the surface film contributes to hysteresis depends on lung volume and the direction of volume change. During inflation, the air-filled lung requires a much larger pressure than the liquid-filled lung; during deflation the difference is less (Fig. 7-4). The molecular mechanisms underlying hysteresis of film and of tissue may be similar.[39] Under some circumstances, smooth muscle contraction may also contribute to hysteresis.[17, 22] Lung tissues in man and in several mammals have similar hysteresis characteristics;[6] hence, basic mechanical properties of lung tissue appear to be independent of species variations. Another consequence of viscoelasticity is *stress relaxation.* When inflated lungs are held at constant volume, the distending pressure decreases with time, which may reflect realignment of tissue fibers and reorientation of the surface film.[39] Conversely, when pressure is constant, lung volume increases slightly with time (*creep* of lung tissue[75]). Opening of previously collapsed alveoli may contribute to stress relaxation and creep.

The difference between deflation and inflation pressure-volume curves in man is consistent with hysteresis-like behavior.[55] Similar characteristics of hysteresis have been found in tissue strips from persons with normal lungs and patients with lung diseases.[72] However, this study did not include tissue from lungs with extensive fibrosis.

Distribution of stress. Isolated strips of tissue, cut in different directions from a lung, are equally distensible.[33, 68, 72] In intact lungs, however, stress is not equally distributed and hence distension is not uniform.[77] In vertical lungs, stress increases downward and laterally, in part because of the force of gravity.[76] As a result, alveoli in the lung tops are more distended than alveoli in dependent zones (Fig. 7-1*B*; Chap. 4). Even during quiet breathing, alveoli near the lung tops may breathe near their maximum volumes. They are stressed considerably in normal conditions, which may explain the predilection of the lung tops for developing emphysema and large tuberculous cavities.[76]

If the lungs and all structures in it (airways, blood vessels) were homogeneous and the lungs were not distorted by the force of gravity, (1) all parts would expand isotropically (Chap. 1); (2) pleural surface pressure would be uniform; and (3) stress (force per unit area, or pressure) would be equal to pleural pressure at all boundaries within this ideal lung. Thus, airways and blood vessels would be subjected to exactly the same distending stresses that exist at the pleural surface. However, many structures within the lung have compliances that deviate from the mean. The dimensions of such structures change more or less than the average during distension, depending on whether they are more or less compliant than the lungs as a whole. Structures that stretch less than the lungs as a whole may be subject to stress magnification[57] since, for the same force at the boundary, they are proportionately more stressed the smaller their surface area. Hence, pressure variations in small lung blood vessels (in excised human lungs) are often greater than elastic recoil pressures.[66] The inverse relation between surface area and distending pressure, in the case of nonisotropic distension and recoil, promotes uniform lung expansion: if one unit is distended more than its neighbor, its surface area becomes larger and its distending pressure consequently decreases.[57]

STATIC PRESSURE-VOLUME CURVE

The lungs' elastic-recoil properties become clear only from a pressure-volume curve. To construct such a curve in man in vivo, one must measure lung volume with a spirometer or a body plethysmograph, which is easy, while simultaneously measuring pleural pressure, which is considerably more difficult.

Pleural Pressure (Ppl)

Because during life the lungs are always distended beyond their resting volume (R in Fig. 7-1*B*), they would collapse if not prevented by their apposition to the chest wall (Fig. 7-2). The collapsing tendency, or recoil force, of the lungs decreases the pressure in the pleural space below atmospheric (Fig. 7-2*C*). In lung mechanics, atmospheric pressure (Patm) is used as a zero reference pressure; the subatmospheric pressure in the pleural space is usually called a negative pressure, i.e., negative with respect to Patm = 0.

If measured by a fluid-filled catheter, the pressure within the intact pleural space is lower than the pressure measured in Figure 7-2*C*[1,3]; the actual pressure includes an additional pleural liquid pressure created by the contact between the pleural membranes. As commonly measured by an air-filled catheter, Ppl is the pleural surface pressure, which is relevant to the elastic recoil of the lungs and chest wall. The interpretation of Ppl measurements is complicated by the fact that the pressure around the lungs is not uniform but increases, becoming less negative from the top to the bottom of vertical lungs. This reflects the distorted shape of the lungs in the thorax, resulting largely from gravity effects.[67] In a healthy, sitting man at FRC, pleural surface pressure is about -8 cm H_2O just below the apex and -2 cm H_2O near the bottom of the lungs; if the vertical height of the lungs is 25 cm, the gradient is about 0.3 cm H_2O/cm height. The effect of gravity on the chest wall and on the abdominal contents appears to contribute to the gradient.[21] The shape and height of the chest, the distribution of muscle force and of stress in the lungs, and the weight of lung tissue and blood are all relevant variables that contribute to the local variations of Ppl.[1]

Measurement of Ppl. The local variations of Ppl and the differences between pleural liquid and surface pressures make it difficult to interpret direct measurements of Ppl in terms of overall lung elastic recoil. Although indirect methods also suffer from limitations, they are at least more practical in man. One indirect method uses the fact that the intrathoracic esophagus is relaxed except during swallowing, and the pressure within its lumen reflects pleural pressure fairly well.[21] Esophageal pressures can be measured by inserting a balloon catheter, a method that depends on precise technical details.[59, 73] Another indirect method uses the retraction of the skin in the suprasternal notch as a measure of lung recoil force.[9]

Determination of Static Lung Recoil Pressure

The difference between pleural surface pressure (Ppl) and Patm equals the sum of two pressure differences: (1) that between the pleural surface and the alveoli (created by lung elastic recoil), and (2) that between alveoli and the atmosphere (the driving pressure for airflow). Thus

$$(\text{Ppl}-\text{Patm}) = (\text{Ppl}-\text{Palv}) + (\text{Palv}-\text{Patm}) \qquad (1)$$

and since $(\text{Ppl}-\text{Palv}) = -\text{Pst}(l)$, and Patm is the zero reference pressure

$$\text{Ppl} = -\text{Pst}(l) + \text{Palv} \qquad (2)$$

where Pst(l) is the static recoil pressure of the lungs and Palv the pressure in the alveoli.

Increased pull of the lungs on the pleural surface [i.e., larger Pst(l)] reduces pleural pressure (makes it more negative), hence the negative sign for Pst(l). Pst(l) depends on lung volume (Figs. 7-1 and 7-5). If the relation between Pst(l) and volume is known, Palv can be determined. Conversely, Pst(l) can be determined from Ppl measurements if Palv is known. For instance, at A (Fig. 7-5), Ppl $= -20$ cm H_2O; Pst(l) $= +10$ cm H_2O. From Eq. (2): $-20 = -10 + \text{Palv}$; hence Palv $= -10$ cm H_2O. Negative, i.e., subatmospheric, alveolar pressures lead to inspiration. Palv is negative at all points left of the curve in Figure 7-5; that area is associated with inspiration. For B in Figure 7-5, Palv $= +20$ cm H_2O.

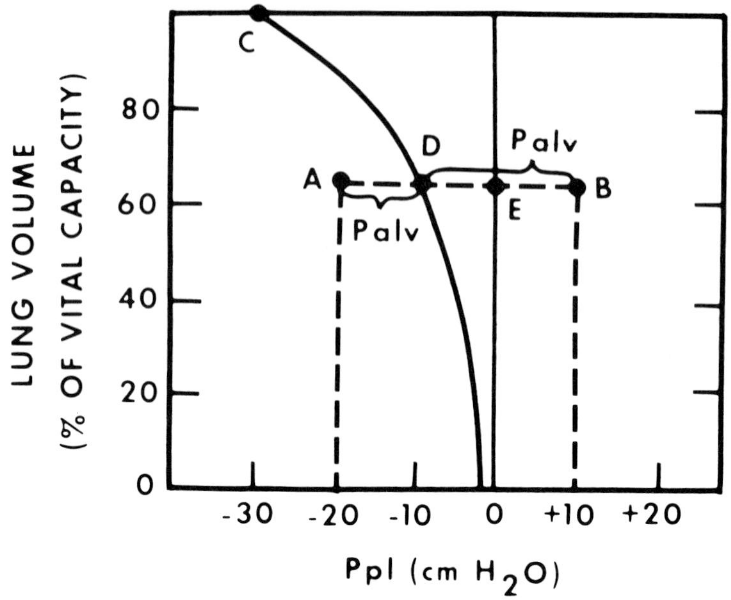

Fig. 7-5. Pressure-volume diagram of lungs in man. Curved line through *C* and *D* is the static recoil curve (see also Fig. 7-1). The diagram shows graphical solutions to Eq. (2). At point *A*, Ppl = −AE and Pst(*l*) = DE. Substituting in Eq. (2), −AE = −DE + Palv; hence, Palv = −AD = −10 cm H_2O. Similarly, at *B*, Palv = +BD = +20 cm H_2O. *C* = static recoil pressure at maximum lung inflation.

Palv is positive for points to the right of the curve; this area is associated with expiration.

When Palv = 0, Ppl = −Pst(*l*) [from Eq. (2)]. The locus of all points where Palv = 0 is the elastic or static recoil curve of the lungs (Figs. 7-1 and 7-5). Palv can be made zero by holding the breath with all airways open; alveolar pressure then equals Patm. Thus, the static recoil curve can be determined experimentally if the subject inspires maximally (to point *C*, Fig. 7-5), and then exhales stepwise, holding the breath with glottis open at several intervals of about 0.5 liters. At each of these points, Palv = 0 and Ppl = −Pst(*l*). The principle of the method can be shown clearly with an experiment on singing (Fig. 7-6). Here, the subject inspired maximally and sang a tone with periodic interruptions. The tone was constant in pitch and loudness and hence required a constant driving pressure (Chap. 11). To provide the pressure for phonation, Palv is elevated each time the note is struck. On the other hand, during each interruption (glottis open), Ppl decreases to the level of Pst(*l*).

The lung static recoil curve is steep at low lung volumes: deflated lungs are highly distensible (Fig. 7-1*B*). As volume increases, the slope of the curve diminishes, indicating that the lungs increasingly resist further inflation. To measure Pst(*l*) by breath holding may require training the subject. Easier methods for use in patients include very slow exhalations with open glottis to achieve nearly static conditions[11] and interruption of airflow at the mouth.[44] Measurement of thoracic gas volume with a body plethysmograph provides data for an absolute

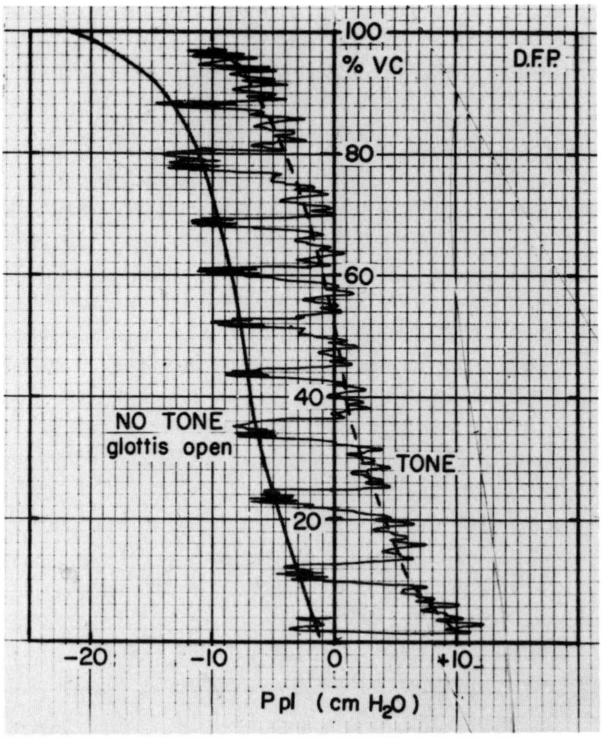

Fig. 7-6. Pleural pressure and lung volume recorded during singing of a tone at constant pitch and loudness. The subject initiated the tone at a lung volume close to 100% of VC and interrupted phonation 10 times. During the brief interruptions he held his breath with his glottis wide open. The noise in the Ppl recording is the result of fluctuations in esophageal pressure caused by the heartbeat. The course of Ppl during phonation is indicated by the dashed line. During the interruptions, Ppl decreases to the value of Pst(l) at the prevailing lung volume. *Solid line.* Static recoil curve of the lungs for this subject. Subglottic pressure = 7.5 cm H_2O at 50% of VC (horizontal distance between solid and dashed lines). From reference 13.

volume scale, as a percentage of TLC (Fig. 7-1). This is important in particular when short-term variations of Pst(l) occur, as in asthma (p. 168).

Lung Compliance

The slope of the Pst(l) versus volume curve reflects lung compliance, or the ease with which the lungs can be expanded. Since the curve is markedly alinear outside the tidal volume range, compliance depends on the breathing level. When lung stiffness increases as a pathological phenomenon, compliance is low; but increased stiffness is also a normal consequence of lung inflation to near TLC.

Only complete static recoil curves give a full picture of lung elastic recoil; compliance values are valid only for the tidal volume range over which they were measured and are generally difficult to interpret.

Dynamic Lung Compliance

In healthy persons who breathe quietly, Palv is zero throughout the lungs at the end-tidal points, i.e., the points of flow reversal between inspiration and expiration. These two points on the pressure-volume loop (Fig. 7-7*C*) therefore coincide with the static recoil curve. Measuring Ppl and volume at these points gives a compliance value, measured during breathing and called dynamic compliance (Cdyn), which is equal to the compliance measured from the static curve (static compliance, Cst). However, Cdyn does not always equal Cst. For instance, when airway obstruction causes some lung regions to fill slowly during inspiration, these areas receive less inspired air as breathing rate increases. The amount of air inspired for a given pleural pressure change thus depends on the duration of inspiration: the shorter the inspiration, the less air inspired. Under such conditions, Cdyn is frequency-dependent and decreases as breathing rate increases.[79] This phenomenon can be used to assess airway obstruction in disease. Its accurate recording requires control of lung volume levels, rapid response of the pressure-sensing device (for use with high breathing rates), and considerable cooperation and training of the subject. Frequency dependence of Cdyn is usually but not always associated with nonuniform inspired gas distribution (N_2 washout [25, 42]).

Variables Influencing Lung Static Recoil

At comparable lung volumes, as a percentage of VC or TLC, mammals with widely different lung sizes have similar static recoil pressures. The same holds true for growing children (Chap. 1). Since in healthy individuals, compliance in absolute units is a measure of lung size rather than of lung-tissue properties, young children and small animals have a small lung compliance. Advancing age is associated with decreased lung recoil,[74] although individual variability is considerable.[45] Whether the rate of aging of elastic structures in the lungs parallels that in other elastic tissues (e.g., the lens or skin) is not clear. Since the amount of elastic and collagen material does not change with age, loss of recoil force is perhaps best explained by degeneration of structure rather than by altered properties of individual elastic fibers.[65] Elastic recoil curves vary individually and are difficult to obtain in large groups of subjects. This limits their usefulness in detecting effects of environmental variables (smoking, air pollutant exposure) on lung recoil. Deep breaths and sighs increase dynamic compliance.[26] Regular deep breaths, perhaps elicited by chemoreceptor stimulation [8] and vagal afferent impulses,[34] may help prevent atelectasis, particularly in small animals that have small, easily collapsible alveoli (p. 7). The sighing mechanism is active in immature animals and may contribute to the events that initiate breathing after birth.[8] Stress distribution in the lungs affects local recoil forces (see p. 153).

STATIC PRESSURE-VOLUME CURVES OF THE LUNGS AND CHEST

This section elaborates on the pressure-volume diagram by adding a curve that represents properties of the chest wall. This allows us to determine how the respiratory bellows generates pleural and alveolar pressures.

Generation of Pleural Pressure

Pleural pressure is actively altered by contraction of respiratory muscles.[19] The action of the muscles is reinforced or opposed by elastic recoil forces in the chest wall. The active and passive forces in the chest wall can be analyzed if one considers Ppl as the pressure difference between the atmosphere (zero reference) and the pleural space, separated by the chest wall

$$\text{Ppl} - \text{Patm} = \text{Ppl} = \text{Pmus} + \text{Pst(w)} \tag{3}$$

where Pmus is the pressure developed by the muscles and Pst(w) the pressure developed by the recoil force of the chest cage. To solve Eq. (3) one measures Ppl at different lung volumes while the subject voluntarily relaxes all respiratory muscles. This maneuver makes Pmus = 0, and thus Ppl = Pst(w). During relaxation, lung volume normally returns to the resting breathing level (FRC). Thus, to measure Ppl during muscle relaxation at volumes other than FRC, one must keep volume at the desired level by closing the airways. To generate the curve of Figure 7-7*A*, the subject inspires maximally and holds the breath momentarily. This is the same maneuver used in Figure 7-5; during breath holding at TLC, Ppl is at point *C* in both figures. Next, a valve in the breathing tube is closed and the subject relaxes all muscles. At TLC, the chest cage tends to collapse through its own recoil and, since no air can escape, this creates a positive pressure in the pleural space. Hence, Ppl becomes positive and volume decreases slightly because of gas compression (point *C′*). At a small lung volume (e.g., at *D*) the chest cage tends to expand when the muscles are relaxed. Ppl then becomes more negative while lung volume increases slightly through decompression (to point *D′*). The reader can perform these maneuvers by closing his mouth and nose manually and relaxing at different lung volumes. If one relaxes near full inspiration, the positive pressure in the chest is transmitted to the mouth. It is more difficult to relax near full expiration; if the maneuver is successful, one notices that the chest tends to inspire air. Between these extremes is a volume where Pst(w) is zero (*E;* at about 60 percent of the VC). This is the resting position of the chest cage, i.e., the volume it would assume if no outside forces (muscle force and lung recoil) acted upon it. The resting volumes of the chest cage and the lungs differ considerably. During life, the properties of the pleural space lead to a resting volume of the lungs and chest that is less than the resting volume of the chest and more than that of the lungs. Since the lungs are more distensible than the chest, the combined resting volume lies closer to that of the chest than to that of the lungs.

Once the Pst(w) versus volume curve is known, Pmus can be determined from Eq. (3) for any value of Ppl. Examples are given in the legend of Figure 7-7*B*. When Ppl is greater than Pst(w), the muscles exert expiratory force and Pmus

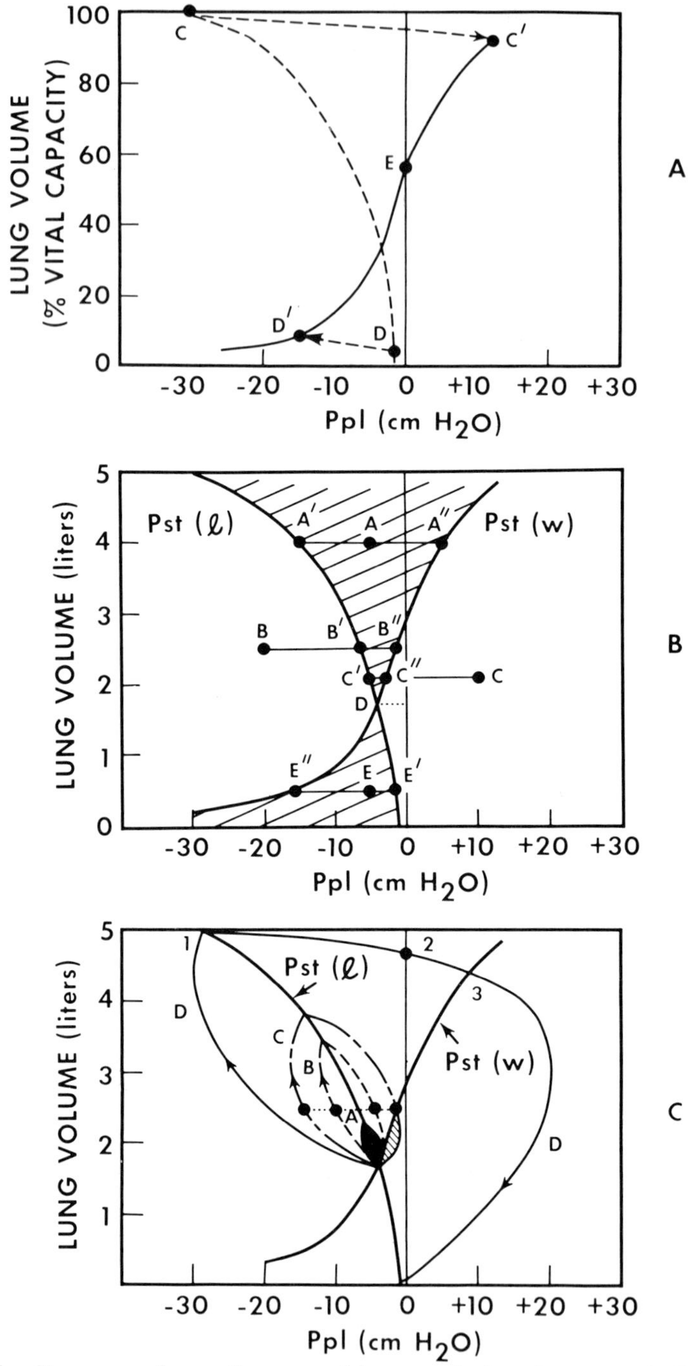

Fig. 7-7. Pressure-volume diagrams of lungs and chest in man. *A*. Dashed curve through *C* and *D* = static lung recoil curve. Drawn curve through *C′* and *D′* = static chest-wall recoil curve. *E* = resting position of the chest cage (volume at which the chest cage exerts no elastic forces on its contents). To obtain the chest wall curve, the subject inspires maximally (to *C*) and relaxes against a closed mouthpiece. The chest wall recoil then compresses the gas in the lungs, and Ppl becomes positive (dashed line

is positive. All points to the right of the Pst(w) curve are associated with expiratory muscle force. When Ppl is less than Pst(w), muscle force is inspiratory and Pmus is negative [all points to the left of the Pst(w) curve].

Any value of Pmus is the net result of contracting different muscles, including agonists and antagonists. Simultaneous contraction of inspiratory and expiratory muscles may result in a net muscle force which is small in comparison to muscular effort. Pmus is zero not only when all muscles are relaxed, but also when agonists and antagonists exert equal forces in opposite directions. The voluntary muscle relaxation used to produce the Pst(w) versus volume curve may not always be complete, and the numerical values of Pmus are then incorrect. Nevertheless, the curve indicates the mechanical behavior of the chest cage accurately, if not in precise quantitative terms.

Generation of Alveolar Pressure

Figure 7-7*B* includes the Pst(*l*) and Pst(w) curves. Five Ppl values are indicated (*A*-*E*); for each of these, equations (2) and (3) can be solved graphically by reading horizontal distances from the Ppl point to the Pst(*l*) and the Pst(w) curve (see legend to Fig. 7-7). At *B,* Palv and Pmus have a negative sign: muscle force is inspiratory, and the negative Palv would lead to inspiration. At *C,* both are positive: expiratory muscle force (with the glottis open) leads to expiration. At *D,* both Pmus and Palv are zero. Here, the elastic recoil of the lungs (pulling inward) and the recoil of the chest (pulling outward) just balance one another. This is the resting, end-expiratory breathing level to which lungs and chest return when all muscles are relaxed and the airways are open. Pmus and Palv have opposite signs at *A* and *E*. Point *A* is associated with expiration (+Palv) and inspiratory muscle force (−Pmus). Point *A* lies in the upper hatched area; points in this area reflect expiratory air movement braked by inspiratory muscle force. Without this brake, relaxing the chest cage would lead to higher pleural and alveolar pressures, e.g., up to +20 cm H_2O (*A*″) at the same volume as for *A*. Conversely, in the lower hatched area, the expiratory muscle force is not strong enough to prevent inspiration. To continue expiration at these small volumes, Pmus needs to be sufficient to increase Ppl to points to the right of the Pst(*l*) curve.

When Palv ≠ 0 and the airways are open, air is inspired or expired and conditions are no longer static (Chap. 8). The development of Palv is, however,

---

CC′). When relaxing at low lung volume, starting at *D*, lung volume expands and Ppl decreases (dashed line *DD*′). *B*. Static lung [Pst(*l*)] and static chest wall [Pst(w)] recoil curves, to show graphical solution of Eqs. (2) and (3). At point *A*, Palv = +*AA*′ and Pmus = −*AA*″. At *B*, Palv = −*BB*′ and Pmus = −*BB*″. At *C*, Palv = +*CC*′ and Pmus = +*CC*″. At *D*, Palv = Pmus = 0. At *E*, Palv = −*EE*′ and Pmus = +*EE*″. *Hatched areas*. See text for discussion. *C*. Pst(*l*) and Pst(w) curves with three pressure-volume loops with different tidal volumes (*A*, *B*, *C*) and a maximum inspiratory and expiratory maneuver (*D*). Hatched area indicates portion of breath *C* where positive expiratory muscle force is used. Dotted horizontal line and points indicate magnitude of resistive pressures on loops *B* and *C*. See text for further discussion.

best discussed on the basis of the pressure-volume diagram. During quiet breathing (loop A in Fig. 7-7*C*), inspiration is associated with inspiratory muscle force. During expiration, Palv is positive but the loop remains to the left of the Pst(w) curve. Expiration results from elastic recoil of the lungs, initially braked by inspiratory muscle force (−Pmus). During a deep and slow breath (loop B) the pattern is similar, but when flow rates are increased the loop widens because higher alveolar pressures are required (loop C). The expiratory portion of loop C crosses the Pst(w) curve, indicating that expiratory muscle force is applied during the last part of the expiration. Loop D represents a rapid inspiration to TLC, followed by a forced expiration to RV. During expiration Palv reaches values up to +30 cm H_2O. Initially, Palv increases because the inspiratory muscles relax (from *1* to *3*). At *2*, Ppl becomes positive; at *3*, Pmus = 0. Beyond point *3*, expiratory muscles contract, further increasing Ppl and Palv. Throughout the expiration Pmus remains positive, while Palv gradually decreases and reaches zero when airflow stops at the residual volume level. Considerable expiratory muscle force is required to maintain lung volume at that level. At each point of all loops, Palv and Pmus can be determined as shown in Figure 7-7*B*. The relations between Palv and airflow rates are discussed in Chapter 8. Special breathing maneuvers (for singing, speech) can also be studied with pressure-volume diagrams (Chap. 11).

WORK OF BREATHING

The product of volume and pressure has the dimensions of work according to its physical definition. Since different muscle efforts may yield the same Pmus, the actual effort for a given amount of work performed on the lungs and chest may vary widely. When agonists and antagonists contract simultaneously, considerable effort is exerted but little work is accomplished. The product of volume and pressure, shown graphically as a surface area on a pressure-volume diagram, indicates only the amount of physical work performed in displacing air at the mouth. This work results partly from muscle force and partly from potential energy stored in the elastic structures of lungs and chest.

The part played by stored energy follows from the Pst(*l*) and Pst(w) curves. At *A′* (Fig. 7-7*B*), the lungs recoil with a pressure of +15 cm H_2O. At the same volume, the chest recoils inward with a pressure of +5 cm H_2O. Thus, the lungs and chest recoil together, in the direction of expiration, with a total pressure of +20 cm H_2O (*A‴* in Fig. 7-8). The different sign accorded to Pst(*l*) in Figures 7-7 and 7-8 may be confusing. In the former figure, pressure is measured outside the recoiling lungs; the lungs tend to pull away from the site of pressure measurement (Fig. 7-2*C*), and lung recoil is measured as a negative pressure. At the same time, lung recoil leads to pressure on the air in the lungs and to expiration. Thus, for the purpose of Figure 7-8, Pst(*l*) has a positive sign. A similar calculation for a point at a low lung volume (*E‴* in Fig. 7-8) shows a net recoil force of lungs and chest in the inspiratory direction—lung elastic recoil is small but the chest cage tends to expand with considerable force. The same calculation at other lung volumes yields the curve through *A‴* and *E‴*

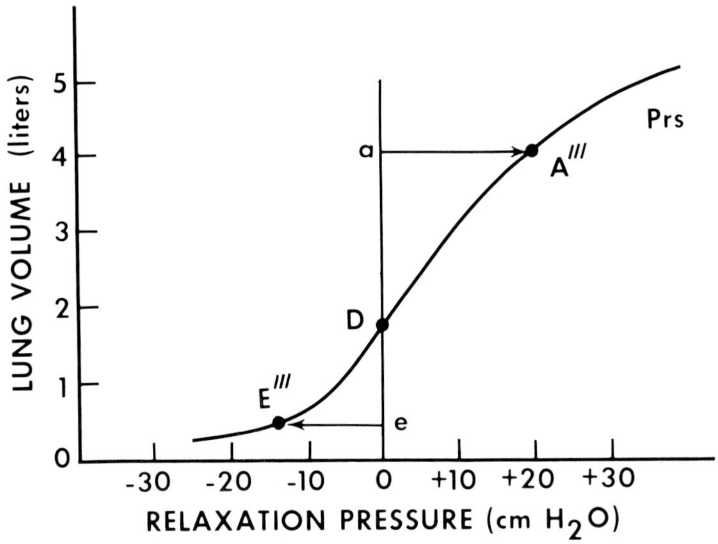

Fig. 7-8. Static pressure-volume curve of lungs and chest together. *Abscissa.* Mouth pressure developed during relaxation against closed airway at different lung volumes. This indicates the total pressure developed by the respiratory system (Prs) under conditions of zero net muscle force. Arrows to *A'''* and *E'''* indicate Prs at volumes equal to those for lines *A' A''* and *E' E''* in Fig. 7-7*B*. See text for derivation of these pressures.

—the relaxation-pressure curve.[69] When one relaxes all muscles during closure of airways at the mouth, pressure within the alveoli and airways equals the values on the curve of Figure 7-8, while Ppl equals Pst(w).

The work of breathing can be analyzed in detail, starting from the relaxation-pressure curve and the Pst(*l*) and Pst(w) curves.[62] When one inspires from FRC, work is needed to increase lung volume; part of this work is provided by chest recoil toward a higher volume. Thus, in addition to that performed actively by the muscles, work is provided by the potential energy in the chest cage. During expiration, some of this work is restored to the chest cage, which returns to a smaller volume where its recoil force is larger. In braking expiration, the inspiratory muscles work while they lengthen (so-called negative work). In addition, work is performed to overcome viscous resistances, primarily those in the airways. This portion of the work of breathing can be measured from the surface area of a pressure-volume loop (e.g., *A* in Fig. 7-7*C*).

The work of respiratory muscles requires oxygen. When ventilation is increased while keeping other muscles at rest, O_2 consumption increases. The increment of O_2 uptake is attributable to the muscles' work of breathing. Thus, the O_2 consumption required for breathing can be measured[52] during inspiration of CO_2-air mixtures (Chap. 10), by increasing the dead space, or by voluntary hyperventilation. However, the experimental errors are large, since the amount of O_2 used for breathing is a small part of the total O_2 consumption. At high ventilation rates, the O_2 uptake of the respiratory muscles increases steeply.[62] When the work of breathing is increased in lung disease, the increased O_2 consumption required for breathing may offset the gain in O_2 consumption derived from increased ventilation rates. Ventilation increases are then useless, since the net supply of O_2 to other working muscles cannot be increased. This limits the exercise performance of patients with ventilatory insufficiency.

The combination of rate and tidal volume chosen to achieve given rates of lung ventilation influences the work of breathing. At low rates, large tidal volumes are required, and as inspiratory lung volume increases, work against elastic recoil increases. Above about 60 percent of VC (Fig. 7-7*A*), chest and lung recoil both oppose inspiration; the work required to expand them then increases markedly, due to the alinearity of the Pst(*l*) and Pst(w) curves. At low lung volumes, considerable muscle force is needed to continue expiration against the increasing recoil of the chest cage. During heavy physical exercise, tidal volume rarely exceeds 50 percent of the VC, probably largely because both volume extremes, near TLC and near RV, require too much work. When ventilation is increased through higher breathing rates, work against flow-resistive forces increases. Here, too, the relation between increased flow and increased work is alinear so that considerable energy is required to increase flows to high values (Chap. 8). Thus, extreme values of tidal volume and rate both greatly increase the work of breathing. During spontaneous breathing, tidal volume and rate values keep respiratory work near a minimum.[58] The adjustment may include setting the rate at a value which also corresponds to minimum muscle force.[54] (See, however, Chap. 10.) Work is a complex result of the forces, but the optimal breathing rates for minimum force and work are similar, and neither optimum is sharply defined.

MAXIMUM STATIC PRESSURES

The physiological limits of the pressure-volume diagram are reached when maximum inspiratory and expiratory pressures are exerted against a closed airway (Fig. 7-9). These limits are set by the force of the respiratory muscles and

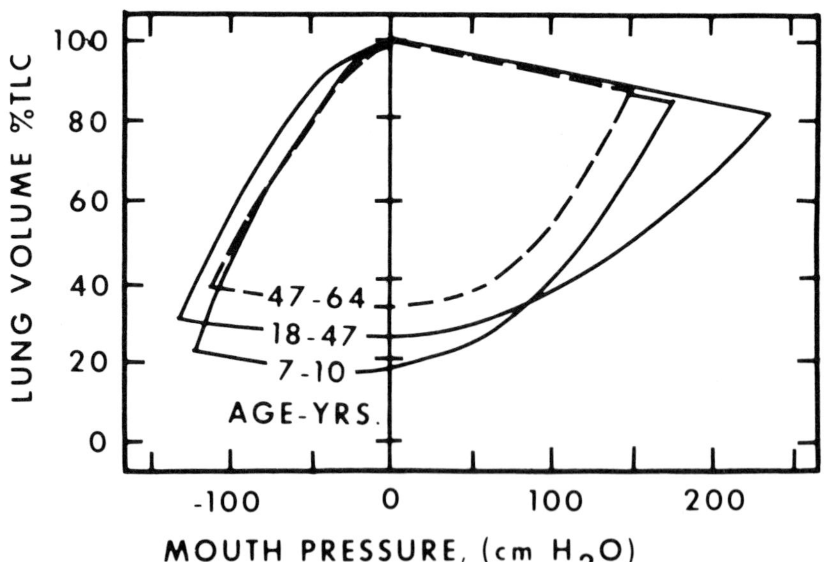

Fig. 7-9. Average maximum inspiratory and expiratory pressures in men of different ages. From reference 23.

the configuration of the chest cage. Near maximum inspiration, the expiratory muscles are stretched and can exert their maximum force. Even at low lung volumes, they can still generate considerable pressure. Optimal conditions for inspiratory muscle contraction exist at lung volumes near RV. As lung volume increases, inspiratory muscle force decreases. In part, this is because the shorter the muscle, the less force it can develop. The muscles probably also work at a mechanical disadvantage near TLC, and contraction of antagonists (particularly abdominal muscles) may further limit their force.

Children can develop high static pressures,[23] and inspiratory pressures can reach 40 to 80 cm H_2O during the newborn's first few breaths.[5] People who use a snorkel during swimming use high inspiratory pressures, too. Prolonged breathing at increased negative pressures in the chest can cause transudation of water from lung blood vessels and may lead to lung edema. Prolonged high expiratory pressures (e.g., during straining movements or when playing wind instruments) may lead to fainting,[29] since the high pressure in the chest hinders venous return of blood to the heart. During exercise, even when ventilation rates are high, the pressures remain below their maximum values.

The large muscle-reserve power permits adequate ventilation even when the muscles are weakened or partially paralyzed. Determination of maximum static pressures is useful to detect respiratory muscle weakness. Since less than maximal pressures are used when performing forced vital capacity maneuvers, VC and expiratory flow rates may be normal while maximum pressures are too low because of muscle weakness.[10]

Breathing efforts against a closed airway do not perform ventilatory work, although the lungs and chest may undergo marked volume changes. The work done in compressing and decompressing gas in the lungs during such maneuvers can be measured with a body plethysmograph.[13] When the airways are partially obstructed, work is spent on gas compression and decompression to the extent that pressures in alveoli behind obstructed airways lag behind those elsewhere. Patients with severe airway obstruction exert considerable effort to breathe, and a large part of this effort is used to generate high alveolar pressures that result in only small flow rates. In such patients, the volume excursions of the chest may be pronounced although tidal volume measured at the mouth may be small. Thus, the observation of chest movements may be misleading.

LIMITS OF INSPIRATION AND EXPIRATION

The limits of maximum inspiratory and expiratory excursions are set by the size of the lungs and chest and by a combination of mechanical factors.

TLC. Near maximum inspiration, compliance of lungs and chest decreases (they become stiffer), while inspiratory muscle force decreases.[56] The limit is reached when the net maximum inspiratory force just balances the combined recoil of lungs and chest. When lung recoil decreases (as in emphysema), the same muscle force can increase volume more; hence, TLC is often increased in emphysema. In addition, long-standing increases in the work of breathing required in emphysema might lead to training of inspiratory muscles; one may speculate that increased inspiratory muscle force may also contribute to increases in TLC.

RV. Near maximum expiration, the alveoli begin to collapse, folding like an accordion (data from cat lungs [47]), but at the end of a maximally forced expiration, the alveoli retain about 20 percent of TLC, the residual volume (RV, Fig. 7-1). Several variables determine whether maximum voluntary expiration is terminated by alveolar collapse,[47] airway closure,[71] or inability to decrease chest cage volume further.[51] Elastic recoil of the chest may set the limit in young persons; their expiratory muscles are unable to compress the chest further, but pressure applied from outside can do so.[51] Contraction of the diaphragm may decrease net muscle force near RV.[4] In older persons and in smokers, airway closure becomes the predominant limiting factor. The two mechanisms—airway closure versus chest recoil and muscle force—can be distinguished from the pattern of MEFV curves (Chap. 9).

In experimental studies, the pressure needed to close small bronchioles is similar to that required to collapse alveoli.[40] Which ones close first depends on the way the lungs are deflated.[20] In dog lungs, airways of about 0.5 mm diameter are likely to close before larger ones; [41] in cat lungs, however, terminal bronchioles, although narrowed and kinked, were not fully closed at low lung volume.[48] Indirect evidence in man suggests that relatively large airways (about 1 mm diameter) may be closed at RV; this results in air trapping, which can be demonstrated by washout of N_2.[16]

CLINICAL APPLICATIONS

The esophageal balloon method for estimating Ppl has been used in many clinical studies on lung elastic recoil. To interpret these data accurately, one should measure thoracic gas volume with a body plethysmograph, so that Pst(*l*) data can be referred to lung volume in absolute terms.

Airway Obstruction

Measurements of Pst(*l*), an important driving force for expiratory airflow (Chap. 8), can be used to interpret changes in airway resistance in patients with airway obstruction. In some patients, elastic recoil is normal while resistances are high, suggesting that the obstruction is caused by changes in the airways themselves (smooth muscle contraction, mucus accumulation, mucosal swelling). In other patients, loss of elastic recoil and the concomitant loss of structural support for the small airways can explain the degree of airway obstruction inferred from measurements of flow rates and airway resistance. Different types of pressure-volume-resistance relations have been described in small groups of patients with airway obstruction in the presence of similar values for conventional spirometric measurements.[46] In hemp workers with byssinosis and ventilatory insufficiency, Pst(*l*) correlated significantly with maximum expiratory flow rates.[36] This suggested that the abnormally low flow rates in these persons were caused, in part, by loss of lung elastic recoil. Thus, measurements of Pst(l) can be used to assess the contribution of reduced elastic recoil to airway obstruction caused by emphysematous lesions.

Emphysema

Loss of elastic lung recoil is a prime feature of the emphysematous lung. The slope of the pressure-volume curve is steep compared to normal, indicating increased lung compliance. Even at maximum inflation, the lungs exert little recoil pressure (Fig. 7-10). Although a low transpulmonary pressure at TLC indicates emphysema,[53] the overlap between normal and abnormal values is considerable, rendering lesser degrees of emphysema undetectable with this method.[46] A genetic abnormality, α_1-antitrypsin deficiency, is associated with an early onset of severe emphysema in young persons.[28] Intermediate degrees of this enzyme deficiency have been attributed to heterozygosity for the relevant gene. Such heterozygous persons have lower Pst(l) values after age 30 than control subjects,[61] which suggests that the more common heterozygous enzyme deficiency may lead to clinical emphysema at a later age.

Lesions similar to those in human emphysema can be produced experimentally in animals with papain, a proteolytic enzyme,[63] and with DL-penicillamine, an agent that inhibits cross-linking between collagen and elastin.[18, 37, 38] Papain acts

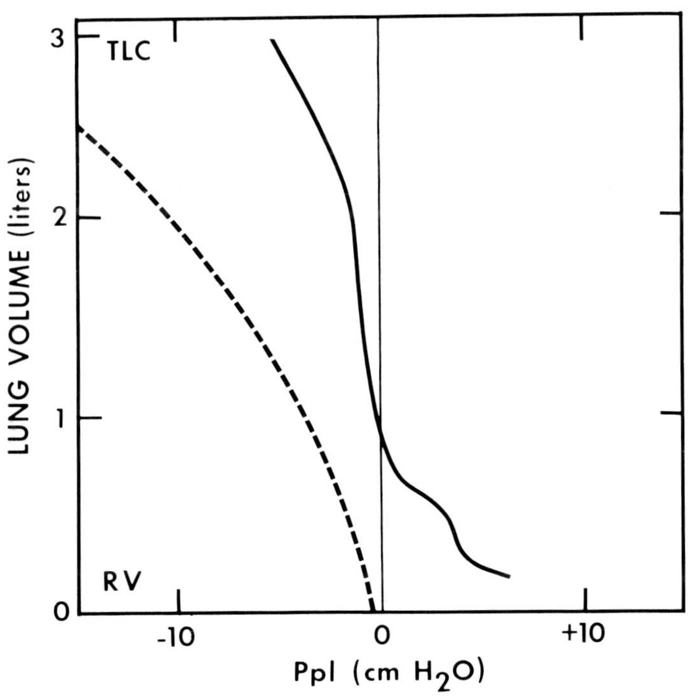

Fig. 7-10. Static lung recoil curve in a patient with emphysema (*drawn curve*) compared to typical normal curve in same volume range (*dashed line*). Static recoil pressure in the patient is minimal even when the lungs are maximally inflated. Lung volume scale in liters above RV.

on the short term, while DL-penicillamine must be administered for 2 or more weeks. The effects of these agents include dilatation of terminal air spaces, increased compliance at small lung volume, and decreased elastic recoil pressures. Such changes also occur in human emphysema, but it is not yet known whether the mode of action of papain or penicillamine is similar to the pathogenetic mechanisms in emphysema. (See also p. 192)

Asthma

Patients with bronchial asthma (see also Chap. 12) often breathe at increased end-expiratory breathing levels. When data obtained during an asthmatic state were compared with data obtained in a symptom-free interval, several studies [30, 35] showed discreet shifts in the static recoil curves of asthmatic patients, in the sense of decreased elastic recoil. The mechanisms of this change are not clear. In part, it may result from changes in the reference volume: when airway obstruction is sèvere, the body plethysmograph may slightly overestimate TGV.[12] However, a similar phenomenon has been induced in animals. Pst(*l*) was decreased and TLC increased in dogs that breathed for 2 weeks with an increased end-expiratory pressure (10–15 cm H_2O). Since liquid-filling of the excised lungs showed no change in pressure-volume curves, the major effect appeared to be on the recoil of the alveolar surface film.[14] In excised dog lungs, a decrease of Pst(*l*) was induced after only 2–3 hours ventilation at end-expiratory pressure of +7 cm H_2O.[70] Thus, it appears that breathing at increased lung volumes, whether induced by asthma or by breathing against an external expiratory resistance, causes loss of lung recoil. Recovery of recoil pressure in asthma appears to be slow; there is no rapid reversal to normal after isoproterenol or other dilator drugs. The loss of recoil in asthma can account for some decrease of expiratory flow rates and is perhaps one reason why flow rates often remain at slightly less than normal levels for some time, even during adequate drug treatment.

Other Conditions

In *mitral stenosis,* Pst(*l*) is low at low lung volumes (probably because of vascular congestion) and high near TLC, perhaps due to lung fibrosis.[78] In *obesity,* chest wall compliance is low and the work of breathing is increased; [60] this can explain the reduced vital capacity of obese persons.

SUMMARY

The movements of the chest cage during breathing transmit forces through the pleural space to the lungs, which passively follow all volume changes of the chest cage. The force required to distend the lungs during inspiration is determined by the viscoelastic behavior of lung tissue, which in turn depends on the extensibility of the elastic and collagen fiber network in the lungs. The elastic recoil of the lungs [Pst(*l*)] can be measured from a pressure-volume curve recorded during stepwise expirations from TLC, relating pleural pressure to lung volume. The elastic recoil of the chest cage [Pst(w)] can be measured from a similar curve recorded during muscular relaxation at different lung volumes. Pst(*l*) and Pst(w) curves together can be used to determine alveolar pressure and the net pressure developed by the respiratory muscles and to analyze the work of breathing. Maximum pressures developed during forceful inspiration and expiration against a closed airway indicate the limits of respiratory muscle force. The limits of lung volume excursions are set by muscle force, by the size of chest and lungs, by their compliance and, at low lung volumes, by alveolar collapse or airway closure. In patients with lung disease, such as emphysema or airway obstruction, Pst(*l*) measurements are used to assess the role of lung elastic recoil in reducing lung function.

REFERENCES

1. Agostoni E: Mechanics of the pleural space. Physiol Rev 52:57–128, 1972
2. Agostoni E, D'Angelo E, Roncoroni G: The thickness of the pleural liquid. Respir Physiol 5:1–13, 1968
3. Agostoni E, Mead J: Statics of the respiratory system, in Fenn WO, Rahn H (eds): Handbook of Physiology, Section 3: Respiration, vol I. Washington, D.C., American Physiological Society, 1964, pp 387–409
4. Agostoni E, Sant'Ambrogio G, del Portillo Carrasco H: Electromyography of the diaphragm in man and transdiaphragmatic pressure. J Appl Physiol 15:1093–1097, 1960
5. Avery ME, Wang N-S, Taeusch HW Jr: The lung of the newborn infant; a disorder of prematurity is combatted. Sci Am 228:74–85, 1973
6. Bachofen H, Hildebrandt J: Area analysis of pressure-volume hysteresis in mammalian lungs. J Appl Physiol 30:493–497, 1971
7. Bachofen H, Hildebrandt J, Bachofen M: Pressure-volume curves of air- and liquid-filled excised lungs—surface tension in situ. J Appl Physiol 29:422–31, 1970
8. Bartlett D Jr: Origin and regulation of spontaneous deep breaths. Respir Physiol 12:230–238, 1971
9. Bevan C, McKerrow CB, Morgan EJ: A method of measuring pulmonary compliance without an oesophageal tube. J Physiol (Lond) 217:10P–11P, 1971
10. Black LF, Hyatt RE: Maximal static respiratory pressures in generalized neuromuscular disease. Am Rev Respir Dis 103:641–650, 1971
11. Bouhuys A: Airflow control by auditory feedback; respiratory mechanics and wind instruments. Science 154:797–799, 1966
12. Bouhuys A, Hunt VR, Kim BM, Zapletal A: Maximum expiratory flow rates in induced bronchoconstriction in man. J Clin Invest 48:1159–1168, 1969
13. Bouhuys A, Proctor DF, Mead J: Kinetic aspects of singing. J Appl Physiol 21: 483–496, 1966
14. Buhain WJ, Brody JS, Fisher AB: Effect of artificial airway obstruction on elastic properties of the lung. J Appl Physiol 33:589–594, 1972
15. Bull HB: Protein structure and elasticity, in Remington JW (ed): Tissue Elasticity. Washington, D.C., American Physiological Society, 1957, pp 33–42
16. Burger EJ Jr, Macklem PT: Airway closure: demonstration by breathing 100% O_2 at low lung volumes and by N_2 washout. J Appl Physiol 25:139–148, 1968
17. But VI: Contraction of smooth muscle of the bronchial tree and its effects on hysteresis of the lungs. Bul Exp Biol Med (USSR) 73:11–13, 1972
18. Caldwell EJ, Bland JH: The effect of penicillamine on the rabbit lung. Am Rev Respir Dis 105:75–84, 1972
19. Campbell EJM, Agostoni E, Newsom Davis J: The Respiratory Muscles: Mechanics and Neural Control. London, Lloyd-Luke, 1970

20. Cavagna GA, Stemmler EJ, DuBois AB: Alveolar resistance to atelectasis. J Appl Physiol 22:441–452, 1967
21. Cherniack RM, Farhi LE, Armstrong BW, Proctor DF: A comparison of esophageal and intrapleural pressure in man. J Appl Physiol 8:203–211, 1955
22. Colebatch HJH, Mitchell CA: Constriction of isolated living liquid-filled dog and cat lungs with histamine. J Appl Physiol 30:691–702, 1971
23. Cook CD, Mead J, Orzalesi MM: Static volume-pressure characteristics of the respiratory system during maximal efforts. J Appl Physiol 19:1016–1022, 1964
24. D'Angelo E, Michelini S, Agostoni E: Partition of factors contributing to the vertical gradient of transpulmonary pressure. Respir Physiol 12:90–101, 1971
25. Defares JG, Donleben PG: Relationship between frequency-dependent compliance and unequal ventilation. J Appl Physiol 15:166–169, 1960
26. Douglas JS, Dennis MW, Ridgway P, Bouhuys A: Airway dilatation and constriction in spontaneously breathing guinea pigs. J Pharmacol Exp Ther 180: 98–109, 1972
27. Einthoven W: Der Donders'sche Druck und die Gasspannungen in der Pleurahöhle. Pfluegers Arch 44:152–174, 1888
28. Eriksson S: Studies of alpha$_1$-antitrypsin deficiency. Acta Med Scand 177 (suppl 432): 1–85, 1965
29. Faulkner M, Sharpey-Schafer EP: Circulatory effects of trumpet playing. Br Med J 1:685–686, 1959
30. Finucane KE, Colebatch HJH: Elastic behavior of the lung in patients with airway obstruction. J Appl Physiol 26: 330–338, 1969
31. Fisher MJ, Wilson MF, Weber KC: Determination of alveolar surface area and tension from *in situ* pressure-volume data. Respir Physiol 10:159–171, 1970
32. Forrest JB: The effect of changes in lung volume on the size and shape of alveoli. J Physiol (Lond) 210:533–547, 1970
33. Fukaya H, Martin CJ, Young AC, Katsura S: Mechanical properties of alveolar walls. J Appl Physiol 25:689–695, 1968
34. Glogowska M, Richardson PS, Widdicombe JG, Winning AJ: The role of the vagus nerves, peripheral chemoreceptors and other afferent pathways in the genesis of augmented breaths in cats and rabbits. Respir Physiol 16:179–196, 1972
35. Gold WM, Kaufman HS, Nadel JA: Elastic recoil of the lungs in chronic asthmatic patients before and after therapy. J Appl Physiol 23:433–438, 1967
36. Guyatt AR, Douglas JS, Zuskin E, Bouhuys A: Lung static recoil and airway obstruction in hemp workers with byssinosis. Am Rev Respir Dis 108:1111–1115, 1973
37. Hoffman L, Blumenfeld OO, Mondshine RB, Park SS: Effect of DL-penicillamine on fibrous proteins of rat lung. J Appl Physiol 33:42–46, 1972
38. Hoffman L, Mondshine RB, Park SS: Effect of DL-penicillamine on elastic properties of rat lung. J Appl Physiol 30:508–511, 1971
39. Horie T, Hildebrandt J: Dynamic compliance, limit cycles and static equilibria of excised cat lung. J Appl Physiol 31: 423–430, 1971
40. Hughes JMB, Rosenzweig DY: Factors affecting trapped gas volume in perfused dog lungs. J Appl Physiol 29:332–339, 1970
41. Hughes JMB, Rosenzweig DY, Kivitz PB: Site of airway closure in excised dog lungs: histologic demonstration. J Appl Physiol 29:340–344, 1970
42. Ingram RH Jr, Schilder DP: Association of a decrease in dynamic compliance with a change in gas distribution. J Appl Physiol 23:911–916, 1967
43. Jaeger MJ, Otis AB: Effects of compressibility of alveolar gas on dynamics and work of breathing. J Appl Physiol 19:83–91, 1964
44. Jonson B: A flow-regulating valve for use in respiratory physiology. Scand J Clin Lab Invest 24:127–130, 1969
45. Jonson B: Pulmonary mechanics in normal men, studied with the flow regulator method. Scand J Clin Lab Invest 25: 363–373, 1970
46. Jonson B: Pulmonary mechanics in patients with pulmonary disease, studied with the flow regulator method. Scand J Clin Lab Invest 25:375–390, 1970
47. Klingele TG, Staub NC: Alveolar shape changes with volume in isolated, air-filled lobes of cat lung. J Appl Physiol 28:411–414, 1970

48. Klingele TG, Staub NC: Terminal bronchiole diameter changes with volume in isolated, air-filled lobes of cat lung. J Appl Physiol 30:224–227, 1971
49. Konno K, Mead J: Static volume-pressure characteristics of the rib cage and abdomen. J Appl Physiol 24:544–548, 1968
50. Landowne M, Stacy RW: Glossary of Terms, in Remington JW (ed): Tissue Elasticity. Washington, D. C., American Physiological Society, 1957, pp 191–201
51. Leith DE, Mead J: Mechanisms determining residual volume of the lungs in normal subjects. J Appl Physiol 23:221–227, 1967
52. Liljestrand G: Untersuchungen über die Atmungsarbeit. Skand Arch Physiol 35: 199–293, 1918
53. Macklem PT, Becklake MR: The relationship between the mechanical and diffusing properties of the lung in health and disease. Am Rev Respir Dis 87: 47–56, 1963
54. Mead J: Control of respiratory frequency. J Appl Physiol 15:325–336, 1960
55. Mead J: Mechanical properties of lungs. Physiol Rev 41:281–330, 1961
56. Mead J, Milic-Emili J, Turner JM: Factors limiting depth of a maximal inspiration in human subjects. J Appl Physiol 18:295–296, 1963
57. Mead J, Takishima T, Leith D: Stress distribution in lungs: a model of pulmonary elasticity. J Appl Physiol 28: 596–608, 1970
58. McIlroy MB, Marshall R, Christie RV: The work of breathing in normal subjects. Clin Sci 13:127–136, 1954
59. Milic-Emili J, Mead J, Turner JM, Glauser EM: Improved technique for estimating pleural pressure from esophageal balloons. J Appl Physiol 19:207–211, 1964
60. Naimark A, Cherniack RM: Compliance of the respiratory system and its components in health and obesity. J Appl Physiol 15:377–382, 1960
61. Ostrow DN, Cherniack RM: The mechanical properties of the lungs in intermediate deficiency of α_1-antitrypsin. Am Rev Respir Dis 106:377–383, 1972
62. Otis AB: The work of breathing, in Fenn WO, Rahn H (eds): Handbook of Physiology, Section 3: Respiration, vol I. Washington, D.C., American Physiological Society, 1964, pp 463–476
63. Park SS, Goldring IP, Shim CS, Williams MH Jr: Mechanical properties of the lung in experimental pulmonary emphysema. J Appl Physiol 26:738–744, 1969
64. Pierce JA: Tensile strength of human lung. J Lab Clin Med 66:652–658, 1965
65. Pierce JA, Ebert RV: Fibrous network of the lung and its change with age. Thorax 20:469–476, 1965
66. Pratt PC: Intrapulmonary radial traction: Measurement, magnitude and mechanics, in Bouhuys A (ed): Airway Dynamics: Physiology and Pharmacology. Springfield, Charles C Thomas Publisher, 1970, pp 109–122
67. Proctor DF, Caldini P, Permutt S: The pressure surrounding the lungs. Respir Physiol 5:130–144, 1968
68. Radford E Jr: Recent studies of mechanical properties of mammalian lungs, in Remington JW (ed): Tissue Elasticity. Washington, D.C., American Physiological Society, 1957, pp 177–190
69. Rahn H, Otis AB, Chadwick LE, Fenn WO: The pressure-volume diagram of the thorax and lung. Am J Physiol 146:161–178, 1946
70. Raimondi AC, Massarella GR, Pride NB: The effects of ventilation on the elastic recoil of excised dogs' lungs. Respir Physiol 12:205–217, 1971
71. Slagter B, Heemstra H: Limiting factors of expiration in normal subjects. Acta Physiol Pharmacol Neerl 4:419–421, 1955
72. Sugihara T, Hildebrandt J, Martin CJ: Viscoelastic properties of alveolar wall. J Appl Physiol 33:93–98, 1972
73. Trop D, Peeters R, van de Woestijne KP: Localization of recording site in the esophagus by means of cardiac artifacts. J Appl Physiol 29:283–287, 1970
74. Turner JM, Mead J, Wohl ME: Elasticity of human lungs in relation to age. J Appl Physiol 25:664–671, 1968
75. van de Woestijne KP: Influence of forced inflations on the creep of lungs and thorax in the dog. Respir Physiol 3:78–89, 1967
76. West JB: Distribution of mechanical stress in the lung, a possible factor in localisation of pulmonary disease. Lancet 1:839–841, 1971

77. West JB, Matthews FL: Stresses, strains, and surface pressures in the lung caused by its weight. J Appl Physiol 32:332–345, 1972
78. Wood TE, McLeod P, Anthonisen NR, Macklem PT: Mechanics of breathing in mitral stenosis. Am Rev Respir Dis 104: 52–60, 1971
79. Woolcock AJ, Vincent NJ, Macklem PT: Frequency dependence of compliance as a test for obstruction in the small airways. J Clin Invest 48:1097–1106, 1969

Chapter 8

Pressure-Flow Relations

Airflow through the airways requires a driving pressure generated by changes in alveolar pressure (Chap. 7). When alveolar pressure is less than atmospheric pressure and the airways are open, air flows in; when Palv is greater than Patm, air flows out. In this chapter we relate Palv to the resulting flows and discuss variables that influence these relations.

PHYSICS OF AIRFLOW

Flow Patterns

Airflow patterns through tubes can be laminar or turbulent; special patterns arise when tube diameter varies (orifice flow) and when the tube branches (Fig. 8-1). In long, straight, smooth-walled, rigid cylindrical tubes, airflow increases in proportion to driving pressure (Fig. 8-2A). But when flow increases, this relationship changes and becomes alinear because flow becomes turbulent beyond a limit set by the Reynolds' number—a dimensionless value that depends upon the linear velocity of the gas, the radius of the tube, and the properties of the gas. Linear gas velocity ($\dot{v}$) relates to $\dot{V}$ (flow rate) and the cross-sectional area of the tube:

$$\dot{V} = \dot{v} \cdot A \tag{1}$$

In the bronchial tree, total cross-sectional area increases greatly toward the periphery (Table 2-1); since flow through each cross section is constant, linear gas velocity decreases and conditions for laminar flow improve.

In the *upper airways,* the complex geometry causes flow patterns that do not fit any of the types shown in Figure 8-1.[25] In the *bronchial tree,* the predominant pattern varies with size (Chap. 3, p. 48): turbulence in trachea and large bronchi,[42] laminar flow in smaller bronchi (down to the 12th generation, approximately), and convective block flow and axial diffusion in the smallest airways. Other patterns

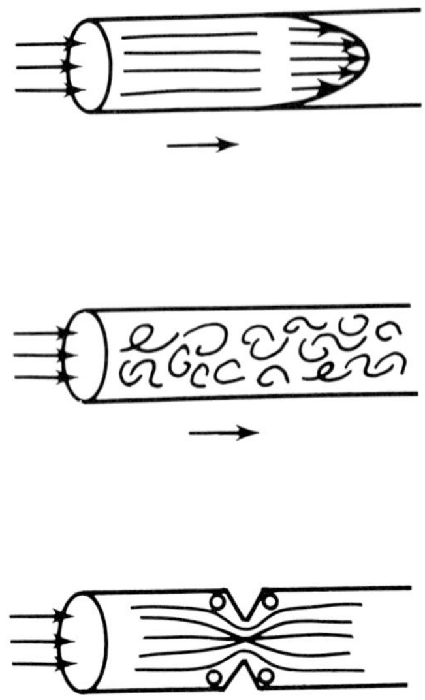

Fig. 8-1. Airflow patterns. *A*. Laminar flow. A flat gas front at the tube entrance is converted to a parabolic velocity front at a point several diameters removed from the entrance of the tube. Length of arrows is proportional to linear gas velocity. Energy is lost in friction between layers of gas; layers nearer to the wall are increasingly slowed down. All molecules move in the direction of flow. *B*. Turbulent flow. Due to increased velocity and a high Reynolds' number, the layers of moving gas (in *A*) have broken up. Gas molecules move in all directions through the lumen of the tube causing extra energy loss. Because of the direction of the driving pressure, there is net motion of gas in the direction of the arrow. *C*. Orifice flow. Gas velocities increase as the lumen of the tube narrows. Vortices may develop in the corners as indicated. In the orifice, kinetic energy of the gas (mv^2) increases and lateral pressure (potential energy) decreases.

are, however, superimposed on these. Vortices, which develop during inspiration and expiration (Fig. 8-3),[52] help mix the gas streams through the cross section of the tubes. In the branchings, the flow profile changes, to a large extent independently of the incoming flow profile (i.e., flat or parabolic). Velocity in the branches is greater near the inside walls (Fig. 8-3). Some authors consider the effect of the branches so important that they see the bronchial tree "as a series of interconnected junctions rather than as a series of branched tubes." [52]

Energy Losses

The relation between driving pressure and flow in tubes depends on the flow pattern. Thus, study of energy losses during flow gives indirect information on the flow pattern. During laminar, or Poiseuille, flow the driving pressure is dissipated in friction between moving layers of air and converted to heat. Airways do not fulfill the strict requirements of laminar flow conditions: they are short, branched, elastic, not quite straight, with uneven wall surfaces, and are not always cylindrical. These deviations from ideal tubes lead to extra losses of energy, in what Rohrer called "extra resistances." [51] Consequently, flow increments decrease as driving pressure increases; the P-$\dot{V}$ relations are curvilinear (Fig. 8-2B).

Laminar flow depends on gas viscosity, while energy losses in vortices, turbulence, and other flow patterns that deviate from laminar flow are influenced by gas density. Since departures from laminar flow are more pronounced in large than in small airways, gas density affects flow through the former more than flow through the latter (see also Chap. 9, p. 207).

In *upper airways* (airway opening to trachea) air flows through channels of relatively fixed geometry (except during speech). The nose is a high-resistance

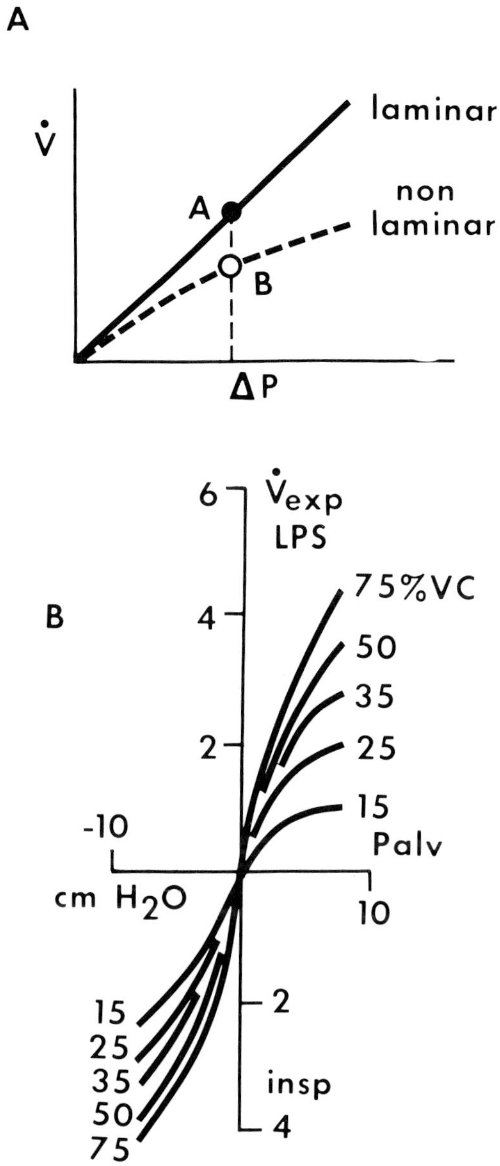

Fig. 8-2. *A*. Linear pressure-flow relation during laminar flow; alinear relation during nonlaminar flow (i.e., turbulence, orifice flow, branching or vortices, etc.). The same driving pressure ΔP yields higher flows during laminar (A) than during nonlaminar (B) flow. *B*. Pressure-flow relations in airways depend on lung volume during inspiration (left lower quadrant) and expiration (right upper quadrant). $\dot{V}_{insp}$ and $\dot{V}_{exp}$ are inspiratory and expiratory flow rates, respectively; Palv = alveolar pressure. From reference 4.

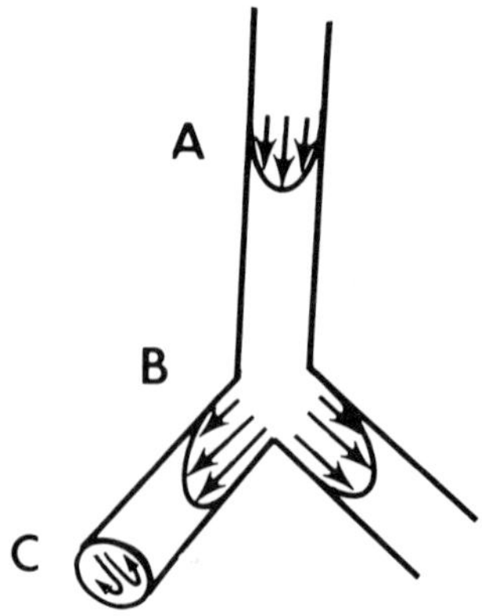

Fig. 8-3. In the daughter branches, a parabolic velocity front (*A*) is converted to an asymmetrical front with high velocities near the inside wall (*B*). Vortices also develop (*C*). Modified from reference 52.

pathway, the mouth a low-resistance one. When the pressure drop across the nasal passages exceeds about 4 cm H_2O, healthy persons begin to breathe through their mouths.[45] Even during mouth breathing, about 50 percent of the total energy loss during breathing (in terms of pressure drop) occurs in the upper airways. Some of this loss is caused by redirection of flow in the pharynx; another part is due to the resistance of the glottal opening to flow. For unclear reasons, both total upper-airway resistance and laryngeal resistance depend on lung volume, increasing as lung volume decreases.[55] Typical pressure drops for 1 liter/sec flow are 0.83 cm H_2O from mouth to trachea, and 0.31 cm H_2O across the larynx, both during quiet breathing at mid-lung volume.[55] The size of the glottal opening decreases with decreasing lung volume and flow rates; it is widest during panting. The mechanisms affecting glottal opening are not clear.[56]

In the *bronchial tree,* about 75 percent of the pressure drop is spent on changing the flow profiles, e.g., from flow with a uniform velocity ("flat front") to a parabolic front.[41] The branches per se and the change in cross-sectional area each account for about 10 percent of the total pressure drop. These losses are not equal in all generations; the largest pressure drop (80 percent of the total) occurs in the first 4 to 6 airway generations, i.e., in the trachea and large bronchi.[41, 47] As air enters the trachea through the narrow glottal chink, secondary turbulences are created in the upper part of the trachea.[42] Otherwise, turbulent flow is not an important source of energy loss. The actual pressure drops are less than would be calculated for turbulent flow; factors related to airway geometry are more important sources of energy loss.[41] During inspiration, gas velocities decrease as gas enters smaller airways with a large total cross-sectional area (divergent flow); during expiration, velocities increase as gas leaves the bronchial tree (convergent flow). The energy losses due to these changes in the kinetic energy of the gas stream are small but increase with flow rate.[23, 41]

Energy losses during flow, other than those in the gas itself, are caused by viscous properties of tissues and by the presence of mucus in airways. Energy losses due to acceleration of the *chest wall* are negligible in healthy persons and are increased in obesity, where they conceivably may limit maximum flows and cough velocities.[53] Viscous losses in *lung tissue* depend more on tidal volume and breathing level than on flow rate.[3] Therefore, lung tissue resistance is in fact a consequence of tissue hysteresis (p. 152). *Airway mucus* is a source of extra energy loss when the thickness of the mucus layer exceeds 300 μm.[12] The shearing forces between air and liquid then agitate the liquid when flow increases, leading to roughness of the liquid surface or even eddies of liquid that may move through the lumen. When this happens, the pressure drop increases sharply since it then depends on the force to move the liquid rather than the air (Fig. 8-4). The liquid's physical properties affect these events: a layer of thin liquid is more easily disturbed than a more tenacious mucus layer. This is an important source of energy loss whenever bronchial secretions are increased, as in bronchitis.

Pressure-Flow Relations

Since energy losses in airways are larger than would be expected if flow were laminar, pressure-flow curves are alinear (Fig. 8-2B). Calculations of pressure drops based on the assumption of laminar flow throughout the bronchial tree [20] yield smaller pressure drops than those actually observed. Equations that correct for nonparabolic flow profiles are more accurate [47] and also account for changes

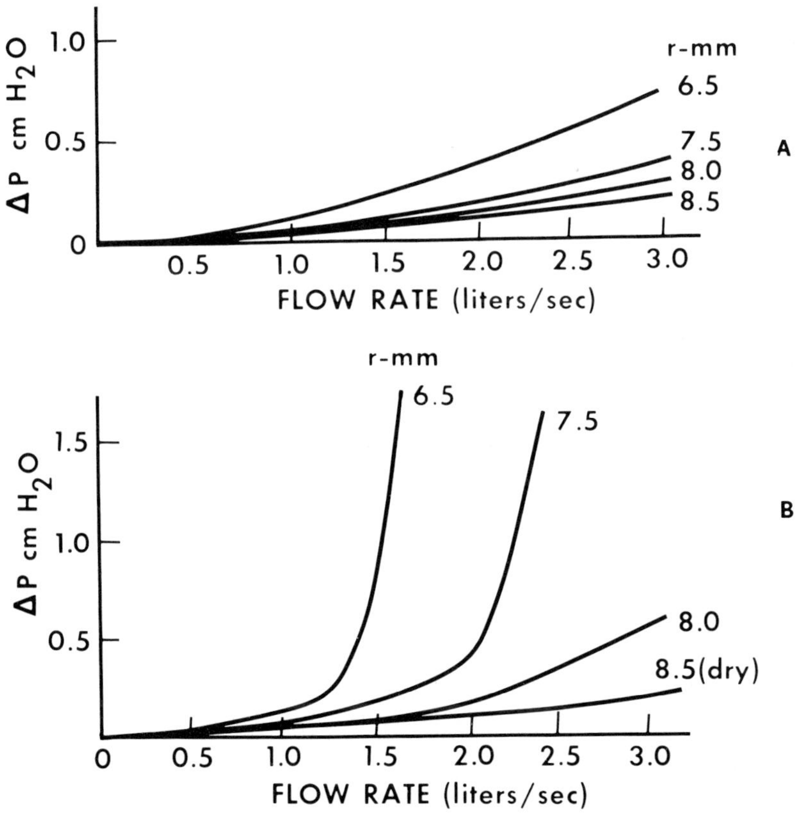

Fig. 8-4. *A, B. Ordinate:* driving pressure for airflow through tubes of different caliber. *Abscissa:* flow rate. The parameter (r) is the radius of several dry tubes (*A*) and the effective radius of a dry tube of 8.5 mm radius in which the caliber is reduced by layers of liquid of varying thickness (*B*). When waves appear in the liquid, resistance increases abruptly. From reference 12.

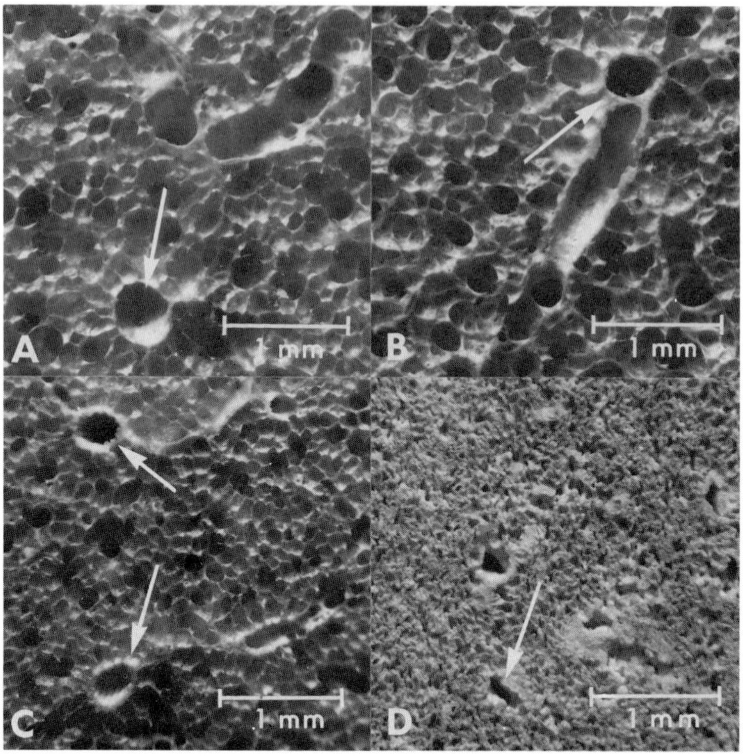

Fig. 8-5. Terminal bronchioles (*arrows*) in freeze-dried cat lungs. Lung volume: *A*, 100%; *B*, 48%; *C*, 23%; *D*, 8% of maximal lobe volume. Airway caliber decreases with lung volume. At the lowest volume (*D*), the terminal bronchioles are thick-walled and kinked but not closed. From reference 29.

in pressure drops when gases of different densities are breathed.[25] Especially in the first 10 airway generations, pressure drops are much greater than would be expected from laminar flow predictions.

Airway caliber increases with lung volume (Fig. 8-5). Therefore, $P\text{-}\dot{V}$ relations cannot be described by a single curve but rather by a family of curves, with lung volume as the parameter (Fig. 8-2*B*). At low driving pressures, inspired and expired flows are similar; as they increase, the $P\text{-}\dot{V}$ curves for inspiration and expiration diverge. Inspiratory flow continues to increase to a limit set mainly by the ability of the inspiratory muscles to contract rapidly (p. 196). Alveolar and pleural pressures are increasingly subatmospheric during inspiration. Hence, the airways in the chest are exposed to an increasing pull on their outside walls, transmitted through the elastic structure of the lungs and through the pleural space. During expiration, however, alveolar and pleural pressures increase, and Ppl exceeds Patm during fast expirations (Fig. 7-7*C*). The high pressures in the chest cage lead to dynamic compression of airways, which narrows them and limits further increases of expiratory flow.

FORCED EXPIRATION

Dynamic Compression

During forced expiration, airway geometry changes radically. A large segment of the trachea and bronchi in the chest cage is compressed when flow is high (hence "dynamic") due to the high pleural pressures that are developed to generate high alveolar pressures. This phenomenon has been described since 1892 (reference 5 gives a historical survey), but accurate observations have only been made recently. The compressed airway segment may occupy several generations of large intrathoracic airways, and its length varies. At large lung volumes the compressed airway segment is short; its length increases as lung volume decreases. It is important to realize that dynamic compression is a physiologic event occurring in all healthy persons during forced expirations and cough maneuvers.

The anatomical extent of dynamic compression can be seen during bronchoscopy or in suitably timed x-ray films of airways lined with contrast medium. The speed at which flow and pressures change during dynamic compression can be shown with the body plethysmograph (Fig. 8-6), which records the sudden compression of alveolar gas that occurs when its pressure rises.[54] When lung volume is known, Palv can be calculated. Near the end of a forced expiration, alveolar pressure increases sharply and suddenly, while airflow decreases. In about 0.2 seconds (between lines *b* and *c* in Fig. 8-6), Palv increases from about +10 to +25 cm H_2O. These events reflect the onset of dynamic compression of large airways.

Models of Pressure-Flow Relations

During forced expiration, dynamic compression is a predominant factor in determining pressure-flow relations, while other factors, such as the effect of branching, become relatively less important. Thus, the altered airway geometry markedly changes the pressure-flow relations from those during quiet breathing.

During dynamic compression of large airways, expiratory flow reaches maximum values, and P-$\dot{V}$ curves therefore show plateaus—further pressure increases do not yield flow increments (see Fig. 8-10*A*). Many variables that affect flow through airways cannot be measured directly (caliber, length, muscle tone, thickness of mucus layer). Analysis of theoretical models allows one to vary these factors one at a time and to examine the effect of each on simulated flow. In this way, hypotheses concerning airflow dynamics can be formulated and compared with experimental data obtained on the total system. Unfortunately, since many variables needed in model studies have been insufficiently quantitated, the results must be interpreted with caution.

Several formal models [17, 44, 60] include a precise description of the system, in simple or complex form, suitable for insertion of experimental data. These models are complete in the sense that they offer a mathematical description of the system. All assumptions and simplifications made in the model design can be clearly defined. Less complete, more intuitive models concentrate on specific character-

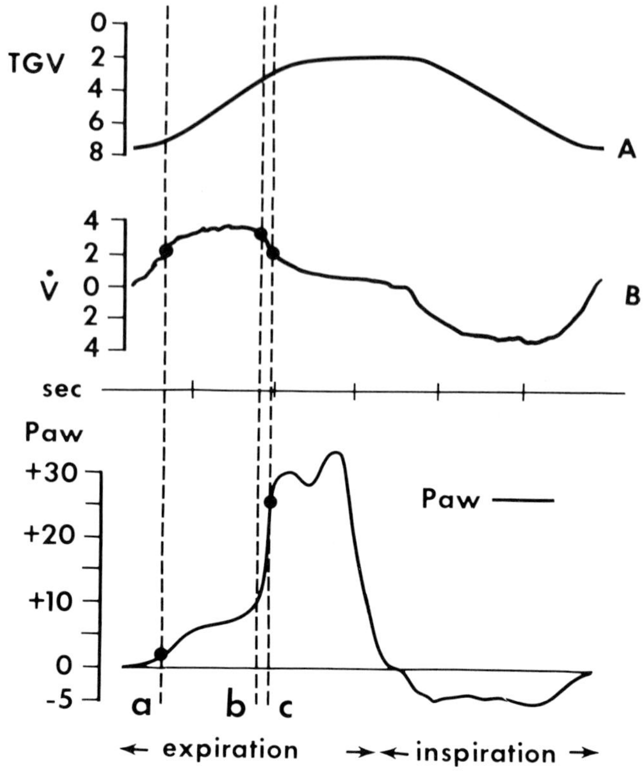

Fig. 8-6. *Upper panel.* From top down, thoracic gas volume (*A*) and airflow rate at mouth (*B*). *Lower panel.* Pressure across airways (alveoli-mouth, Paw, cm H_2O) measured with body plethysmograph. *Abscissa.* Time in seconds. During *inspiration,* the pressure (Paw) and flow (*B*) traces are similar in shape; pressure and flow change in the same direction. During *expiration* this is only true in the initial phase (*a–b*). From *b* to *c,* pressure (Paw) increases sharply, while flow rate decreases. This reflects the onset of dynamic compression of large airways. Modified from reference 6.

istics of the system and use these to derive a theory concerning the whole.[34, 50] Each of these models illustrates important physiological principles.

Many features of pressure-flow curves can be explained with a simple model of airway geometry (Fig. 8-7).[60] The peripheral airways, suspended without cartilage in the structure of the lungs, are represented by a distal airway segment (1); its resistance to flow is a function of lung volume.[29] The intermediate segment (2) is dynamically compressed during forced expirations, and has a resistance determined primarily by the pressure difference across its walls. Finally, the upper airways form a proximal segment (3) with a fixed resistance. In this model [60] the critical variable is the pressure at which segment 2 begins to compress, or the critical transmural pressure, Ptm′.[50] With different values of Ptm′, the model predicts many physiological features of pressure-flow relations. Palv is the independent variable that drives the model. Although the model is simple, it can simulate the main features of IVPF curves (p. 184) and MEFV curves (Chap. 9), and it allows qualitative estimates of effects of airway obstruction and loss of lung recoil force.

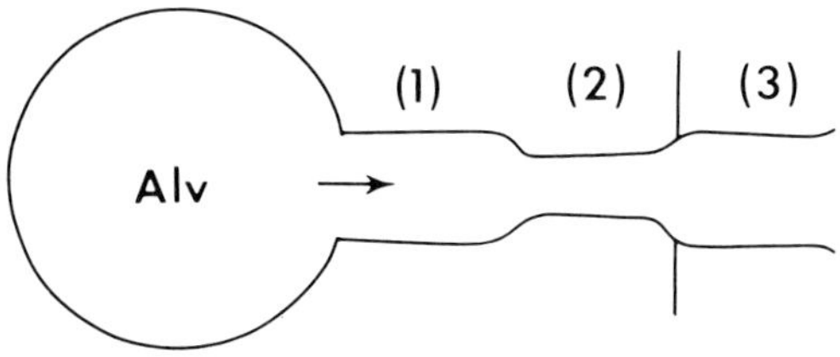

Fig. 8-7. Simple model of expiratory airflow. See text for description of segments 1, 2, and 3. A formal description of this model has been given by Yamabayashi et al.[60]

A much more complex model[44] calculates pressure drops associated with flow based on airway geometry, gas properties, and energy losses in airways. It simulates IVPF and MEFV curves more accurately than the simple model of Figure 8-7. As in other models, lung elastic recoil and airway wall compliance are the main variables affecting pressure-flow relations during forced expirations. Also, beyond a critical driving pressure, corresponding to the pressure at which maximum flows are reached, airways become unstable in this model.[44]

In Fry's model[17] the precise description of transmural stress across the airway walls is crucial in determining the pressure-flow relations. In particular the final configuration of the compliant airways is important, as shown for plastic tubes in Figure 8-8. If the tube closes at infinitely high pressures (1 in Fig. 8-8), the P-$\dot{V}$ curve reaches a plateau. If the tube does not close completely at any pressure, flow first levels off to a plateau, but as driving pressure increases further, flow resumes its increase; this represents flow through a maximally narrowed tube which cannot be further compressed (2 in Fig. 8-8). Finally, if the tube closes at a finite compressing pressure (3 in Fig. 8-8), flow reaches a maximum and then becomes unstable. When the tube closes, flow stops; as a result, dynamic compression is reduced and flow resumes. Hence, airflow oscillates, and conditions in the tube depend on time as an additional variable. Experimental data in man have also suggested unstable airway behavior during maximum flow,[6] similar to that of the plastic tube of Figure 8-8, 3.

Equal Pressure Point Theory

In the airways, pressure decreases in the direction of flow. During expiration at high flow rates, somewhere inside the airways the pressure must equal Ppl (Fig. 8-9). This is because Palv is always greater than Ppl by the amount of Pst(l) (Eq. 7-2, p. 155). The pressure difference between the alveoli and the equal pressure point (EPP) equals Palv−Ppl=Pst(l). Hence, the driving pressure for flow from alveoli to the EPP equals the static lung recoil pressure.[34] The flow rate through the upstream airway segment (U in Fig. 8-9) must equal flow through the downstream segment (D) and the upper airways because the three are in series. Since the model applies to conditions of maximum flow, this flow rate equals $\dot{V}_{max}$. Therefore, the flow resistance of the upstream segment is given by Rus=Pst(l)/$\dot{V}_{max}$[34] and can thus be calculated from two measurable quantities, Pst(l) and $\dot{V}_{max}$.

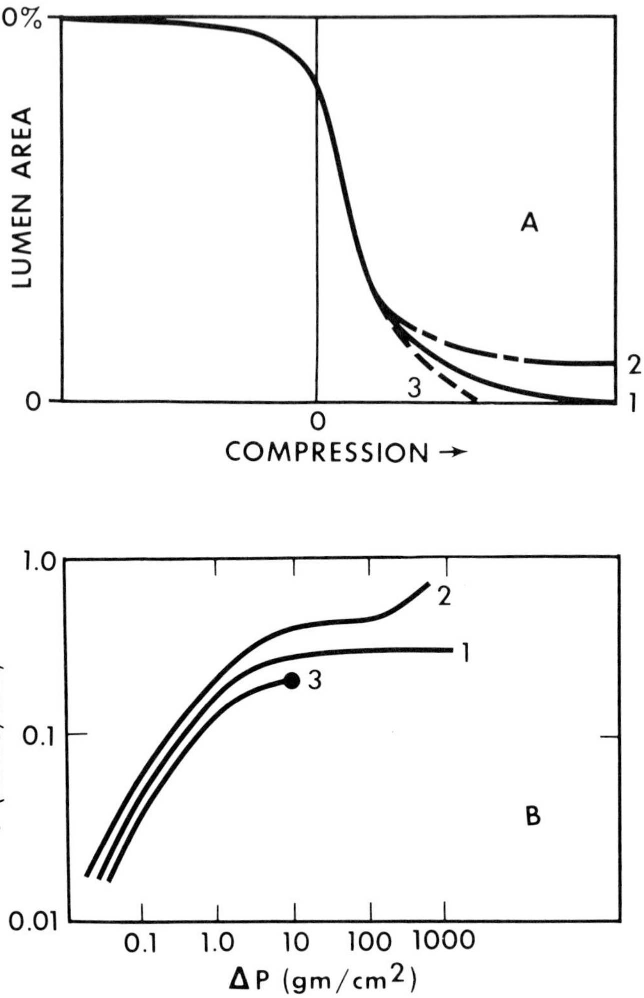

Fig. 8-8. Behavior of plastic tubes (Penrose tubing) at high flow rates. *A*. Pressure-lumen area diagram (100% = wide open; 0% = closed). Zero ordinate = resting position of tube. Lines 1, 2, and 3 indicate different tube configurations under compressing pressures, corresponding to the pressure-flow curves 1, 2, and 3 in *B*. Curve 3 terminates at the black dot; at higher pressures, pressure-flow relations are unstable and cannot be described by a line. See also text. Modified from reference 17.

The EPP model directs attention to the important role of Pst(l) as a driving pressure for airflow. It explains why $\dot{V}_{max}$ decreases when the lungs have lost elastic recoil or when peripheral airways are obstructed (Chap. 9). Confusion can arise, though, from unwarranted extensions of the concept. For instance, while the pressure relations show clearly that there must be an EPP somewhere along the airway, its location cannot be determined accurately in anatomical terms. The EPP does not separate the uncompressed and the compressed airway segment. Dynamic compression probably begins somewhere downstream from the EPP, where a sufficiently strong transmural compressing pressure develops during forced expiration.

As Ppl and Palv increase at a given volume, the EPP travels upstream, begin-

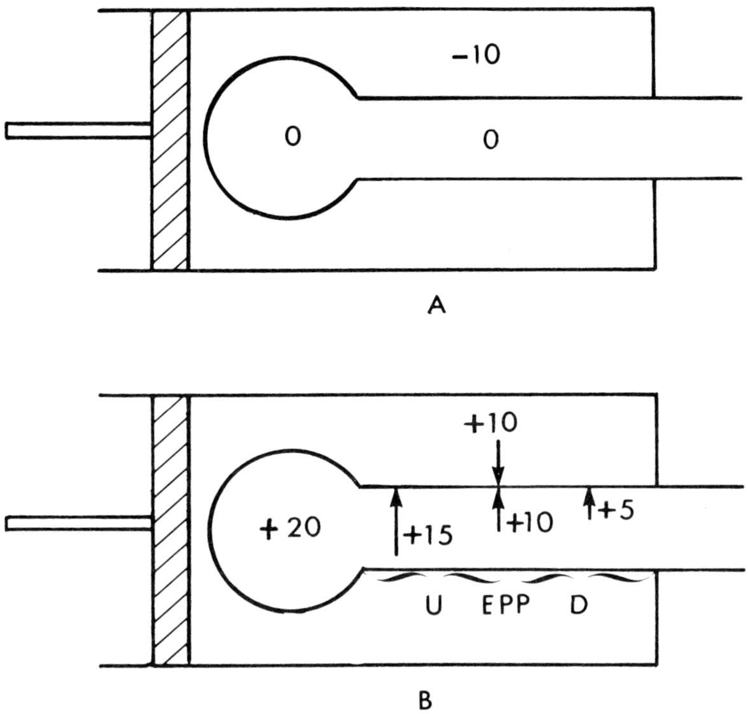

Fig. 8-9. The equal pressure point (EPP) model.[34] *A*. No airflow. Ppl=Pst(l) =−10 cm H_2O. Palv = 0. *B*. Maximum expiratory flow. Palv = +20 cm H_2O. Ppl= −10+20= +10 cm H_2O [Eq. (2), Chap. 7]. At EPP, pressure in airway=Ppl= +10 cm H_2O. U=upstream, D=downstream segment. A more complete set of similar diagrams has been discussed elsewhere.[4, 57]

ning in the trachea at the chest cage inlet. It stops when dynamic compression is fully established and flow has reached its maximum value at that volume. As lung volume decreases, Pst(l) decreases and Ppl for the same Palv must increase (see Fig. 7-6, p. 157). Unless the compressed airway segment is highly compliant, the EPP moves toward the periphery with decreasing lung volume. At the same time, the compressed airway segment lengthens, as can be observed directly in excised lungs where the pressure outside the extrapulmonary airways is known.[31]

The Flow-Limiting Segment

Once the large airways are dynamically compressed, upstream pressure variations no longer affect flow. Rather, flow is determined by the difference between the extrabronchial (compressing) pressure and the pressure at the airway opening. This behavior is that of a Starling resistor.[50] However, the compressed segment is unstable and vibrates,[6, 18] and its behavior is highly complex. Wheezing during forced expirations probably results from the vibrations in the compressed airway segment as well as in the larynx. The concept of a critical transmural pressure at which compression begins is elusive—it is difficult to define in an oscillating airway segment and depends on airway wall compliance. The latter varies as a function of cartilage content and structure and of smooth muscle tone.[40, 43] The Starling resistor theory predicts increased maximum flow after smooth muscle relaxation;[50] in fact, flow rates may remain the same or increase or decrease in healthy persons.[7, 59]

Airway Wall Compliance

During quiet breathing, movements of airway walls are minimal. During deep and forced breathing, their caliber changes to an extent determined by airway wall stiffness. The pressure-diameter curve of isolated airways is S shaped (as in the tubes of Fig. 8-8); most of the caliber change occurs in a narrow range of pressures. In small airways, smooth muscle tone, attachments to lung tissue, and perhaps surface forces in the epithelial lining are the principal factors affecting wall compliance.[36] In large airways, cartilage and muscle tone are its principal determinants. Smooth muscle contraction can change the trachea into a nearly rigid tube, protected against compression by overlapping cartilage edges.[40] Muscle tone itself also changes tracheal compliance, and graded increases in tracheal stiffness can be achieved by electrical stimulation of the nerve in an isolated preparation.[43] Thus, tracheal compressibility might be subject to physiological regulation.

Relaxing muscle tone makes large airways more flaccid and compressible and may lead to decreased maximum expiratory flows in healthy persons.[7] In contrast, reducing muscle tone in small airways leads to increased caliber and higher maximum expiratory flows. An operational definition of small and large airways can be based on this difference in the consequences of muscle tone changes.[4] *Small airways* are unprotected by cartilage and have a thick layer of smooth muscle. Their caliber decreases with increasing muscle tone. *Large airways,* however, are protected against caliber changes by cartilage—during quiet breathing, muscle tone does not greatly affect their caliber; during dynamic compression, their tone provides wall rigidity and thus prevents compression and enhances maximum flows. During dynamic compression, the effects of muscle tone on airway caliber and maximum flows are opposite in small and large airways.[4, 7]

EXPERIMENTAL MEASUREMENTS

Isovolume Pressure-Flow (IVPF) Curves

Since pressure-flow relations depend on lung volume, they cannot be described by a single curve, but rather by a family of curves, with lung volume as the parameter (Fig. 8-2*B*). These curves differ during inspiration and expiration; they show flow limitation during expiration, and they can be altered by changing the density of the inspired gas.[19]

The three variables (volume, pressure, flow) can be measured with different methods. Flow is recorded with a flowmeter at the mouth; this signal can be integrated to obtain lung volume changes. Alternatively, volume changes can be measured with a body plethysmograph,[14] which can provide lung volume in absolute terms if thoracic gas volume is also measured.[28] Palv can be measured from esophageal pressure (Pes) records or from plethysmographic recordings. The shape of IVPF curves differs when volume is recorded at the mouth or with a body plethysmograph: the latter "sees" the volume change due to both the volume of the gas expired and the volume of the gas compressed, while an instrument at the mouth measures only volume changes due to the volume of expired gas. The two volumes differ whenever Palv is not equal to zero; the difference is important when Palv is high.[6, 24] Measurements of Palv with the esophageal balloon[19, 34] or with the body plethysmograph[6] result in similar curves. The IVPF curves recorded with one method can be transferred into diagrams valid for another method by using the static recoil curve to relate Pes to Palv, and by using Boyle's law to calculate lung volume at Palv from volume measured at the mouth.[6] The choice between volume measurements at the mouth and plethysmographic volume measurements is discussed further in Chapter 9 (p. 212).

Volume-pressure-flow relations are described in graphs with two variables on the *x* and *y* axis and the third variable as the parameter. Pressure-flow (Fig. 8-10*A*) and flow-volume (Fig. 8-10*B*) diagrams are commonly used; in the first, volume is the parameter, and in the second, pressure. Diagram *A* is a set of IVPF curves; diagram *B* includes the MEFV curve (Chap. 9).

Inspiratory IVPF curves depend less on volume than expiratory IVPF curves (Fig. 8-10*A*). Due to dynamic compression, the expiratory curves have flow plateaus at low volumes. At large volumes, expiratory flow is limited by the velocity of muscle contraction (see below). In normal subjects, plateaus are observed at lung volumes up to about 80% of VC (range, 57–93 percent[58]). As lung volume decreases, the pressure needed to reach maximum flow decreases. At

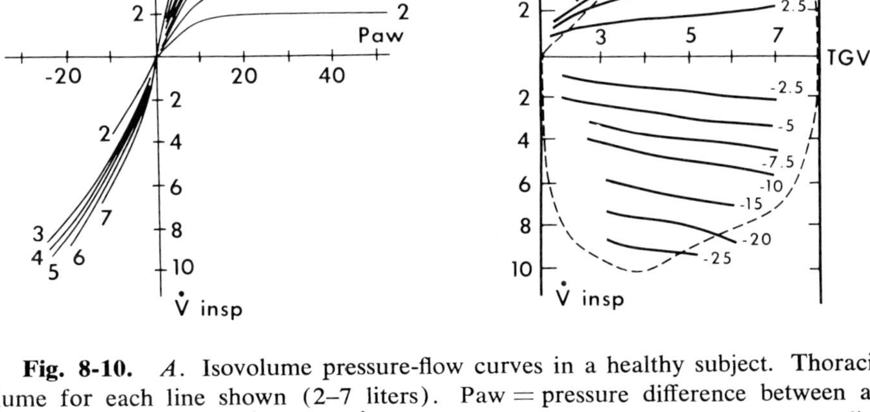

Fig. 8-10. *A*. Isovolume pressure-flow curves in a healthy subject. Thoracic gas volume for each line shown (2–7 liters). Paw = pressure difference between alveoli and mouth (cm H_2O). $\dot{V}_{exp}$ and $\dot{V}_{insp}$ in liters per second. *B*. Flow-volume diagram from same data as *A*. *Ordinate*. Same as *A*. *Abscissa*. Thoracic gas volume (TGV) in liters. Isobars for Paw in cm H_2O. *Dashed line*. Single forced inspiratory (below abscissa) and expiratory (above abscissa) vital capacity maneuvers. Modified from reference 6.

small lung volumes, very small alveolar pressures will lead to maximum flow rates. This can also be seen in diagram *B,* where pressure isobars indicate Palv values at different flows and volumes. The slope of these isobars, in particular during expiration, reflects the increased airway resistance (see below) as lung volume decreases.

A more detailed diagram of experimental points on IVPF curves is given in Figure 8-11. During inspiration and during expiration at low flows, the points are grouped closely together around the lines, which were drawn freehand. These data were obtained from large series of breaths recorded at different times and with varying breathing patterns. Thus, these pressure-flow relations appear to vary little with time or breathing pattern. When expiratory flow rates reach maximum values, the variability increases, as indicated by the hatched areas in Figure 8-11. Standardizing volume history (i.e., all expirations made from TLC) does not reduce this variability.[27, 58] Previous flow rates are important—during forced expirations maximum flows are often lower than during more relaxed expirations, with lower initial flows (see also Fig. 9-5, p. 209). In Figure 8-11, optimal IVPF curves were drawn through the highest flow points at each volume. Similar data

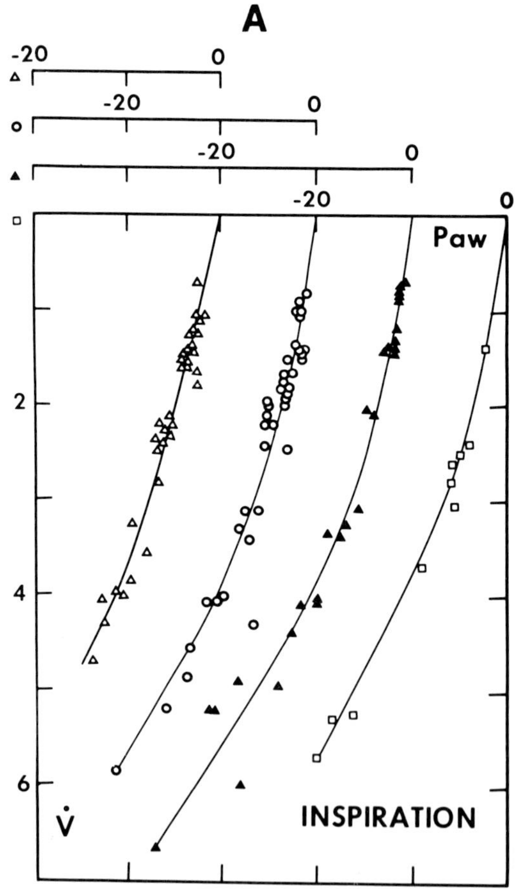

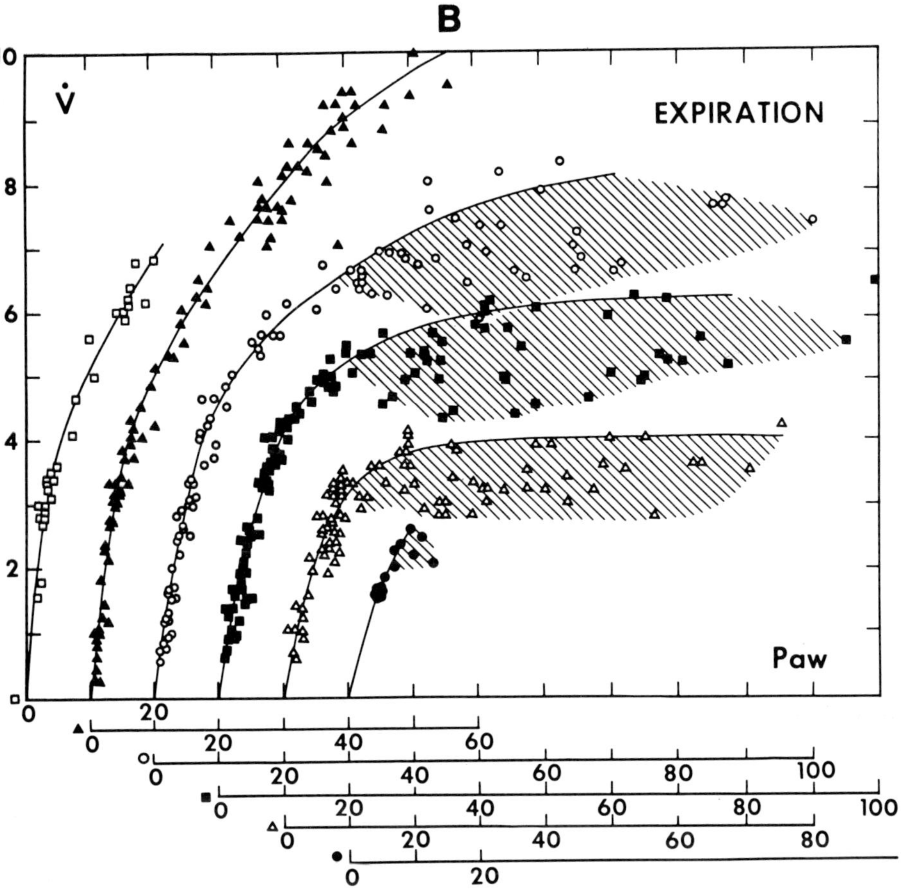

Fig. 8-11. Experimental isovolume pressure-flow data in a healthy subject. Zero points for Paw (see legend to Fig. 8-10) on abscissa are different for each IVPF curve, as indicated by the appropriate symbol next to each zero line, to avoid overlapping curves. Parameter: volume; □ = 6 liters, ▲ = 5 liters, ○ = 4 liters, ■ = 3.5 liters, △ = 3 liters, ● = 2.5 liters (thoracic gas volume at alveolar pressure). From reference 6.

are also shown as Paw isobars in the flow-volume diagram of Figure 8-10. These optimal isobars reach higher maximum flows, at a given volume, than were actually obtained during forced expirations.

Consequently, flow rates are often less than optimal during forced expirations[34] (see also Chap. 9, p. 205). In some subjects there may be a true "negative effort-dependence" of flow. That is, the IVPF curve goes through a maximum flow value and flow decreases when pressure increases further. However, this phenomenon occurs only in a few subjects.[34, 48] Time charts of the same data (e.g., Fig. 8-6) show that optimal flow rates always occur before dynamic compression becomes obvious (i.e., before *b* in Fig. 8-6). Suboptimal flows occur later. It appears that the onset of dynamic compression can vary, perhaps because of subtle differences in airway compliance or in the time course of transmural pressure changes. Thus, the mechanical behavior of large airways may vary subtly from breath to breath. Accurate information on transmural pressure changes during dynamic compression along the airway is not available and the precise course of the mechanical events is difficult to analyze.[48] Models of expiratory flow also suggest unstable conditions during maximum flow (p. 181). In addition, the shape of the compressed segment may vary.[46]

Equations Describing IVPF Curves

Two types of equations have been proposed

$$\text{Palv} = K_1 \cdot \dot{V} + K_2 \cdot \dot{V}^2 \qquad \text{(Rohrer's equation)}^{51}$$

$$\text{Palv} = k \cdot \dot{V}^n \qquad \text{(Ainsworth and Eveleigh's equation)}^{2}$$

Both describe pressure-flow relations accurately at low flows but underestimate Palv as flows increase, particularly for expiratory curves.[6] The constants in both equations vary with lung volume. Therefore, calculations of these constants from pressure-flow curves which have not been obtained under isovolume conditions carry little meaning. The constants have no physiological meaning but can serve to summarize portions of the curves as an empirical description.

Airway Resistance (Raw)

Airway resistance, the ratio of driving pressure to flow rate at any point on an IVPF curve, varies with lung volume and flow rate. The nearly linear initial parts of IVPF curves, near zero flow, represent values for resistance at low flow rates. Their slopes are, however, affected by the variable resistance of the glottis and depend on the exact maneuvers used.[56] Also, these slopes vary with volume and flow, and hence Raw depends on volume. At higher driving pressures, Raw increases owing to the alinearity of IVPF curves. A set of relations between Raw, lung volume, and flow rate is shown in Figure 8-12. Inspiratory resistance depends much less on volume than expiratory resistance, which increases sharply as dynamic compression narrows the large airways. The higher the flow rate, the larger the volume at which Raw begins to increase steeply. This steep increase reflects the plateau of IVPF curves.

Raw and its reciprocal, airway conductance (Gaw), can be measured with a body plethysmograph[14] using either panting breaths[13] or a rebreathing technique.[26, 28] Flow-resistive pressure differences can also be derived from Ppl measurements (Fig. 7-7*C*, p. 160); the result is then called pulmonary resistance (R1) rather than airway resistance. The total resistance (Rt) of the respiratory system (including chest wall) can be estimated by imposing oscillating flow patterns upon spontaneous breaths, e.g., with a loudspeaker placed in series with a mouthpiece. Like other methods, this technique requires careful control of lung volume levels;[16] it is not sensitive to small variations in resistance.[15]

Measurement of Raw during panting in the body plethysmograph at inspiratory flow rates of 0.5–1.0 liters/sec, and with simultaneous determination of thoracic gas volume (TGV), is the preferred method. The effect of lung volume on Raw is often taken into account by calculating specific conductance (SGaw), i.e., the Gaw/TGV ratio. Although this is sometimes useful for summarizing Gaw data,

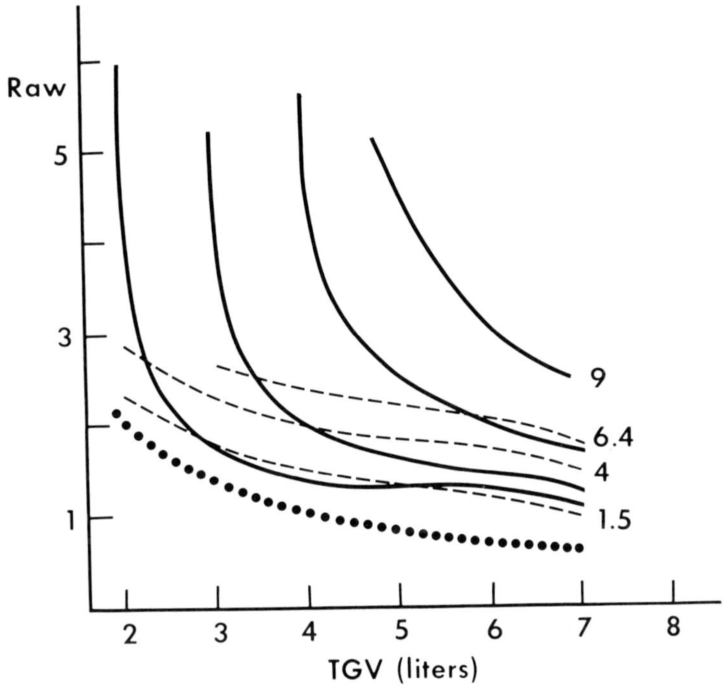

Fig. 8-12. Raw (cm H_2O/liter/sec) as a function of lung volume, with flow rate (1.5–9 liters/sec) as the parameter. *Drawn lines:* expiration; *dashed lines:* inspiration. These data were obtained with a rebreathing method.[28] Typical data for panting Raw (at lower flows) are indicated by the dotted line. After reference 6.

it may be misleading if the slopes and positions of Gaw-TGV curves differ (Fig. 8-13). Measurement of Gaw at different volumes is the preferred method for describing changes in Raw, e.g., after bronchodilator drugs.[4, 7]

Measurements of Raw in man in vivo include the resistance of all airways between airway opening and alveoli. By measuring pressures at points in between, one can partition Raw into portions corresponding to different parts of the airways. For instance, measurement of the pressure below the glottis (Ps [25, 59]) allows determination of the pressure differences (Palv – Ps) and (Ps – Pao) [Pao = pressure at airway opening]. Thus, the resistance of the lower (alveoli to subglottic area) and upper (from there to airway opening) airways can be measured. At large lung volumes, upper airway resistance is minimal (Fig. 8-14); it increases during deflation. Within the bronchial tree, further partitioning of Raw is possible with catheters placed in different bronchi. Such measurements have been performed in patients with lung diseases and in healthy persons.[21, 33] More elaborate experiments are feasible in animal experiments and also in excised human lungs where the pressure outside the airways can be controlled. In dog lungs, the airways of the fourth to ninth generation contribute most to total lower airway resistance.[30] In excised human lungs, pressure measurements in small airways have shown that airways smaller than 2 mm internal diameter contribute little to the resistance of the bronchial tree.[32] These findings agree with theoretical calculations on the distribution of flow resistance in the bronchial tree.[20, 41]

The site of resistance is important for interpretating Raw measurements. Raw

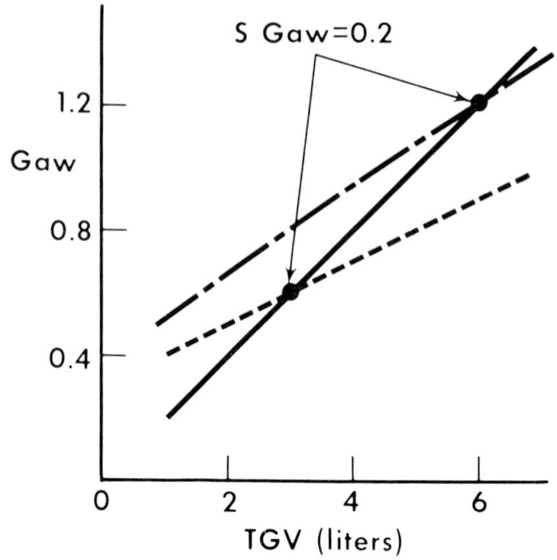

Fig. 8-13. Airway conductance (Gaw, liters/sec/cm H_2O) as a function of thoracic gas volume, TGV. Three Gaw-TGV graphs are shown. Gaw at a given lung volume may differ even though the Gaw/TGV ratio (SGaw) is equal (= 0.2) on selected points of each curve.

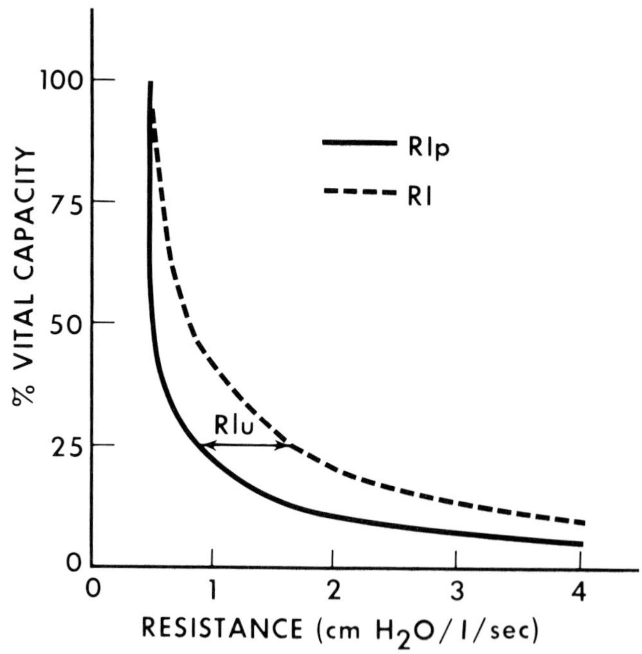

Fig. 8-14. Total lung resistance (Rl), resistance of lower airways (below glottis) and lungs (Rlp), and resistance of upper airways (Rlu) as a function of lung volume (*ordinate*). Deflation curves for healthy subject; data from reference 59.

is chiefly determined by the resistance of upper airways, glottis, trachea, and large bronchi. Thus, resistance changes in more peripheral airways must be large and extensive in order to affect total Raw. Measurements of maximum expiratory flow rates detect small airway obstruction better than Raw measurements[4, 8, 59] (Chap. 9). When Raw changes without significant alterations of maximum flows, the resistance changes probably occur in upper or large airways.

Maximum Expiratory Flow-Volume Curves

These curves are derived from IVPF curves (Fig. 8-10) and are described in Chapter 9.

VARIATION IN AIRWAY CALIBER

Experimental Changes in Airway Caliber

Asthma and several other lung diseases (Chap. 12) are characterized by airway obstruction, often developing slowly over the course of years. Acute changes of airway caliber can be induced by drugs (histamine, choline esters), by dust exposure, and by reflex actions. In vivo, acute changes of airway caliber are usually assessed with indirect measurements, e.g., of Raw or maximum flows. Recently,

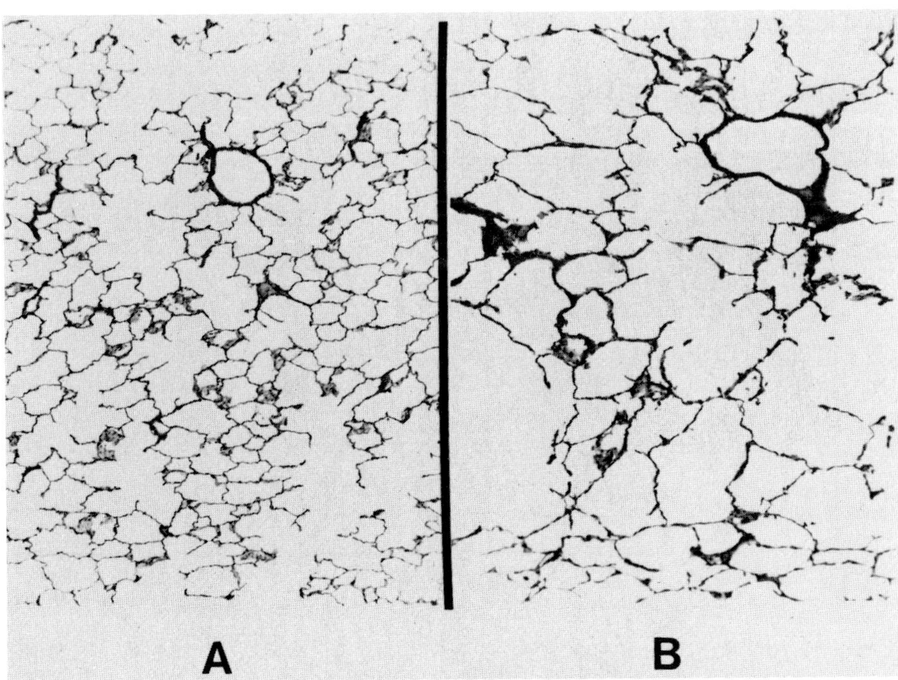

Fig. 8-15. *A*. Control rabbit lung; *B*. lung of rabbit treated with papain (same magnification as *A*). The mean number of alveolar attachments to small airways (< 1.25 mm internal circumference) was 10.1 in the controls and 8.5 in the papain-treated animals. Alveolar and alveolar duct sizes are increased after papain administration. Figure and data from reference 10.

improved radiological techniques using tantalum,[11] or without any contrast medium,[35, 36] have led to direct visualization of airway caliber changes in experimental animals. These methods can demonstrate the site as well as the extent of airway narrowing under various experimental conditions.[11, 35, 37]

The decreased caliber of small airways in emphysema is usually attributed to loss of recoil in the lungs (p. 167). Emphysema can be simulated in rabbits treated with papain, a proteolytic enzyme (p. 167). This treatment resulted in decreased maximum flow rates on IVPF curves in rabbits in which structural lung damage was minimal and lung compliance was normal.[10] The flow decrement appeared to be due to a loss of tethering of small airways by surrounding alveolar attachments (Fig. 8-15). After papain administration, alveolar size increased moderately, but

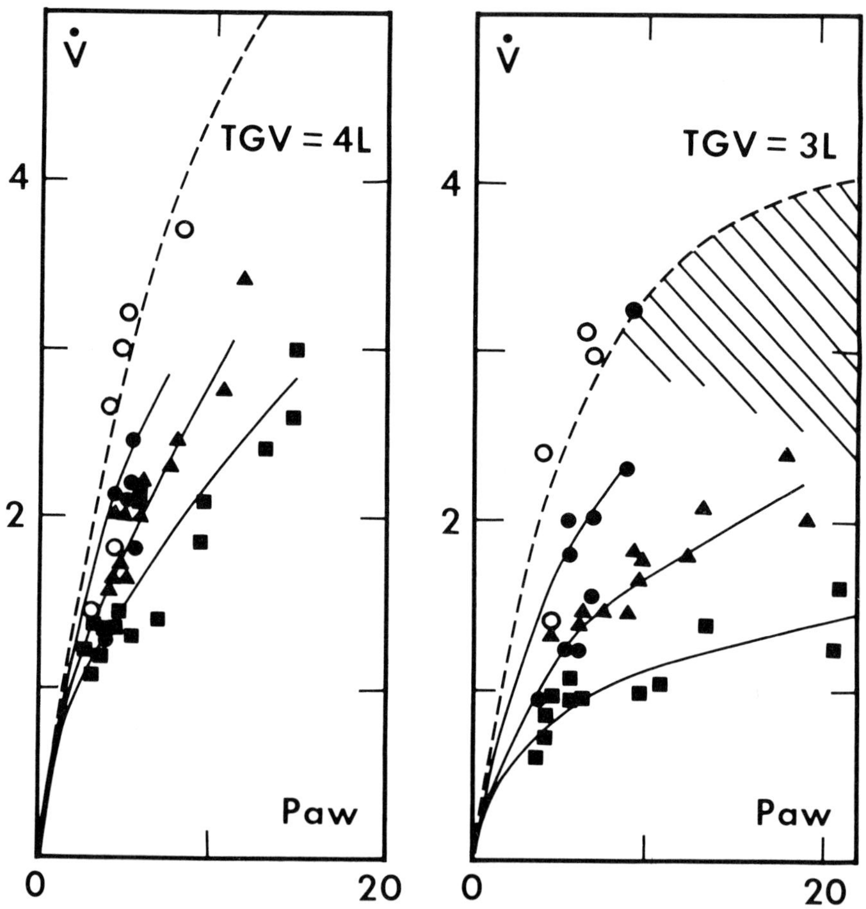

Fig. 8-16. Effect of histamine inhalation on expiratory IVPF data in a healthy subject, at two values of TGV. Paw (see legend to Fig. 8-10) in cm H_2O; $\dot{V}$ in liters per second. Symbols: control inhalation ○; 10 mg histamine base per ml ●; 20 mg histamine base per ml ▲; 30 mg histamine base per ml ■. Hatched area similar to those in Figure 8-11. After histamine inhalation, maximum flow rates at TGV = 3 liters are depressed, in dose-related fashion. The effect is less marked at the higher lung volume. From reference 6.

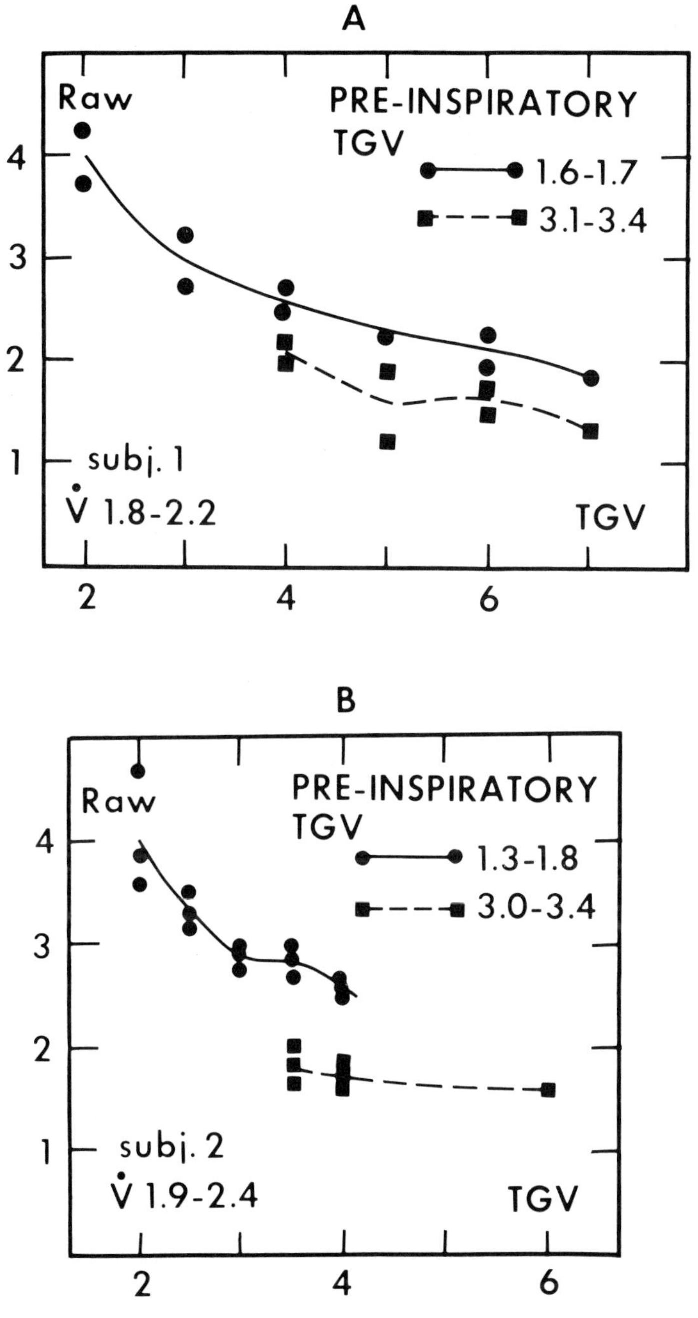

Fig. 8-17. Effect of preinspiratory lung volume on Raw. *Drawn lines.* Inspiration from near RV. *Dashed lines.* Inspiration from higher volumes, as shown in graph. Range of flow rates shown for each subject; the difference between drawn and dashed lines cannot be explained by pressure-flow alinearity. From reference 6.

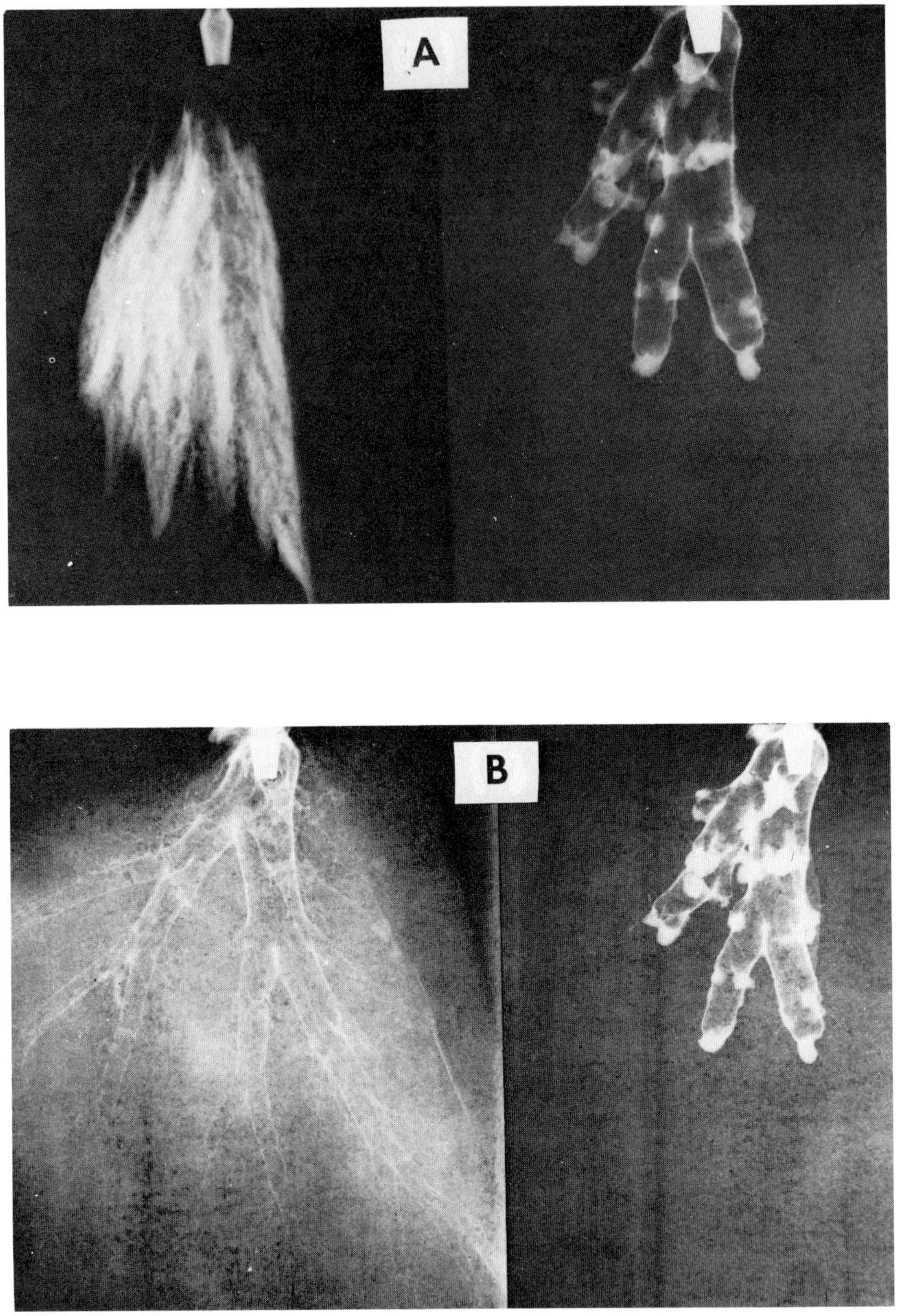

Fig. 8-18. *A*. Roentgenogram of intact dog lung lobe inflated to Ptp = 15 cm H_2O (*left*) and dissected bronchial tree at same Ptp (*right*). The airways are much wider when lung tissue is removed. *B*. Inflated dog lung lobe (*left*) and dissected airways (*right*), both at Ptp = 40 cm H_2O. At this high inflation pressure, airway caliber is similar in lobe and dissected airways. No contrast medium used. From reference 36.

the airways showed no anatomical changes that could explain the decreased flows. Decreased maximum flows, therefore, may reflect damage to lung structure when more direct measurements of lung elastic recoil do not yet pick up any change (see also Chap. 7, p. 158). Maximum flows on IVPF curves are also sensitive indices of drug-induced small airway obstruction, especially when flows are measured at small lung volumes[4, 6] (Fig. 8-16). The initial slope of IVPF curves may also change, indicating increased resistance at low flows, but this usually happens at higher dose levels of airway constrictor drugs.

Airway Caliber and Lung Volume History

Airway caliber and resistance to flow depend on both momentary conditions and previous history. For instance, at a given volume, Raw is higher if the preceding expiration was to RV than if expiration was less complete[6] (Fig. 8-17). This hysteresis (p. 152) of Raw can be abolished by atropine;[59] it is, therefore, probably caused by smooth muscle tone. However, when breathing at low lung volumes is prolonged, atelectasis appears to develop, and under these conditions Raw decreases during lung inflation.[9] In animal lungs, the state of the tissue surrounding airways affects their caliber. At the same inflation pressure, lobar and segmental bronchi in dog lungs have a smaller caliber when the lobe is atelectatic than during deflation from an inflated condition.[36] When surrounding atelectatic lung tissue is removed, airway caliber increases[36] (Fig. 8-18*A*); this does not happen with an inflated lobe (*B*). How atelectatic tissue compresses the airways is not quite clear, but the phenomenon illustrates the important effect of lung inflation on airway caliber. Muscle tone modifies the effect of the surrounding tissue.[36]

MUSCULAR EFFORT

Force-Velocity Relations

The pressures required to produce maximum flows during expiration are far less than those that can be developed during either static or dynamic breathing maneuvers (Fig. 8-19). Some 40 cm H_2O is enough to reach peak flows at large volumes, although the muscles can easily develop much higher pressures. Peak pressures during maximum exercise average -30 cm H_2O during inspiration and $+6$ cm H_2O during expiration in healthy persons.[39] In patients with airway obstruction, maximum flows are lower, while expiratory pressures during exercise are much higher than the levels required to produce maximum flow rates.[49] In addition, these patients usually require less pressure to achieve $\dot{V}_{max}$ at similar lung volumes than normal persons do. They breathe uneconomically during exercise, exerting much expiratory effort but achieving only low flows.

Potter et al.[49] proposed that this inefficient effort pattern results from an inappropriate motor drive to the expiratory muscles. The IVPF diagram of Figure 8-20 contains force-velocity curves for the expiratory muscles,[22] which indicate that the muscles' ability to produce expiratory pressure increases as the speed of contraction (i.e., flow rate) decreases. When flow rate is zero, muscle force is largest (static effort; Fig. 8-19). This inverse relation between flow rate and

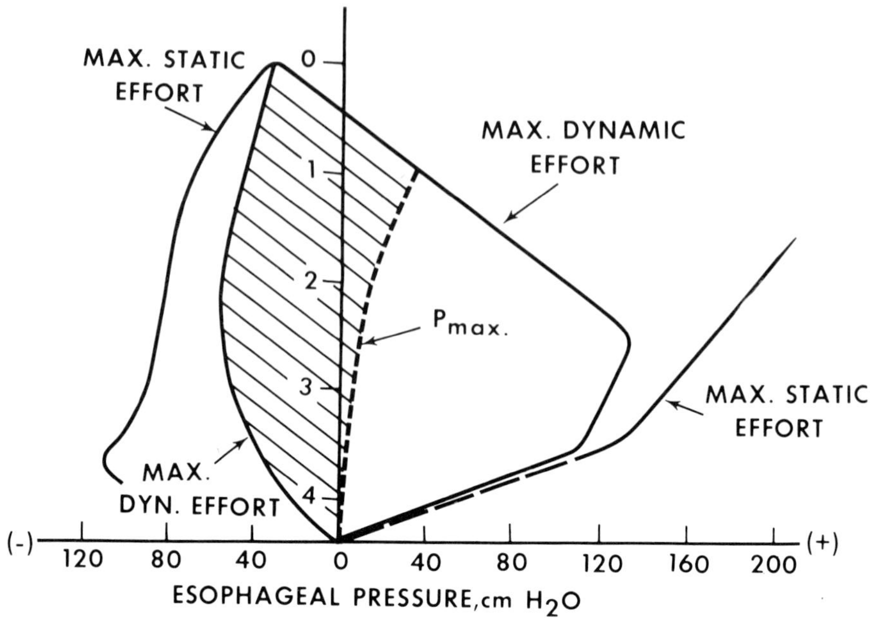

Fig. 8-19. Maximum static and dynamic pressures as a function of lung volume. Static effort = against closed airway. Dynamic effort = during forced vital capacity maneuvers. P_{max} = pressures needed to reach maximum expiratory flow rates. *Ordinate:* lung volume (liters from TLC). *Abscissa:* esophageal pressure, cm H_2O. From reference 22.

pressure is inherent to the physiological properties of striated muscles.[1] During inspiration and at large volumes during expiration, the rate of expiratory flow is limited by the muscles' ability to develop force during rapid contractions.[1, 22] If persons with airway obstruction continued to develop the same muscle force as during health, they would use higher pressures and achieve lower flows (compare points *A* and *B* in Fig. 8-20). If they increased muscle force, in a vain attempt to increase flow, breathing would become even more uneconomical (e.g., point *B* might move to *C*).

Indirect support for this hypothesis comes from acute experiments with unloading of the respiratory system.[38] When healthy subjects breathe a helium-oxygen mixture (80 percent He, 20 percent O_2), their expiratory flow rates increase, and IVPF curves are shifted upward (Fig. 8-20). For the same oxygen uptake, exercise ventilation increases, while peak expiratory pressure decreases. Breathing of helium, a light gas, unloads the respiratory system because less energy is lost in turbulence and other nonlaminar flow patterns, which are density-dependent. This response to unloading is largely a consequence of the force-velocity curve of the muscles.[38] Apparently, respiratory motor drive is only incompletely adapted to the lesser energy losses, since flow increases and P_{CO_2} decreases. Thus, the regulation of breathing fails to keep P_{CO_2} constant (see also Chap. 10, p. 254). Similarly, regulation may fail to decrease motor drive in patients with airway obstruction who seem to continue to use a motor drive appropriate for healthy

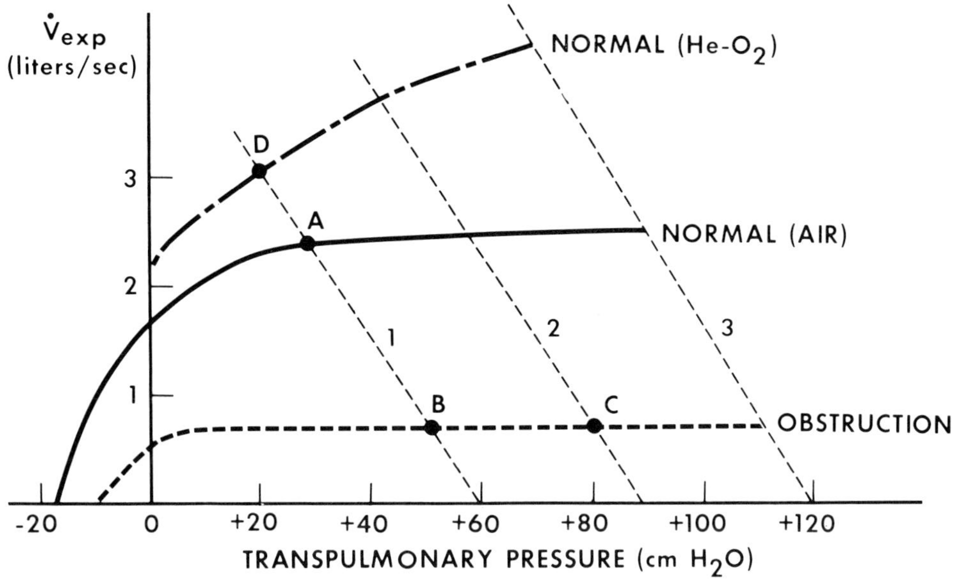

Fig. 8-20. IVPF curves in normal subject breathing air (——) or He-O_2 (— — —), and in a patient with airway obstruction (- - -). Force-velocity curves of respiratory muscles 1, 2, and 3 describe increasing levels of muscular effort, corresponding to static transpulmonary pressures of +60, +90, and +120 cm H_2O. When the system is loaded by airway obstruction, flow decreases and pressure increases for the same effort (compare points *A* and *B* on force-velocity curve 1). When the system is unloaded by He-O_2 breathing, flow increases and pressure decreases, again for the same effort, e.g., from *A* to *D*. Modified from reference 49; the He-O_2 curve indicates the direction of changes observed by Nattie and Tenney.[38]

lungs. Training these patients to decrease their uneconomical breathing patterns might result in less energy spent on respiratory muscles and hence more energy available for physical work by other muscles.

Work Rate of Breathing

The power dissipated during airflow is given by

$$\dot{W} = 0.1 \ P \cdot \dot{V} \qquad (2)$$

where $\dot{W}$ = power (rate of work) in watts, P = driving pressure in cm H_2O and $\dot{V}$ = flow rate in liters per second. The equation is strictly valid only when pressure and flow rate are in phase. In a logarithmic pressure-flow diagram (Fig. 8-21) instantaneous power values can be read from the diagonal lines of equal power. During maximally forced expirations, power may reach more than 20 watts for brief instants. During quiet breathing, power is minimal, and even during heavy exercise the rate of work remains small. In patients with airway obstruction, it is usually said that the work of breathing is large. This is true if one looks at pressure-volume loops (discussed in Chap. 7). However, here we consider only the power exerted to drive airflow, not the overall effort of breathing. Expiratory

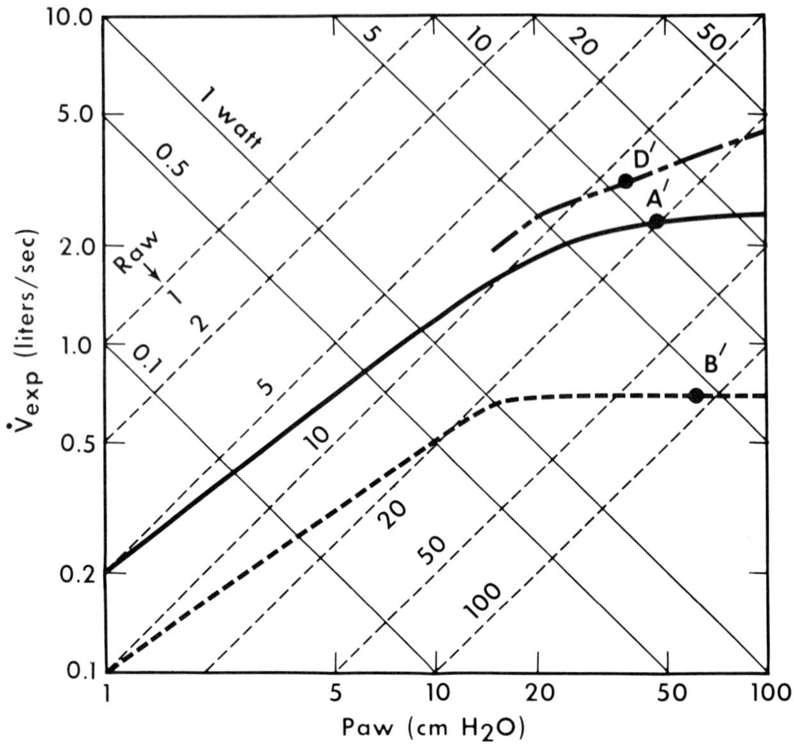

Fig. 8-21. Pressure-flow diagram on logarithmic coordinates. IVPF curves are those also shown in Figure 8-20. Points A', B', and D' correspond to points A, B, and D in Figure 8-20. Drawn diagonal lines are isobars for equal power output [from Eq. (2)]. Dashed diagonal lines are lines for equal Raw ($=$Paw/$\dot{V}_{exp}$).

power remains low in obstructed patients even though high pressures are used in an effort to overcome the high airway resistance (B') Unloading the system with helium increases expiratory power only slightly; flows and pressure change reciprocally (e.g., from A' to D' in Fig. 8-21).

SUMMARY

Airflow patterns in airways are complex and do not fit a simple physical model. Pressure-flow relations are alinear and much energy is lost in transforming flow patterns (entrance effects; branches). During forced expiration, the geometry of large airways in the chest is profoundly changed by dynamic compression, which limits expiratory flow rates. The dynamically compressed airways are unstable and vibrate; the degree of compression depends on wall stiffness and smooth muscle tone. Experimentally, pressure-flow relations can be assessed with IVPF and MEFV curves and with airway resistance measurements. Airway-constrictor drugs decrease airway caliber, and this also happens when alveolar structure is damaged with a proteolytic enzyme, papain. Both actions result in lower flow rates on IVPF curves. Muscular effort limits inspiratory flow and, at large lung volumes, expiratory flow. Force-velocity relations of the respiratory muscles can account for the inappropriately high expiratory pressures used by patients with airway obstruction who exert much effort but achieve only a low expiratory flow and a low external work rate of breathing.

REFERENCES

1. Agostoni E, Fenn WO: Velocity of muscle shortening as a limiting factor in respiratory air flow. J Appl Physiol 15: 349–353, 1960
2. Ainsworth M, and Eveleigh JW: A method of estimating lung resistance in humans. Porton, Wiltshire, England, Ministry of Supply, Chemical Defense Experimental Establishment, Porton Tech. Paper No. 320, 1952
3. Bachofen H, Scherrer M: Lung tissue resistance in healthy subjects and in patients with lung disease, in Bouhuys A (ed): Airway Dynamics; Physiology and Pharmacology. Springfield, Charles C Thomas, 1970, pp 123–134
4. Bouhuys A: Airway dynamics and bronchoactive agents in man, in Bouhuys A (ed): Airway Dynamics; Physiology and Pharmacology. Springfield, Charles C Thomas, 1970, pp 263–282
5. Bouhuys A: Relation entre le débit expiratoire maximum et le volume pulmonaire (Maximum flow/volume relationships). Bull Physiopathol Respir (Nancy) 7:303–311, 1971
6. Bouhuys A, Jonson B: Alveolar pressure, airflow rate, and lung inflation in man. J Appl Physiol 22:1086–1100, 1967
7. Bouhuys A, van de Woestijne KP: Mechanical consequences of airway smooth muscle relaxation. J Appl Physiol 30:670–676, 1971
8. Bouhuys A, van de Woestijne KP: Respiratory mechanics and dust exposure in byssinosis. J Clin Invest 49:106–118, 1970
9. Butler J, Caro CG, Alcala R, DuBois AB: Physiological factors affecting airway resistance in normal subjects and in patients with obstructive respiratory disease. J Clin Invest 39:584–591, 1960
10. Caldwell EJ: Physiologic and anatomic effects of papain on the rabbit lung. J Appl Physiol 31:458–465, 1971
11. Clarke SW, Graf PD, Nadel JA: In vivo visualization of small-airway constriction after pulmonary microembolism in cats and dogs. J Appl Physiol 29: 646–650, 1970
12. Clarke SW, Jones JG, Oliver BR: Resistance to two-phase gas-liquid flow in airways. J Appl Physiol 29: 464–471, 1970
13. DuBois AB, Botelho SY, Comroe JH Jr: A new method for measuring airway resistance in man using a body plethysmograph: values in normal subjects and in patients with respiratory disease. J Clin Invest 35:327–335, 1956
14. DuBois AB, van de Woestijne KP (eds): Body Plethysmography, Progress in Respiration Research, 4; Herzog H, Series Editor. Basel, S Karger, 1968
15. Ferris BG Jr: Use of pulmonary function tests in epidemiologic surveys. Bull Physiopathol Respir (Nancy) 6:579–594, 1970
16. Fisher AB, DuBois AB, Hyde RW: Evaluation of the forced oscillation technique for the determination of resistance to breathing. J Clin Invest 47:2045–2057, 1968
17. Fry DL: A preliminary lung model for simulating the aerodynamics of the bronchial tree. Comput Biomed Res 2: 111–134, 1968
18. Fry DL: Theoretical considerations of the bronchial pressure-flow-volume relationships with particular reference to the maximum expiratory flow-volume curve. Phys Med Biol 3:174–194, 1958
19. Fry DL, Hyatt RE: Pulmonary mechanics. A unified analysis of the relationship between pressure, volume and gas flow in the lungs of normal and diseased human subjects. Am J Med 29:672–689, 1960
20. Green M: How big are the bronchioles?, St. Thomas' Hosp Gazette 63:136–139, 1965
21. Herzog H, Keller R, Maurer W, Baumann HR, Nadjafi A: Distribution of bronchial resistance in obstructive pul-

monary disease and in dogs with artificially induced tracheal collapse. Respiration 25:361–394, 1968
22. Hyatt RE, Flath RE: Relationship of airflow to pressure during maximal respiratory effort in man. J Appl Physiol 21:477–482, 1966
23. Hyatt RE, Wilcox RE: The pressure-flow relationships of the intrathoracic airway in man. J Clin Invest 42:29–39, 1963
24. Ingram RH Jr, Schilder DP: Effect of gas compression on pulmonary pressure, flow, and volume relationships. J Appl Physiol 21:1821–1826, 1966
25. Jaeger MJ, Matthys H: The pressure flow characteristics of the human airways, in Bouhuys A (ed): Airway Dynamics; Physiology and Pharmacology. Springfield, Charles C Thomas, 1970, pp 21–32
26. Jaeger MJ, Otis AB: Measurement of airway resistance with a volume displacement body plethysmograph. J Appl Physiol 19:813–820, 1964
27. Jonson B: Pulmonary mechanics in normal men, studied with the flow regulator method. Scand J Clin Lab Invest 25: 363–373, 1970
28. Jonson B, Bouhuys A: Measurement of alveolar pressure. J Appl Physiol 22: 1081–1085, 1967
29. Klingele TG, Staub NC: Terminal bronchiole diameter changes with volume in isolated, air-filled lobes of cat lung. J Appl Physiol 30:224–227, 1971
30. Macklem PT: Partitioning of the pressure drop in the airways, in Bouhuys A (ed): Airway Dynamics; Physiology and Pharmacology. Springfield, Charles C Thomas, 1970, pp 85–97
31. Macklem PT, Mead J: Factors determining maximum expiratory flow in dogs. J Appl Physiol 25:159–169, 1968
32. Macklem PT, Mead J: Resistance of central and peripheral airways measured by a retrograde catheter. J Appl Physiol 22:395–401, 1967
33. Macklem PT, Wilson NJ: Measurement of intrabronchial pressure in man. J Appl Physiol 20: 653–663, 1965
34. Mead J, Turner JM, Macklem PT, Little JB: Significance of the relationship between lung recoil and maximum expiratory flow. J Appl Physiol 22:95–108, 1967
35. Murtagh PS, Proctor DF, Permutt S, Kelly B, Evering S: Bronchial closure with mecholyl in excised dog lobes. J Appl Physiol 31:409–415, 1971
36. Murtagh PS, Proctor DF, Permutt S, Kelly BL, Evering S: Bronchial mechanics in excised dog lobes. J Appl Physiol 31:403–408, 1971
37. Nadel JA: New technique for studying structural changes of airways in vivo using powdered tantalum, in Bouhuys A (ed): Airway Dynamics; Physiology and Pharmacology. Springfield, Charles C Thomas, 1970, pp 73–83
38. Nattie EE, Tenney SM: The ventilatory response to resistance unloading during muscular exercise. Respir Physiol 10: 249–262, 1970
39. Olafsson S, Hyatt RE: Ventilatory mechanics and expiratory flow limitation during exercise in normal subjects. J Clin Invest 48:564–573, 1969
40. Olsen CR, Stevens AE, McIlroy MB: Rigidity of tracheae and bronchi during muscular constriction. J Appl Physiol 23:27–34, 1967
41. Olson DE, Dart GA, Filley GF: Pressure drop and fluid flow regime of air inspired into the human lung. J Appl Physiol 28:482–494, 1970
42. Owen PR: Turbulent flow and particle deposition in the trachea, in Wolstenholme GEW, Knight J (eds): Circulatory and Respiratory Mass Transport, Ciba Foundation Symposium. Boston, Little, Brown and Company, 1969, pp 236–252
43. Palombini B, Coburn RF: Control of the compressibility of the canine trachea. Respir Physiol 15:365–383, 1972
44. Pardaens J, van de Woestijne KP, Clément J: A physical model of expiration. J Appl Physiol 33:479–490, 1972
45. Patrick GA, Sharp GR: Oronasal distribution of inspiratory flow during various activities. J Physiol (London) 206: 22P–23P, 1970
46. Pedersen OF: Relation entre le débit expiratoire maximum et le volume pulmonaire (Maximum flow/volume relationships). Bull Physiopathol Respir (Nancy) 7:327–331, 1971
47. Pedley TJ, Schroter RC, Sudlow MF: The prediction of pressure drop and variation of resistance within the human bronchial airways. Respir Physiol 9:387–405, 1970
48. Peslin R: Relation entre le débit expira-

toire maximum et le volume pulmonaire (Maximum flow/volume relationships). Bull Physiopathol Respir (Nancy) 7: 348–351, 1971

49. Potter WA, Olafsson S, Hyatt RE: Ventilatory mechanics and expiratory flow limitation during exercise in patients with obstructive lung disease. J Clin Invest 50:910–919, 1971
50. Pride NB, Permutt S, Riley RL, Bromberger-Barnea B: Determinants of maximal expiratory flow from the lungs. J Appl Physiol 23:646–662, 1967
51. Rohrer F: Der Strömungswiderstand in den menschlichen Atemwegen und der Einfluss der unregelmässigen Verzweigung des Bronchial-systems auf den Atmungsverlauf in verschiedenen Lungenbezirken. Pflueger's Arch 162:225–299, 1915
52. Schroter RC, Sudlow MF: Flow patterns in models of the human bronchial airways. Respir Physiol 7:341–355, 1969
53. Sharp JT, Henry JP, Sweany SK, Meadows WR, Pietras RJ: Total respiratory inertance and its gas and tissue components in normal and obese men. J Clin Invest 43:503–509, 1964
54. Sonne C: Untersuchungen über die relative Weite der Bronchiolen bei der verschiedenen Luftspannung der Lungen. Beitrag zur Kenntnis der Pathogenese des Bronchial-Asthmas. Acta Med Scand 58:313–341, 1923
55. Spann RW, Hyatt RE: Factors affecting upper airway resistance in conscious man. J Appl Physiol 31:708–712, 1971
56. Stănescu DC, Pattijn J, Clément J, van de Woestijne KP: Glottis opening and airway resistance. J Appl Physiol 32:460–466, 1972
57. van de Woestijne KP, Afschrift M, Bouhuys A: Pressions, débits et volumes pulmonaires pendant la respiration forcée. Poumon Coeur 24:969–987, 1968
58. van de Woestijne KP, Zapletal A: The maximum expiratory flow-volume curve: peak flow and effort-independent portion, in Bouhuys A (ed): Airway Dynamics; Physiology and Pharmacology. Springfield, Charles C Thomas, 1970, pp 61–72
59. Vincent NJ, Knudson R, Leith DE, Macklem PT, Mead J: Factors influencing pulmonary resistance. J Appl Physiol 29:236–243, 1970
60. Yamabayashi H, Takahashi T, Tonomura S, Takahashi H: An analog model of the mechanical properties of the lung and airway, in Bouhuys A (ed): Airway Dynamics; Physiology and Pharmacology. Charles C Thomas, 1970, pp. 33–41

Chapter 9

Flow Volume Curves

The derivation of maximum expiratory flow-volume (MEFV) curves from isovolume pressure-flow (IVPF) curves, discussed in the previous chapter, is shown in the schematic diagram of Figure 9-1. Over a large portion of the vital capacity (VC), MEFV curves represent flows that correspond to plateaus on IVPF curves. MEFV curves can be recorded simply during a forced expiration and do not require pressure measurements in a plethysmograph or with an esophageal balloon. MEFV curves were first used by Dayman [14] and by Fry and Hyatt.[19, 23] In recent years they have been used in many experimental and clinical studies. Maximum flow rates on MEFV curves depend on many physiological and mechanical factors, any one of which can alter the curve's configuration. Since the mechanical events during forced expiration are complex and insufficiently understood, interpretation of MEFV curves in terms of lung mechanics is limited.[23] This limitation does not detract, however, from the value of flow-volume curves in detecting and quantitating acute changes in lung function that result from drugs, pollutants, or disease. For this purpose, the partial expiratory flow-volume (PEFV) curve [6] is particularly suitable.

DETERMINANTS OF MAXIMUM FLOW RATES

The dynamics of forced expirations have been described in Chapter 8. Here we discuss these mechanical events as they affect maximum flows and determine the size and shape of the MEFV curve.

Airway Resistance

Increased resistance in upper airways or an added resistance placed at the mouth decreases flow rates. This decrease occurs first at large lung volumes and extends to lower volumes as the resistance increases [Fig. 9-4 (*5*)].[26, 37a, 41] At high lung volumes, expiratory muscle power sets the limit on expiratory flow; peak

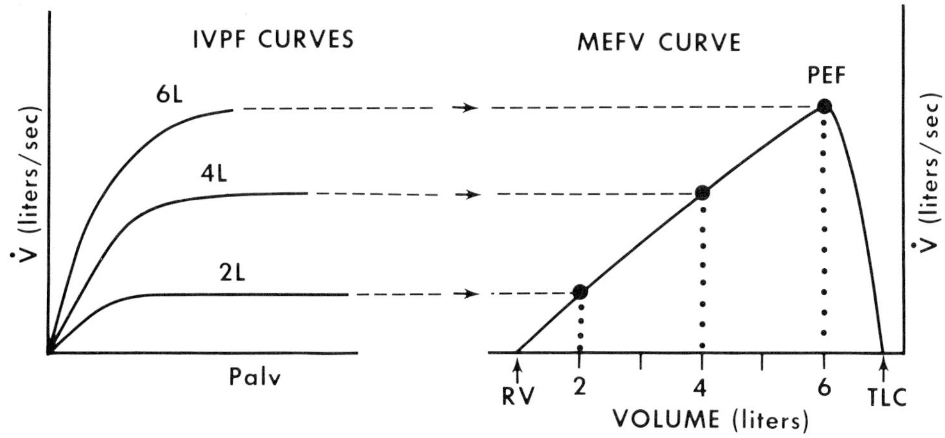

Fig. 9-1. Schematic diagram to illustrate derivation of maximum expiratory flow-volume (MEFV) curve from a family of isovolume pressure-flow (IVPF) curves. *Ordinates:* expiratory flow rate. *Abscissa:* (left) alveolar pressure; (right) lung volume. From reference 2.

flows are determined chiefly by upper airway resistance and muscle power. When, as in tracheal stenosis, upper airway resistance is markedly increased, it limits flow to values lower than those that result from the normal flow-limiting mechanism. The MEFV curve then only reaches its normal contour at volumes where the physiological mechanism sets a lower limit than the resistance in the upper airways. However, upper airway resistance must be significantly increased in order to affect the MEFV curve.

In the upper third of the VC, expiratory effort has a pronounced effect on flow rates (Fig. 9-5). Below about 80 percent of the VC (Chap. 8, p. 185), the MEFV curve represents flows that correspond to plateaus on IVPF curves (Fig. 9-1). The analysis in the previous chapter has shown that maximum flows at these volumes are chiefly determined by the flow resistance of peripheral airways and by lung elastic recoil. Since measurements of airway resistance during quiet breathing or panting primarily reflect the resistance of large and extrathoracic airways (p. 189), it is not surprising that data on airway resistance and MEFV curves may disagree. The discrepancies arise because resistance is chiefly determined by large-airway caliber, while maximum flow mainly reflects the caliber of small airways. Airway resistance increases only when there is extensive narrowing of small airways (Chap. 8).

These discrepancies between resistance and flow rates occur, for instance, when airways are dilated with drugs that relax airway smooth muscle.[9] In healthy persons, these drugs nearly always decrease airway resistance while maximum flows increase slightly, if at all, and may even decrease. The reduced resistance probably reflects an increased large-airway caliber, measured when airflow rates are low and no dynamic compression occurs. Maximum flow changes result from two opposing factors: (1) increased caliber of small airways, leading to increased flow, and (2) decreased stiffness of large airways through smooth muscle relaxation (p. 184), leading to increased dynamic compression and lower flows. Depending on the balance between these opposing factors, maximum flow may increase, decrease, or remain constant. In asthma the increased small-airway caliber following administration of dilator drugs is the preponderant factor and maximum flows usually increase markedly.

Lung Elastic Recoil

Lung elastic recoil is the principal driving force for expiratory flow at low lung volumes (p. 182). The relation between maximum flow and elastic recoil can be assessed graphically (Fig. 9-2); their ratio $[Pst(l)/\dot{V}_{max}]$ equals the resistance of the upstream airway segment in Mead's theory (p. 181). In the experiment of Figure 9-2, a constrictor drug decreased maximum flow at equal values of Pst(l). Since Pst(l) did not change, this result indicates a decrease in small airway caliber by smooth muscle contraction.[6] In other conditions, maximum flow and elastic recoil both change while their ratio remains constant. For example, when elastic recoil in hamsters is reduced by a proteolytic enzyme (papain), Pst(l) decreases

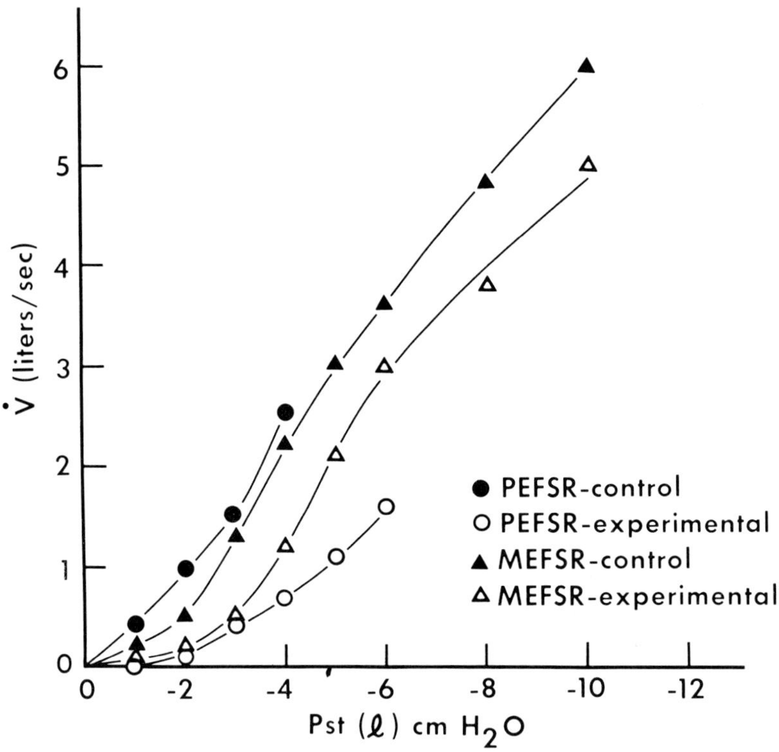

Fig. 9-2. Maximum flow-static recoil curves in a healthy subject, before and after histamine aerosol inhalation. *Abscissa:* static lung recoil pressure [Pst (l)]; *ordinate:* expiratory flow rate. PEFSR = partial expiratory flow-static recoil curve, corresponding to PEFV maneuver. MEFSR = maximum expiratory flow-static recoil curve, corresponding to MEFV maneuver. After inhalation of the constrictor aerosol, maximum flows at equal Pst(l) are decreased, indicating small-airway narrowing. The difference is greater on the partial (PEFSR) than on the maximum (MEFSR) curves. From reference 6.

but the ratio between maximum flow and Pst(*l*) is unchanged.[42] In man, chest strapping increases Pst(*l*) as well as maximum flow, again leaving the relationship between the two unchanged.[49] In these instances, as in parenchymal lung disease, the changes in maximum flow result from changes in lung elastic recoil. In diffuse lung fibrosis, high static recoil pressures are often associated with high maximum flows.[28, 31] In emphysema, low maximum flows are associated with loss of elastic recoil and low values of Pst(*l*).[14, 50] Since small airways are embedded in the lung parenchyma (Fig. 2-2*B*; p. 32), parenchymal elastic-recoil forces are transmitted to these airway walls. In this manner, lung structure provides the conditions in which an increase or decrease of elastic recoil force can lead to passive changes in airway caliber and hence to changes in maximum expiratory flow.

Acceleration of Gas

The total cross section of the airways decreases from the alveoli to the trachea (p. 31). Therefore, gas velocity rises as expired gas travels from the alveoli through the increasingly narrow bronchial tree. The acceleration of expired gas may affect maximum flows at high lung volumes;[36] at lower volumes, when flows decrease, this factor is minor.

Limits to Inspiration and Expiration

These limits determine VC, the volume axis of the MEFV curve. When airway closure limits expiration, flow gradually decreases toward the residual volume (RV) point (the "tail" of curve *3* in Fig. 9-4). When chest wall recoil limits expiration, the curve terminates abruptly, as in Figure 9-4, *1* (see also Chap. 7, p. 166).

Flow History

The variability of maximum flows on IVPF curves is discussed on p. 186 (Fig. 8-11). At a given volume, maximum flow is a function of previous flow rates (Fig. 9-5*A* and *C*): the lower the preceding flow, the higher the maximum flow. A precise explanation of this phenomenon is not available. The development of dynamic compression probably varies as a function of initial flows during more or less forced expirations.[7, 44] When initial flows are low, dynamic compression is still in progress at low lung volumes. The compression contributes to increased flow but cannot fully explain it.[44] Gas flow from compressing large airways can also lead to short-lasting bursts of flows above the contour of the MEFV curve, e.g., during a cough.[27] Since these transients do not reflect gas expired from alveoli, they should be ignored when assessing maximum flows as an index of ventilatory capacity. In emphysema, alternating compression and decompression of large airways can lead to spuriously high flow rates during maximum breathing capacity maneuvers, thereby overestimating the true capacity of the patient to ventilate the alveoli. Much of the volume displaced during such maneuvers may shuttle back and forth between the atmosphere and the large airways.[50]

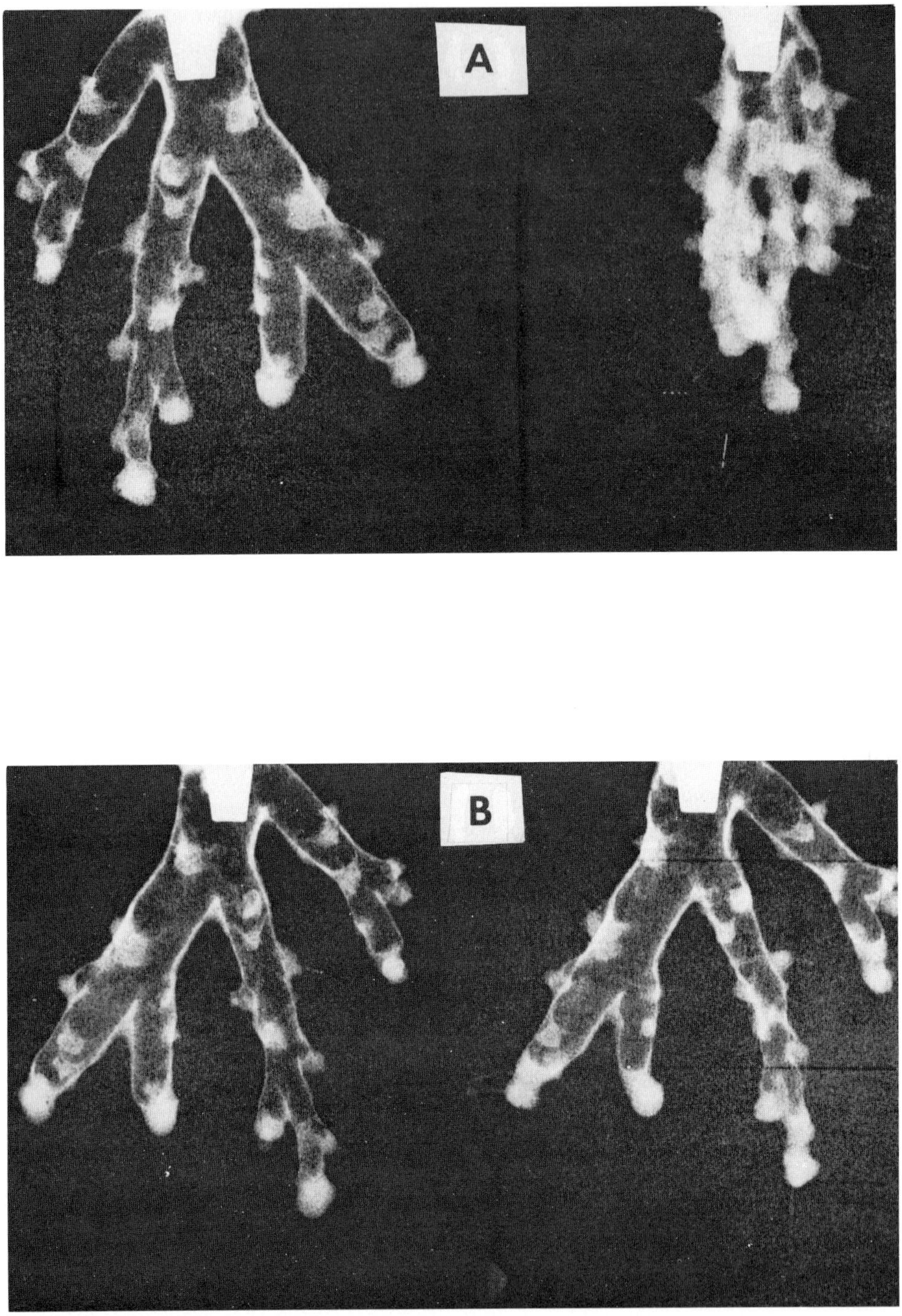

Fig. 9-3. Dissected bronchial tree of dog lung lobe. Left: control; right: after mecholyl. *A:* Inflation to 20 cm H_2O transpulmonary pressure. Mecholyl causes marked airway constriction. *B:* Inflation to 40 cm H_2O transpulmonary pressure. A similar administration of mecholyl causes no discernible constriction of the passively distended airways. From Murtagh et al.[40]

Inspired Gas Composition

Maximum flow rates on MEFV curves increase with the inspiration of a light gas (80 percent He-20 percent O_2) and decrease as gas density increases.[47] Viscosity of the inspired gas has only a minor effect. With a light gas, the flow increase is most pronounced at large lung volumes. These flows are determined largely by effort and by the caliber of large airways, where the flow pattern is consistent with a major effect of gas density (p. 174). In some patients with airway obstruction, the absence of a flow rate increase upon breathing He-O_2[15] suggests a decreased dependence of expired gas flow on density. In part, this reduced dependence may result from low flow rates and hence a decrease in turbulence and other density-dependent energy losses. The lack of density dependence in these patients' maximum flows might also be explained by small-airway narrowing.[15] In the lower-volume portion of the MEFV curve, the portion most sensitive to small-airway obstruction, breathing He-O_2 has little effect on maximum flow.[15, 47]

Airway Muscle Tone

In isolated dog lung lobes, the effect of constrictor drugs on airway caliber can be observed directly.[40] Figure 9-3 shows that this effect depends markedly on lung inflation. At a low inflation pressure (*A*), airway narrowing and closure are pronounced, while the length of these lobar and segmental bronchi changes much less. High inflation pressures are required to open the airways again. Surface tension of the mucosa may contribute to closure once caliber is reduced. At a high inflation pressure (*B*), almost no narrowing occurs after the constrictor drug is applied. This experiment demonstrates phenomena quite similar to those seen in flow-volume curves in man (Figs. 9-8, 9-9): constrictor agents lead to much more significant reductions of airway caliber at low lung volumes than at high volumes. In addition, airway closure in man may occur at an increased volume (e.g., the increased RV after histamine exposure on the PEFV curves in Fig. 9-8), and a maximum inspiration can reopen these airways, at least temporarily (RV is lower at the end of the MEFV curves in Fig. 9-8). The effects of changes in smooth muscle tone in man are described in more detail on p. 227.

For practical purposes, the most important determinants of maximum flows on MEFV curves, at lung volumes less than about 70 percent of VC, are small-airway caliber and lung static recoil pressure. In several instances, increased or decreased elastic recoil leads to changes in maximum flows. In other conditions, small-airway caliber is the principal variable.

PATTERNS OF MEFV CURVES

The shape and size of the MEFV curve vary considerably among normal subjects and patients with lung disease—in fact, no simple mathematical expression fits all the variations.[12] Three main patterns account for the majority (Fig. 9-4). In healthy young persons, the descending portion of the curve is approximately linear (*2*) or concave to the volume axis (*1*). In older persons, the tail end of the curve, near RV, is often convex to the volume axis (*3*). Some subjects have

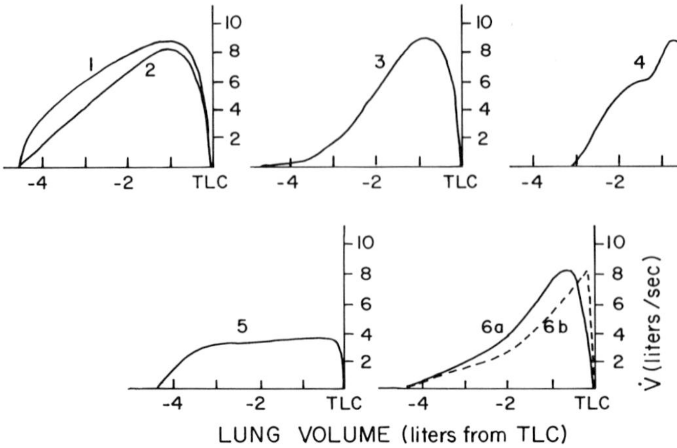

Fig. 9-4. MEFV curve patterns. *1* and *2*. Healthy young subjects. *3*. Older subject; this pattern is also frequent among young smokers.[48] *4*. Curve with intermediate plateau ("shoulder"). *5*. Typical curve pattern in upper airway obstruction, e.g., tracheal stenosis. *6*. A slow response of the volume-recording instrument distorts the true form of the curve (*a*) into the pattern of curve *b*.

an intermediate plateau ("shoulder") on the curve (*4*). MEFV curve patterns in growing children have been discussed in Chapter 1 (p. 16 and Fig. 1-9). The shape of MEFV curves may be distorted by technical factors, e.g., when the response time of the flow channel exceeds that of the volume-recording channel (Fig. 9-4, *6*).

In series of successive blows, the shape of the MEFV curve varies as a function of effort (Fig. 9-5*A*). Flow rates at lower lung volumes are often similar in spite of considerable variation in initial effort (Fig. 9-5*B*). Although this phenomenon has prompted the description of the descending portion of the curve as effort-independent, this term should not be taken literally, as the example of Figure 9-5*A* indicates. At any volume, a certain minimal effort is required to achieve maximum flow, but at low lung volumes flow is independent of further effort once this minimum has been attained. At high volumes, IVPF curves do not show plateaus, and flow continues to increase until the limit of expiratory muscle power has been reached.

Fig. 9-5. MEFV curves recorded with computer system (Fig. 9-7). Each graph shows five consecutive blows. The dashed lines in *A* and *C* indicate the maximum flow contour (see text). The examples chosen are from subjects whose expiratory effort varied considerably, as appears from the large differences in PEF between individual blows. The $FEV_{1.0}$ is less sensitive to differences in effort than PEF, partly because flows at midlung volumes are often higher when effort is less (see *C*). This phenomenon is observed also when lung volume changes are measured with a body plethysmograph.[7] In *C*, $FEV_{1.0}$ varied only between 1.88 and 2.00 liters in the five blows shown, in spite of large differences in peak flow between the blows.

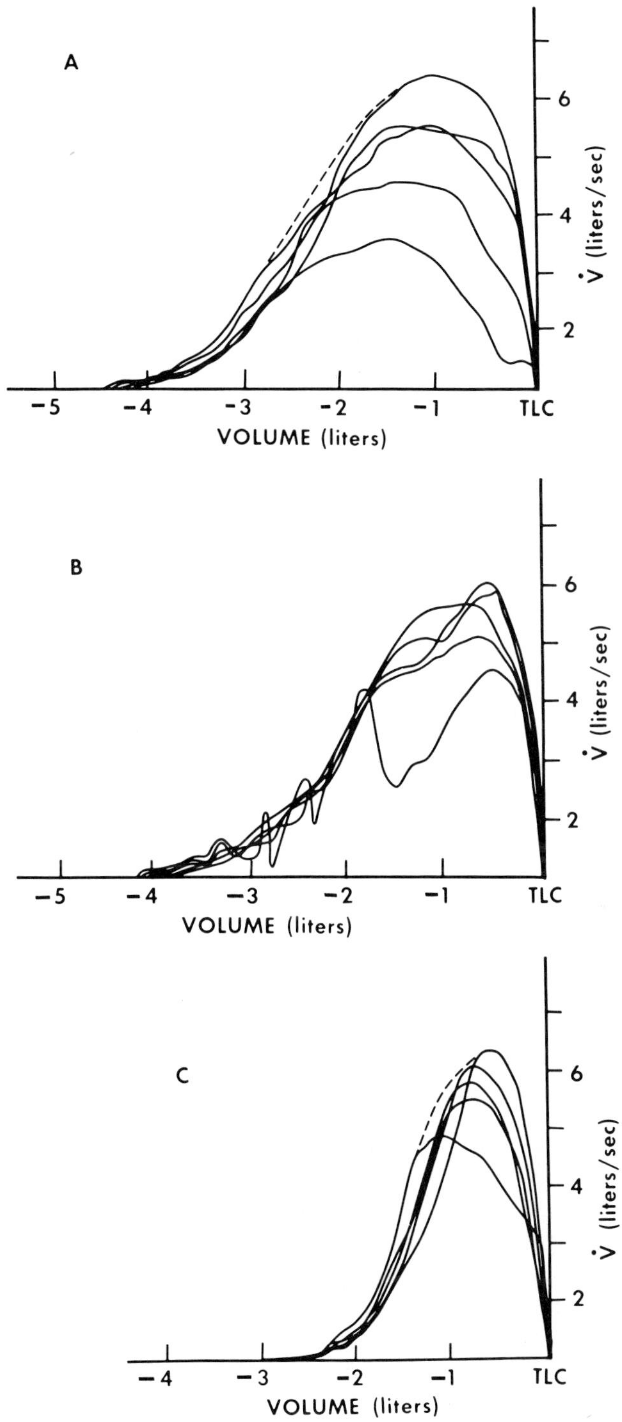
A
6
4
2
V̇ (liters/sec)
−5 −4 −3 −2 −1 TLC
VOLUME (liters)
B
6
4
2
V̇ (liters/sec)
−5 −4 −3 −2 −1 TLC
VOLUME (liters)
C
6
4
2
V̇ (liters/sec)
−4 −3 −2 −1 TLC
VOLUME (liters)

Maximum flows at lower lung volumes often show reverse effort-dependence, with a reduction in flows following an increase in initial effort and initial flow rates (Fig. 9-5*A* and *C*). In these instances, the curve recorded during maximally forced expiration shows lower flows than the curve obtained by superimposing a number of curves recorded during less forced expirations.[24] The contour of this set of curves is indicated by the dashed lines in Figure 9-5*A* and *C*. For practical purposes, the maximum-effort curve is easier to perform and to standardize.

Gross changes in MEFV curve patterns occur in obstructive as well as restrictive lung diseases (Fig. 9-6*A*). In obstructive disease, flow rates are low, especially near RV, and the curve is convex to the volume axis. In restrictive function loss, VC is decreased and flow rates are relatively high, resulting in a pronounced concave descending portion of the curve. Comparison of these curves with the normal pattern should take TLC into account. In obstructive disease, TLC is often abnormally large, while it is decreased in restrictive disease. Comparison on an absolute volume scale (Fig. 9-6*B*) shows better how much the mechanical characteristics of airways and lungs differ in the two types of patients. The patient with restrictive disease reaches high flow rates at thoracic gas volumes less than the residual volume of the patient with severe airway obstruction.

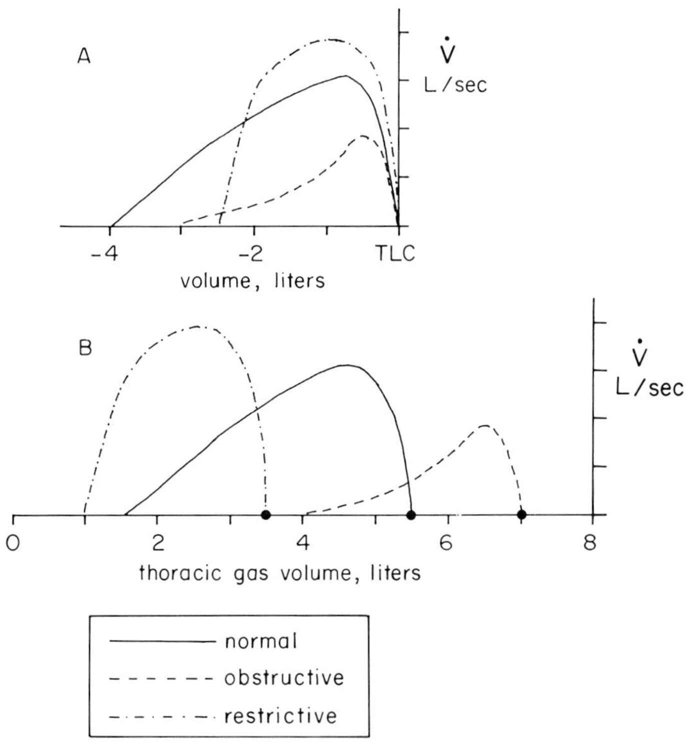

Fig. 9-6. *A*. MEFV curves plotted on volume scale relative to total lung capacity (TLC). Typical curves of a healthy person, a patient with severe airway obstruction, and a patient with restrictive function loss. *B*. The same curves plotted on an absolute lung volume scale, based on measurements of thoracic gas volume; ● = TLC for each curve. From reference 5. Used with permission of McGraw-Hill Book Co. (copyright 1974).

The visual pattern of MEFV curves allows major changes, in the sense of obstruction or restriction, to be recognized at a glance. Observer error in distinguishing the three main shapes is infrequent.[48] Recognition of inconsistent or faulty "blowers" is easy. Since the curve provides a picture of ventilatory reserves that can be understood without much explanation, it is often helpful in the clinical management of patients with lung disease. In asthma patients, the curves can be used to demonstrate effects of drugs, and a smoker's obstructive curve pattern can help convince him to stop smoking. In these respects, the MEFV curve is superior to the spirogram, which does not facilitate visualization of flow rates. Because MEFV curves are increasingly used as lung function tests in clinical and epidemiological studies, the following sections of this chapter focus on the methods for recording the curves, the measurements provided, and the clinical applications.

METHODS FOR RECORDING MEFV CURVES

Recordings of maximum expiratory flow versus lung volume can be obtained with respiratory flowmeters (pneumotachographs), or with spirometers, or with a combination of the two.

SPIROMETERS

Spirometers provide a record of expired volume versus time. By differentiating this record with respect to time, one can obtain flow rates, but this is a laborious, error-prone task when done manually.[3] Although electrical differentiating circuits can simplify the job, they suffer from low signal-to-noise ratios and signal distortion.[1] A specially designed spirometer[46] records MEFV curves directly, but its insufficient response characteristics distort the high initial flows.

PNEUMOTACHOGRAPHS

A pneumotachograph consists of a mechanical resistance placed in the airstream (a wire mesh screen, orifice, or, in Fleisch's instrument, a bundle of narrow tubes). To avoid instrumental reduction of flow rates, its resistance should be minimal, yet sufficient to produce a measurable pressure difference as a function of flow rate. This pressure difference is sensed by a transducer and amplified to a voltage suitable to drive a pen recorder or oscilloscope beam. The output should be a linear function of flow rate; otherwise the flow recording requires correction for alinearity. In addition, the instrument needs to have adequate frequency response and minimal phase shift. With Fleisch pneumotachographs,[18] frequency response is adequate and phase shift minimal up to frequencies of about 20 Hz.[45] This is sufficient since higher frequencies are insignificant during forced expirations.[32] The tubing attached to Fleisch pneumotachographs can affect their calibration;[17] hence, they should be calibrated and used with the same tube configuration.

VOLUME EXPIRED VERSUS PLETHYSMOGRAPHIC VOLUME CHANGES

The volume measurement needed for the MEFV curve can be obtained with (1) a spirometer at the mouth, (2) integration of expiratory airflow rate to volume, or (3) a body plethysmograph. The choice is a matter of principle as well as practice. The simplest method is to measure the volume expired at the mouth (methods 1 or 2) under atmospheric pressure. During a forced expiration, alveolar gas is compressed from atmospheric to a higher pressure. Consequently, the alveolar gas volume decreases (according to Boyle's law) even if no air is expired. The body plethysmograph measures the chest's volume decrease, which during flow exceeds the amount of gas expired; the difference is the volume decrement of alveolar gas that results from gas compression.[25] Therefore, MEFV curves obtained with methods 1 or 2 differ from those obtained with the plethysmograph. Peak flows are closer to TLC on the former. In healthy persons the difference is small, and MEFV curves recorded with the plethysmograph and a spirometer at the mouth, from the same expiration, can almost be superimposed.[10] In patients with airway obstruction the difference is larger, since alveolar pressures are often high.[25]

The choice of method depends on one's purpose. To relate maximum flow rates to lung static recoil, one needs plethysmographic volume measurements since static recoil pressure depends on the actual lung volume, regardless of alveolar gas compression. The plethysmograph is also preferable if one wants to compare flow rates measured under conditions in which gas compression may vary markedly, e.g., when comparing spontaneous flow rates during exercise with forced expiratory flows.[20] However, to assess airway obstruction, volume measurement at the mouth may be preferable. The "compression artifact" in MEFV curves recorded at the mouth [23] is in fact a consequence of airway obstruction. At apparently equal lung volumes, volume measurement at the mouth yields lower flow rates because of alveolar gas compression, which increases with the degree of airway obstruction. Hence, this method reflects airway obstruction more completely than the plethysmographic method.[59] In restrictive lung disease, high flows are reached with minimal effort and the effect of gas compression should therefore be minimal. For assessing maximum expiratory flow rates in lung disease, measuring volume changes at the mouth is a valid procedure. We have adopted this procedure in routine recording of MEFV curves in the laboratory and in epidemiological studies; the plethysmographic procedures used in our laboratory have been described previously.[4]

INTEGRATION OF FLOW

For measuring volume changes at the mouth we favor integration of a flow signal (method 2) over volume recording with a spirometer (method 1). In method 2 a single signal (flow rate) acts as input to obtain both volume and flow at the output; furthermore, there are no mechanical moving parts, maintenance is minimal, and the electronic signal is easy to handle. Integration can be done by digital computer or with stable integrating circuits. The inaccuracies of differentiating circuits are thus avoided, as is the need to match the response characteristics of a separate flowmeter and spirometer. A compact and portable instrument using integrating circuitry has been developed in our laboratory.[53] The instrument provides internal digital outputs of forced vital capacity (FVC), peak expiratory flow rate (PEF), and timed forced expiratory volumes ($FEV_{0.5}$, $FEV_{1.0}$, and $FEV_{3.0}$), as well as flow and volume outputs for MEFV curve display on a storage oscilloscope or XY-recorder. For measuring $FEV_{0.5}$, $FEV_{1.0}$, and $FEV_{3.0}$, it is useful to superimpose time pulses on the recording.[21]

REFERENCE VOLUMES

Measurement of total lung capacity is often required for a comparison of MEFV curves on an absolute volume scale rather than relative to the point of maximum inspiration (Fig. 9-6*B*). Absolute lung volumes are used for comparing MEFV curves in some patients with asthma whose TLC (determined with the plethysmograph) decreases during treatment with bronchodilator drugs (see Fig. 7 in Bouhuys et al., reference 6). RV is less satisfactory as a reference volume,[26] since it varies more than TLC breath-to-breath during a series of forced expirations. When absolute volume data are not available, it is better to superimpose curves of an individual subject on the assumption that TLC is constant, as in Figures 9-5 and 9-10.

COMPUTER SYSTEM

For routine clinical use and for epidemiological studies, processing MEFV curve data with a digital computer allows integration of flow to volume, standardization of recording and data processing, and immediate availability of numerical values and computer-compatible data output. The system * used in our mobile facility for epidemiological studies (Fig. 9-7) employs a Fleisch #4 pneumotachograph as the flow sensor and a pressure transducer and electronic hardware to

SYSTEM CONFIGURATION FOR THE MOBILE LABORATORY

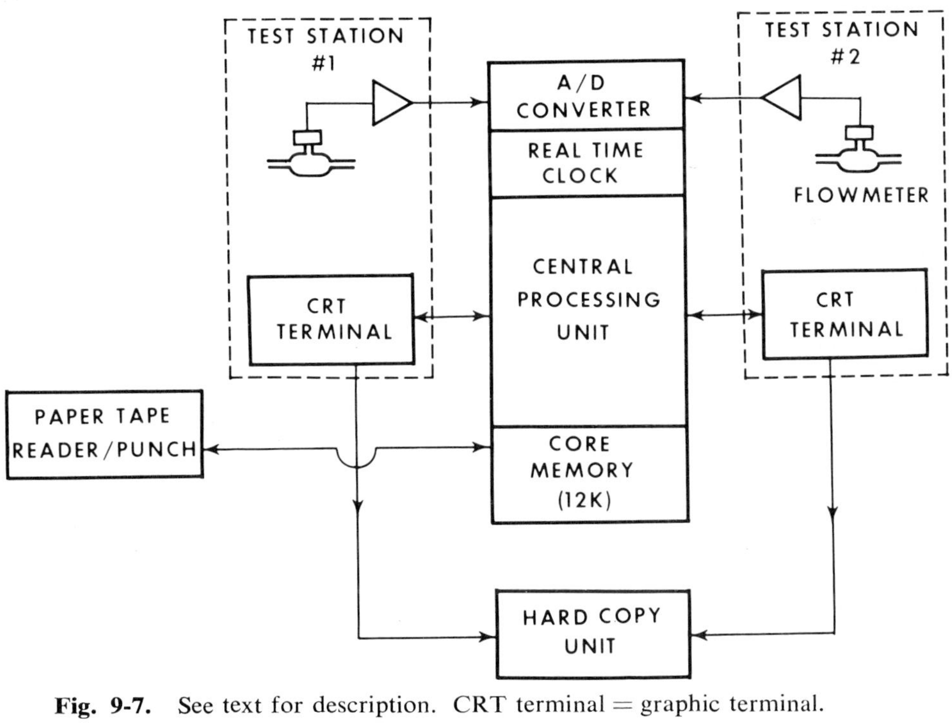

Fig. 9-7. See text for description. CRT terminal = graphic terminal.

* Bouhuys A, Mitchell CA, Tuttle RW: On-line computer system for recording of respiratory questionnaires and MEFV curves. Biosci Commun 1:219–236, 1975

generate a signal suitable for analog-to-digital conversion. Two such systems are linked to a PDP-8E computer via an analog-digital converter. Two graphic terminals suitable for oscilloscopic display of alphanumeric data and graphs are also linked to the computer in an interactive mode. A time-sharing program allows simultaneous use of both terminals with minimum waiting times for data processing. The software includes special calibration and zero drift correction subroutines. In using the system, the test operator first enters identification data and administers a questionnaire (Chap. 12). Next, the subject is instructed to perform the MEFV curve test. Upon command from the operator, the computer starts sampling flow signals to establish a zero flow baseline. Flow is sampled every 5 msec, and the baseline value is subtracted from each sample. When expiratory flow exceeds 0.5 liters/sec, all counting elements in the computer are set at zero and accumulation of expiratory flow data begins. All successive flow signals, at 5-msec intervals, are added to obtain volume change; at each 50-ml volume increment, the corresponding flow value is stored. The number of 50-ml volume increments is counted. Special subroutines are used to store values for PEF, $FEV_{1.0}$, and $FEV_{3.0}$ during the forced expiration. (For definitions of these terms see Table 9-1). Flow sampling continues as long as flow exceeds 0.05 liters/sec. At the end of the blow the total volume expired is added up and stored (FVC). Thus, at the end of the first blow the computer has stored FVC, PEF, $FEV_{1.0}$, and $FEV_{3.0}$, as well as instantaneous flow points at 50-ml intervals over the full FVC range. Immediately after the blow, both the key data (FVC, $FEV_{1.0}$) and the MEFV curve are displayed on the terminal. The process is started anew for the following blows with the same data storage. After the third blow, a subroutine compares the $FEV_{1.0}$ values of the three blows and eliminates the data from the blow with the lowest $FEV_{1.0}$ from the computer memory. This comparison is repeated after the fourth and fifth blows. At the end of five blows, the terminal displays all five MEFV curves and their FVC and $FEV_{1.0}$, values, while the computer memory contains an array of flow points, at 50-ml intervals, for the two blows with the highest $FEV_{1.0}$, as well as the FVC, PEF, $FEV_{1.0}$, and $FEV_{3.0}$ values for these two blows. Next, the operator initiates a computation routine that uses all data from the two blows with the highest $FEV_{1.0}$ values. Their average FVC, PEF, $FEV_{1.0}$, and $FEV_{3.0}$ are computed, and the stored flow points are averaged at each 50-ml interval. These points are displayed as an average MEFV curve on the terminal, and MEF50% and MEF25% (Table 9-1) are computed and displayed. From prediction equations stored in the computer, predicted values for FVC, $FEV_{1.0}$, and flow rates are computed and used to display the actual data as a percentage of the predicted values.

The software includes several quality-control features. A blow is automatically rejected if it lasts 1 second or less. If a blow was delivered in a faulty manner, the operator may reject it, thereby eliminating the data from the computer memory. So that the operator can monitor the consistency of blows, the percentage difference between the highest and next highest $FEV_{1.0}$ is displayed on the terminal. At the end of the test all data are displayed on the terminal screen. The operator then activates (1) a hard copy unit that produces a sheet with all data and the MEFV curve as they appear on the screen (Fig. 12-2), and (2) a paper tape punch unit that stores the same data in computer-compatible format for later processing. The hard copy makes possible immediate review of data and, if necessary, initiation of medical care; the paper tape is essential for processing grouped data. A somewhat simpler system used in our clinical routine function laboratory since 1970 provides a condensed output report on a Polaroid ® print, which is convenient for permanent filing in a patient's record.

PARTIAL EXPIRATORY FLOW-VOLUME (PEFV) CURVE

In studies of airway constrictor and dilator agents, the measurement of flow rates at low lung volumes is of special interest (p. 195). The PEFV curve is a recording of maximum expiratory flow rates at volumes less than about 50 percent of VC, during a forced expiration starting at about 60 percent VC rather than at TLC (Figs. 9-8 and 9-9). Thus, the PEFV curve records maximum flows at low lung volumes without a previous inspiration to TLC. To compare PEFV curves before and after drugs or environmental inhalants, one needs a reference volume. Residual volume (RV) is not suitable, since it often increases during airway obstruction and is therefore not constant. TLC is more suitable since it usually remains constant unless constriction is severe. If the subject inspires to TLC

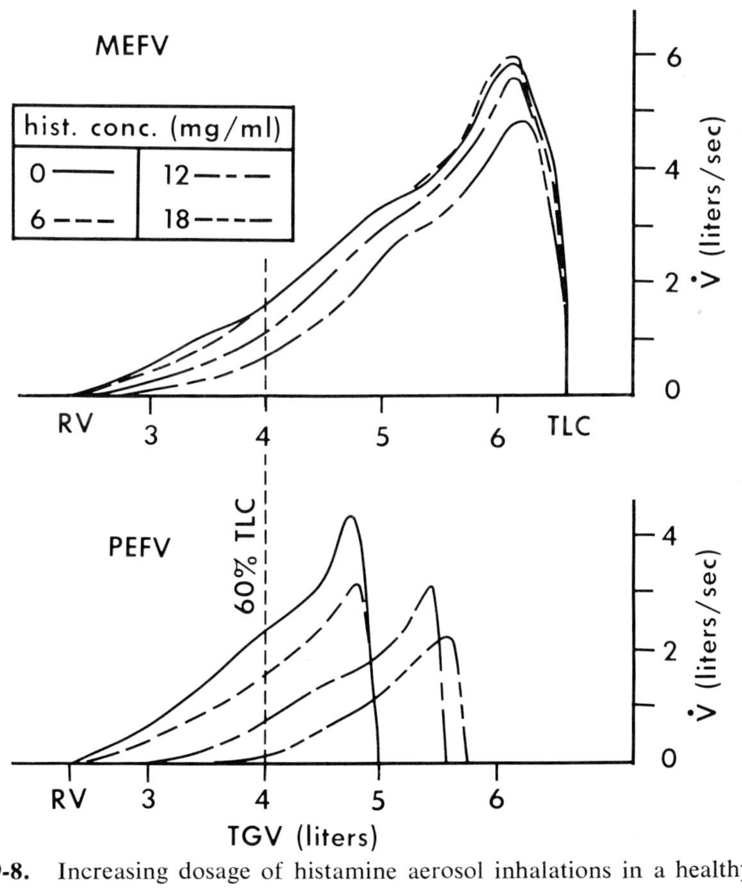

Fig. 9-8. Increasing dosage of histamine aerosol inhalations in a healthy subject. *Ordinate:* expiratory flow rate; *abscissa:* thoracic gas volume (TGV). Upper curves: MEFV curves; lower curves: PEFV curves. Flow measurements at 60% TLC can be used to quantitate the response (vertical dashed line; 60% TLC = 4 liters). From reference 6.

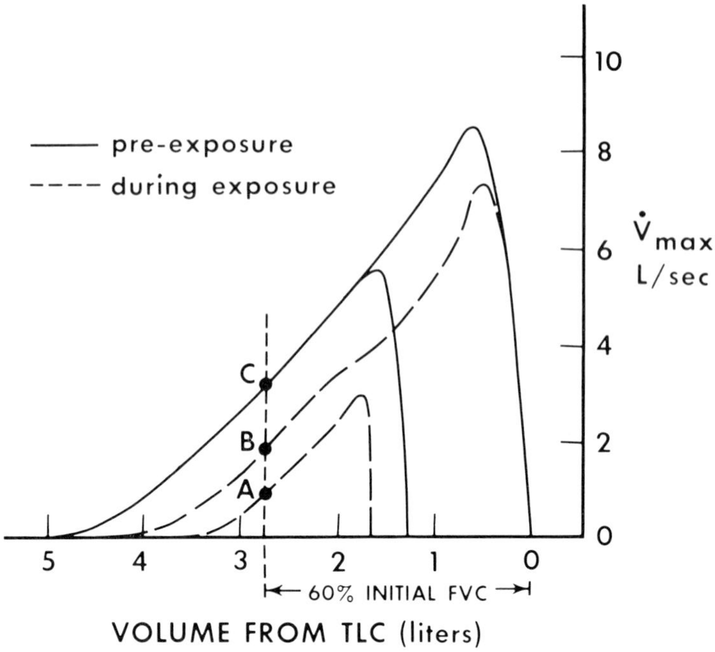

Fig. 9-9. MEFV and PEFV curve in a healthy subject before and during exposure to flax dust. The vertical dashed line indicates MEF40% (at TLC —60% of the initial FVC). MEF40% decreases from *C* to *A* on the PEFV curve and from *C* to *B* on the MEFV curve. From reference 8.

directly after the PEFV curve recording, TLC can be established as a reference volume point on the record. This procedure allows serial PEFV curves to be superimposed, using TLC as a common reference (Fig. 9-9). Separate determinations of TLC with the body plethysmograph can be used to demonstrate whether the assumption of a constant TLC is valid. Alternatively, one can record PEFV curves with the subject in the body plethysmograph and determine thoracic gas volume (TGV) at the beginning of each PEFV curve (Fig. 9-8).[6] For this procedure the subject inspires to about 60 percent VC; a shutter in the mouthpiece is then closed and TGV determined while the subject pants against the closed shutter.[16] Next, the shutter is opened and the subject expires forcefully to RV to record the PEFV curve. Although we used this method initially, later work has confirmed the validity of the simpler procedure, using TLC as the reference volume, under different experimental conditions.[8, 38, 56, 57, 58]

MEASUREMENTS FROM MEFV AND PEFV CURVES

All conventional spirometric measurements (FVC, $FEV_{1.0}$, and $FEV_{3.0}$) can be obtained from MEFV curve recordings. The definitions and preferred abbreviations of these terms are given in Table 9-1. As a single measurement of ventilatory capacity, the $FEV_{1.0}$ has several advantages.[22] It is relatively independent of effort (see Fig. 9-5 and its legend), and it includes sufficient flows at low lung volumes to be sensitive to airway obstruction. In contrast, $FEV_{0.5}$ is too effort-dependent,

Table 9-1.
Nomenclature and Definitions

Measurements	Recommended Name	Abbreviations	Comments and Synonyms
1. Maximum volume measured on expiration after the deepest inspiration	Vital capacity	VC	
(a) during a slow expiration	Slow vital capacity	SVC	
(b) during a forced expiration	Forced vital capacity	FVC	Fast vital capacity; forced expiratory vital capacity
2. Volume of gas expired over a given time interval during a forced expiration	Forced expiratory volume	FEV_T* ($_T$ = time interval in sec)	Timed vital capacity; fast vital capacity; forced expiratory vital capacity
3. Peak expiratory flow	Peak expiratory flow	PEF	
4. Mean expired flow during specified segments of the forced expiratory volume; e.g., between 25% and 75% of FVC †	Mean maximum expiratory flow, qualified by volume range	MMEF MMEF 25%–75%	
5. Instantaneous maximum expiratory flow at specified lung volumes, e.g.:	Maximum expiratory flow, qualified by volume at which measured	MEF	
(a) at 50% FVC ‡		MEF 50% §	
(b) at 25% FVC ‡		MEF 25% §	
(c) at TGV = 5 liters		MEF 5 liters	
(d) at 60% TLC		MEF 60% TLC	
6. Instantaneous maximum expiratory flow rates at specified lung volumes, from PEFV curves, e.g., at 40% FVC ‡	As 5	As 5 a-d, add (P) MEF 40% (P) §	

* When computing the FEV_T/VC ratio, specify whether SVC or FVC is used in the denominator, e.g., $FEV_{1.0}/FVC$. Use of FVC is preferred since it is obtained from the same blow as $FEV_{1.0}$.

† Percentages of VC are expressed on a scale where TLC=100% and RV=0%; use FVC to determine volume segments.

‡ I.e., TLC-50% FVC (5a), TLC-75% FVC (5b), and TLC-60% FVC (6). In serial experiments where FVC varies, control FVC values should be used to determine volume levels for all flow measurements (see Fig. 9-9).

§ The abbreviation presumes that percentage FVC is the most common volume reference; further qualification is only needed when another reference is used, as in 5c and d.

This table is a modified and expanded version of Hyatt's table.[22]

while $FEV_{2.0}$ and $FEV_{3.0}$ always include low flows near the end of the FVC and are therefore less sensitive to airway obstruction than the $FEV_{1.0}$. From spirometric recordings of forced expirations, one can calculate the mean mid-expiratory flow rate (MMFR [29]), i.e., the average flow rate between 25 and 75 percent of the FVC. This excludes the flows at large lung volumes, which are high even in patients with airway obstruction, as well as those near RV which are usually low even in normal subjects. Hence, the MMFR averages flow over a portion of the MEFV curve that is most sensitive to airway obstruction. However, the MEFV curve allows more detailed interpretation of these flow rates. Now that accurate flowmeters are widely available, there seems little reason to continue the use of average flows like the MMFR.

The slope of the effort-independent portion of the MEFV curve shows individual differences related to lung disease—it is steep in patients with restrictive disease and flat in patients with airway obstruction. Early studies concluded that this slope contains the most useful clinical information, since it reflects the time constants of the peripheral portions of the airways and lungs.[47] The slope of the effort-independent portion is, however, often nonlinear. It can be expressed quantitatively by taking the average slope over a defined portion of the curve, e.g., between 50 and 75 percent of VC, or between 50 and 25 percent of VC [28] (Fig. 9-10). These slope indices discriminate between healthy subjects and persons with airway obstruction,[28] but they are not sensitive to minor changes in airway caliber. In many experiments with constrictor and dilator drugs, we have found that the slope remains unchanged even though maximum flows at a given lung volume decrease.[6] Figures 9-8, 9-9, and 9-10 show examples. Measurement of flow rates at 1 liter above RV has also been proposed,[30] but this procedure is unsatisfactory because it uses RV as a reference volume (see p. 213). In our

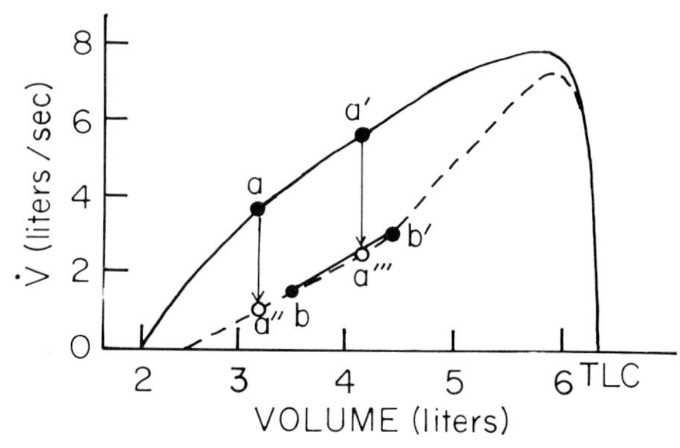

Fig. 9-10. Quantitation of MEFV curve data. A straight line *aa′* is the slope of the drawn MEFV curve between 25% and 50% of FVC. *bb′* is the slope over the same volume segment, after airway constriction, on the dashed curve. The slope remains nearly unchanged (*bb′* parallels *ad′*), while MEF25% (at TLC − 75% control FVC) decreases from a to a″ and MEF50% (at TLC − 50% control FVC) decreases from *a′* to *a‴*. The change of peak flow is minimal.

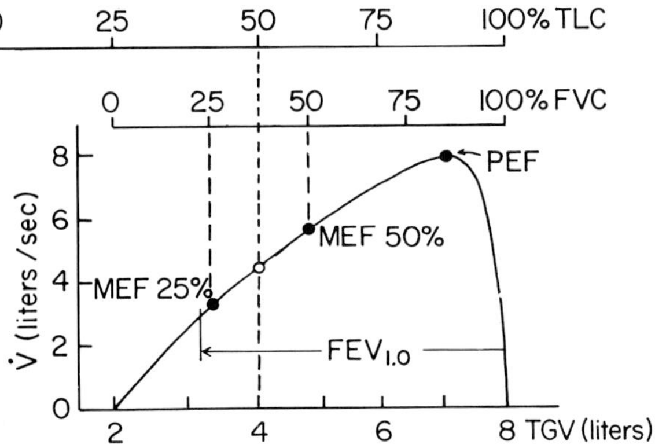

Fig. 9-11. Quantitation of MEFV curve data. One-second mark on the curve indicates the end point of the $FEV_{1.0}$. Maximum flows are referred to three different lung volume scales: %TLC, %FVC, and liters thoracic gas volume. PEF, MEF25%, MEF50%, MEF50% TLC, and MEF 4 liters are indicated on the curve; the last two are identical. See Table 9-1 for definition and nomenclature of these measurements.

experience this index does not reflect changes in airway caliber with sufficient sensitivity.[6] Any measurement based on the last portion of the curve depends on the endpoint of vital capacity, which is often variable and difficult to determine, especially in patients with airway obstruction.

Measuring instantaneous flow rates is more satisfactory than assessing the slopes of MEFV curves. Since inhalation of low doses of histamine aerosol decreases plateau flow rates on IVPF curves (Fig. 8-16), particularly at low lung volumes,[7] we studied these flow rates on MEFV and PEFV curves.[6] First, we had to decide what volume levels were suitable for flow measurements. Figure 9-11 indicates the main choices. A volume level in terms of percentage of VC is most practical, since this value is always available. Measuring MEF values at different percentages of FVC and of TLC has been useful in clinical studies where patients were compared with healthy subjects (p. 225). For assessing airway obstruction on MEFV curves we have found useful MEF50%, MEF40%, and MEF25%. On PEFV curves we usually measure MEF40% (P) (i.e., flow at TLC minus 60 percent of the control FVC), which avoids the transients that may be present near the peak of the PEFV curve.

The most commonly measured flow rate on the MEFV curve is the peak expiratory flow rate (PEF). Since it can be measured with simple devices, the PEF is often used as a separate lung function test. Unfortunately, PEF is highly sensitive to effort (Fig. 9-5) and varies considerably within the same subject.[3] In addition, PEF reflects the conductance of large and upper airways rather than that of small airways; in fact, PEF may depend largely on the size of the subject's trachea.[36] It is insensitive to slight degrees of airway obstruction (Fig. 9-10). Thus, a normal PEF does not exclude significant lung disease, and PEF underestimates airway obstruction. In patients with severe airway obstruction, PEF may include significant contributions of transients (p. 205) which do not reflect

Table 9–2.
Prediction Equations

Measurement	Males	Females	Coefficients for Height in cm *	
			Males	Females
FVC	0.12102H† − 0.01357A‡ − 3.18373	0.07833H − 0.01539A − 1.04912	0.04765	0.03084
$FEV_{1.0}$	0.09107H − 0.02320A − 1.50723	0.06029H − 0.01936A − 0.18693	0.03585	0.02374
MEF75%	0.09030H − 0.01987A + 2.72554	0.06876H − 0.01926A + 2.14653	0.03555	0.02707
MEF50%	0.06526H − 0.03049A + 2.40337	0.06220H − 0.02344A + 1.42640	0.02569	0.02449
MEF25%	0.03583H − 0.04142A + 1.98361	0.02334H − 0.03450A + 2.21596	0.01411	0.00919
PEF	0.14393H − 0.02403A + 0.22544	0.09130H − 0.01776A + 1.13160	0.05666	0.03594

* Insert in corresponding equation if height is measured in cm.
† Height in inches.
‡ Age in years.
From Cherniack and Raber,[11] based on data from 859 nonsmoking men and 452 nonsmoking women. FVC and $FEV_{1.0}$ in liters. BTPS; flow rates in liters per second, ATPS.

airflow from alveoli. For these reasons, PEF should be discarded as a separate lung function test.

In studies in which each subject serves as his own control, one needs to compare flows at a constant lung volume under different conditions. MEF50% is not suitable for this purpose since its volume level varies with the vital capacity. If TLC is constant, it can be used as the reference volume, and MEF can be measured at TLC minus a constant volume (e.g., 60 percent of the control FVC: Fig. 9-9). If thoracic gas volume measurements are available for all measurements, serial curves can be superimposed on an absolute lung volume scale (Fig. 9-8). When comparing changes of flow rates, e.g., after drugs, in different subjects, the results can be expressed in terms of percentage change (Fig. 9-16). One can also use a correction factor for lung size, e.g., by expressing flow rates in units of TLC/sec (Fig. 1-9, p. 16) or of FVC/sec.

NORMAL VALUES

Prediction equations for flows on MEFV curves based on a study of non-smoking residents of a low-pollution area (Manitoba, Canada [11]) are shown in Table 9-2. Average normal MEFV curves constructed from these equations are shown in Figure 9-12. To emphasize the similarity in the shape of the curve's descending portions in all women and in young men, these curves have been superimposed at RV. Only the curve for older men is markedly convex toward

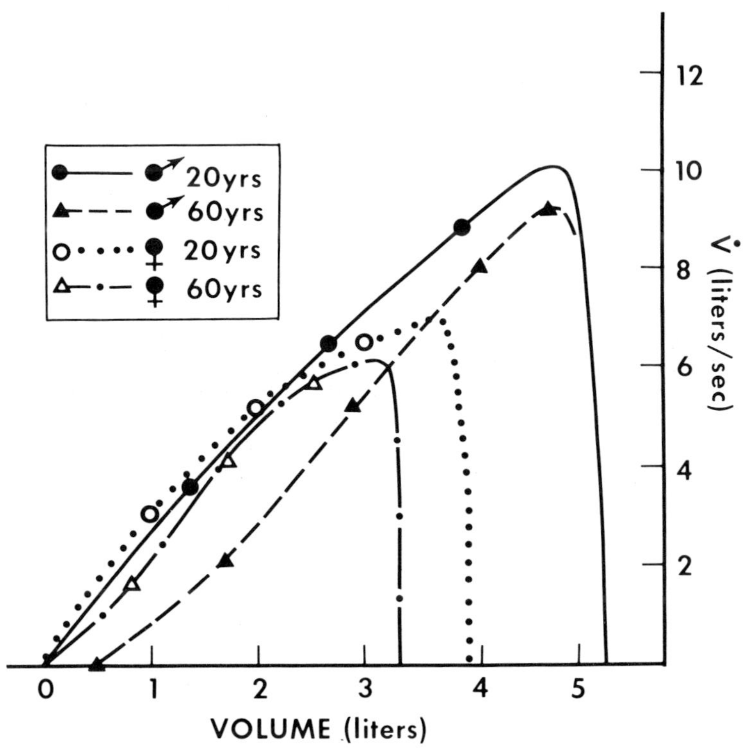

Fig. 9-12. Normal MEFV curves computed from the prediction equations in Table 9-2 [11] using height = 72 in. for men and 68 in. for women. See text for discussion.

Table 9–3.
Variability of Maximum Expiratory Flow Rates in Healthy Subjects

	Subject 1	Subject 2	Subject 3	Subject 4
FVC (liters)				
n	50	52	50	23
$\bar{x}$	6.35	2.94	3.90	4.60
S.D.	0.148	0.242	0.161	0.164
C.O.V.(%)	2.3	8.2	4.1	3.6
S.E.	0.020	0.034	0.022	0.034
S.E./$\bar{x}$(%)	0.3	1.2	0.6	0.7
$FEV_{1.0}$ (liters)				
n	28	—	17	10
$\bar{x}$	5.31	—	3.04	3.66
S.D.	0.141	—	0.151	0.109
C.O.V. (%)	2.7	—	5.0	3.0
S.E.	0.026	—	0.036	0.035
S.E./$\bar{x}$ (%)	0.5	—	1.2	1.0
MEF40% (liters per second)				
n	50	52	50	23
$\bar{x}$	5.16	1.74	2.54	3.22
S.D.	0.420	0.228	0.292	0.301
C.O.V. (%)	8.1	13.1	11.5	9.3
S.E.	0.059	0.032	0.041	0.063
S.E./$\bar{x}$ (%)	1.1	1.8	1.6	2.0
MEF40% (P) (liters per second)				
n	48	51	51	15
$\bar{x}$	4.66	1.98	2.24	3.32
S.D.	0.738	0.420	0.348	0.347
C.O.V. (%)	15.8	21.2	15.5	10.5
S.E.	0.106	0.059	0.049	0.090
S.E./$\bar{x}$ (%)	2.3	3.0	2.2	2.7

Data from control experiments over a period of several months in laboratory workers (subjects 1–3) and in one untrained subject (4) on a single day. All were nonsmokers. The timemarker on MEFV curves (for $FEV_{1.0}$ determination) was used only part of the time, and not at all in subject 2; hence the smaller number of $FEV_{1.0}$ values. n=number of blows; $\bar{x}$= mean values; S.D.=standard deviation; C.O.V.=coefficient of variation (=S.D.×100/$\bar{x}$); S.E. =standard error. The variability of FVC and $FEV_{1.0}$ values (C.O.V. 2.3%–8.2% and S.E. 0.3%–1.2% of mean) is less than that of MEF values (C.O.V. 8.1%–21.2% and S.E. 1.1%–3.0% of mean). Unpublished material, Yale University Lung Research Center.

the volume axis. This difference between older men and women is unexplained, especially since the men did not include persons with known occupational exposures (R.M. Cherniack, personal communication, 1973). It may reflect differences in the aging process in male and female lungs, or undetected environmental exposures in the men. Since the methods to obtain MEFV curves are as yet insufficiently standardized, these data still need to be confirmed by results from other population groups.

VARIABILITY OF MAXIMUM EXPIRATORY FLOW RATES

The between-blows variability of MEF measurements has been discussed on p. 208; it is largely a function of flow history and effort. If all data are taken from maximum-effort blows, this source of variability can be reduced. Data on a large number of forced expirations were obtained in healthy persons (Table 9-3). The MEF40% and MEF40%(P) values varied more than $FEV_{1.0}$ and FVC. Although such variations may not be random (e.g., some values might be low because of an undetected pollutant exposure), in practice, they constitute "noise" in the measurement. The method's ability to detect changes depends on the signal-to-noise ratio, rather than on the variability of control values per se, as Table 9-4 illustrates. MEFV curves were recorded in 17 teen-age smokers, before and after smoking a cigarette.[57] The standard error of the mean MEF50% was about twice that of the mean FVC and $FEV_{1.0}$, both before and after smoking. However, the decrease in MEF50% after smoking was much larger than the decrease in FVC and $FEV_{1.0}$, both as a percentage of the mean control value and as a percentage of the standard error of the mean control value. The latter percentage relates the effect of smoking (the signal) to the variability of the control data (the noise) and is hence analogous to a signal-to-noise ratio. Thus, even though the MEF values vary more than FVC and $FEV_{1.0}$, they are more sensitive to changes even in the presence of this variability.

Under less controlled conditions, as when comparing individual results to an average norm derived from group data in healthy persons, there are additional sources of variability. It is likely that known or unknown pollutants subtly but significantly affect flow rates and influence the data from any normal group of persons. Data from one large group of male and female nonsmokers in a low-pollution area (Table 9-2 [11]) show standard errors for the estimate of MEF50% and MEF25%, from their multiple regressions on age and height, which are 1.7 to 2.6 times larger than those for $FEV_{1.0}$. Extension of such studies to persons in urban environments may show whether MEFV curves are able to quantitate pollutant effects against the background of the other variables involved.

CLINICAL APPLICATIONS

Functional Assessment of Lung Disease

MEFV curves, which can detect obstructive as well as restrictive lung function changes,[28, 31] provide a quantitative assessment of ventilatory function suitable for routine use in any person capable of delivering a few forced expirations. The curves can be used (1) as a diagnostic test in individual patients, (2) to provide objective data on the effects of treatment, (3) to study the natural course of disease, (4) to detect subclinical function disturbances, and (5) to assist in the assessment of ventilatory limitations on exercise performance.

Use of MEFV curves in diagnosing asthma, bronchitis, emphysema, and other obstructive diseases is based on recognition of the obstructive curve pattern (Fig. 9-6) and on measurement of flow rates. In children and adolescents, an MEFV curve which is convex to the volume axis is nearly always associated with

Table 9–4.
Changes in Lung Function After Cigarette Smoking

Measurement	Mean ± S.E.		Difference (liters or liters per sec)	Difference (% of mean control)	Difference (% of S.E.)
	Before	After			
FVC (liters)	5.38 ± 0.15 (2.8%) *	5.37 ± 0.17 (3.2%)	−0.01 (NS)	−0.2	7%
$FEV_{1.0}$ (liters)	4.57 ± 0.13 (2.8%)	4.51 ± 0.12 (2.7%)	−0.06 (NS)	−1.3	46%
MEF50% (liters per sec)	5.8 ± 0.34 (5.9%)	5.4 ± 0.31 (5.7%)	−0.40 ($p < 0.001$)	−6.9	118%

* In parentheses: S.E. as a percentage of mean value (columns 2 and 3). Difference between before and after values in absolute units (column 4), as a percentage of the mean control value (column 5), and as a percentage of the standard error of the control data before smoking (column 6). NS=not significant.

Data from 17 teenagers before and after smoking one cigarette (from reference 57).

a history of smoking, asthma, or other lung disease. Recognition of the restrictive curve pattern assists in the diagnosis of different forms of lung fibrosis. Treatment procedures (drugs, mist therapy) can be assessed from curves recorded before and after treatment, using appropriate controls.[6, 9, 34, 35, 37, 54, 56] If a standardized method is used, MEFV curves can help define the natural course of lung function changes in such diseases as sarcoidosis and cystic fibrosis, and in long-term observations of groups of patients during periods on and off therapy. MEFV curves are particularly appropriate for detecting subclinical disease in epidemiological studies on population groups outside hospitals (Chap. 12). The use of MEFV curves to assess limits on exercise performance is shown in Figure 12-4 (p. 306) and its legend. Many patients with emphysema reach maximum expiratory flow rates during tidal breathing at rest.[50] Such persons have little or no reserve for ventilation increases during exercise, and attempts to increase ventilation result in unduly high expiratory pressures (Chap. 8, p. 196). Although this does not explain the subjective symptom of dyspnea, it does provide an objective explanation of severely limited exercise tolerance. Other applications of MEFV and PEFV curves are discussed in Chapter 12. Clinical studies in our laboratories have used MEFV curves to assess lung function in cancer patients treated with bleomycin [43] and in children with congenital heart disease.[39] The use of MEFV and PEFV curves in the assessment of small airway obstruction warrants a more detailed discussion.

Assessment of Small-Airway Obstruction

Maximum flow rates at low lung volumes are decreased when small-airway caliber is reduced by drugs or dust [6, 52] and in bronchial asthma and cystic fibrosis.[54] In experiments with drugs, cigarette smoke, or textile dust, maximum flow rates decrease more on PEFV than on MEFV curves [6, 38, 56, 57] (Figs. 9-8, 9-9, 9-16). In patients with asthma, maximum flows on MEFV curves are often decreased at a time that airway resistance is within normal limits.[6, 41] The improvement of asthma patients after treatment with dilator drugs is best seen in the increase of flow rates in the lower half of the VC.[37] It is not yet possible to draw a definite conclusion concerning the relative sensitivity of different function tests in detecting small-airway obstruction. Several studies suggest, however, that maximum flows at low lung volumes are highly sensitive to changes in small-airway caliber. In smokers, maximum flows at low lung volumes often decrease when other tests (nitrogen washout, "closing volume," and frequency dependence of dynamic compliance) show normal results or less significant changes.[13, 33] In a group of 10 men, measurable closing volumes were found in only 5 men with "tails" on the MEFV curve.[51] The relation between closing volume and flow rates on MEFV curves is further discussed on page 71 (Fig. 4-9).

Figure 9-13 illustrates the difference between measurements of peak flow and of MEF25% in children with cystic fibrosis or asthma; MEF25% was much more frequently abnormal than PEF. Measurements of MEF also correlated with an independent assessment of the children's condition, as expressed in a clinical score (Fig. 9-14). An example of airway obstruction in a cotton cardroom worker, partially reversed by inhalation of an isoproterenol aerosol, is shown in

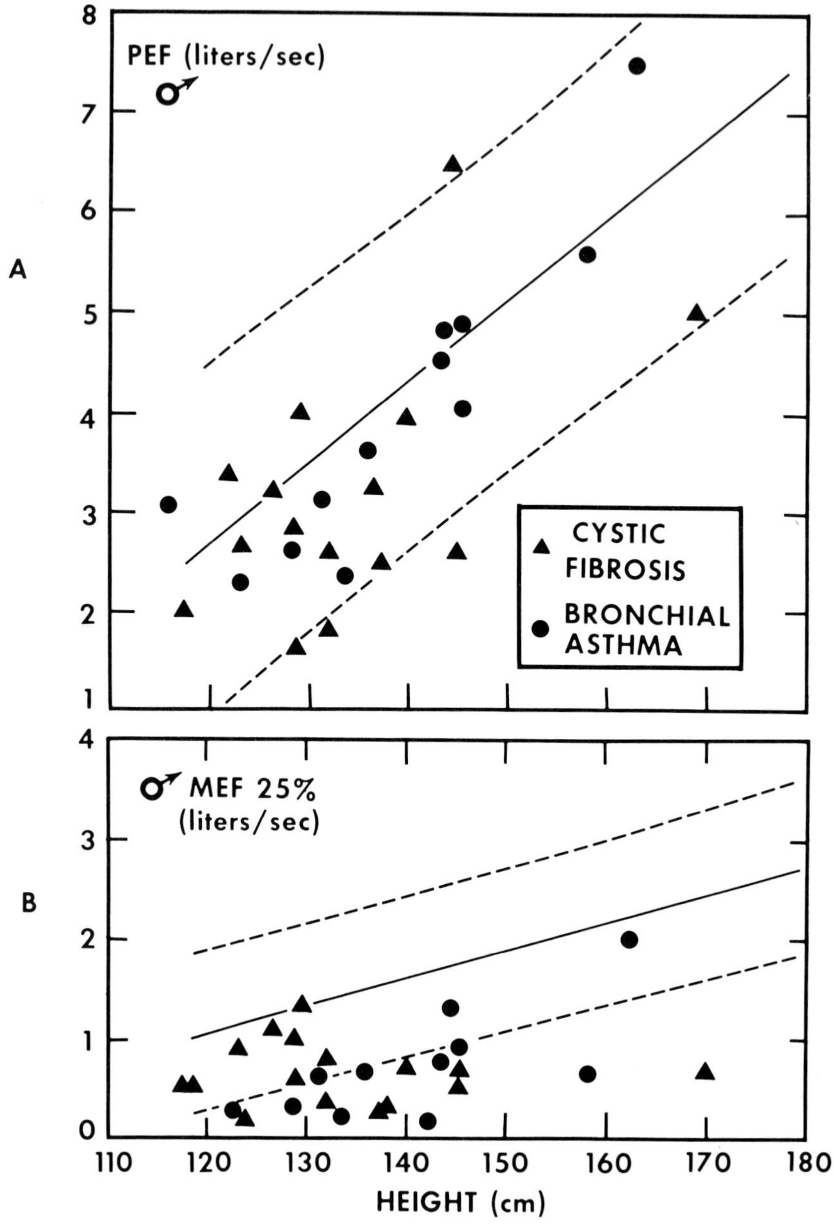

Fig. 9-13. MEFV curve data in children with cystic fibrosis or asthma. Drawn and dashed lines: mean normal values ± standard error.[55] *A*. Only a few patients have abnormally low peak flows; *B*. many more have abnormally low flow rates at 25% VC. Modified from reference 54.

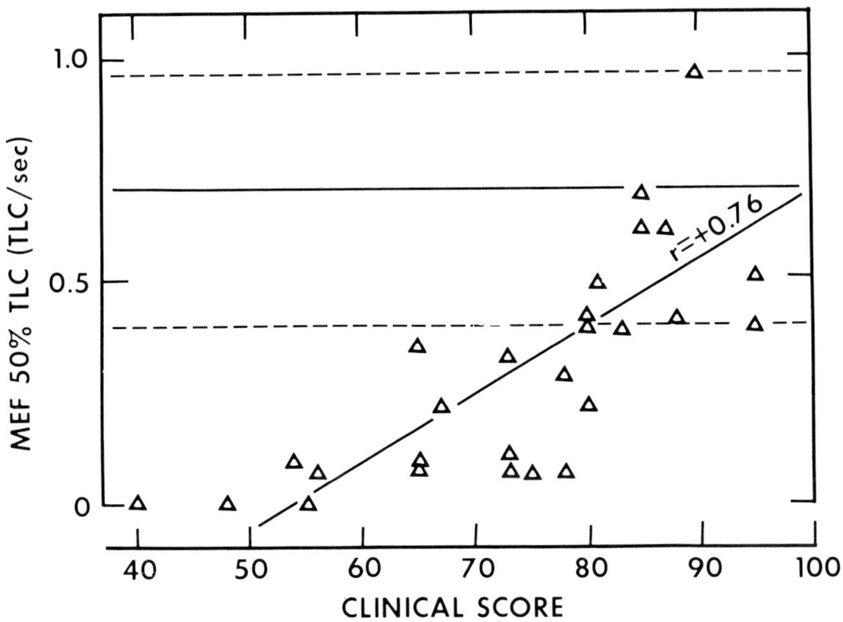

Fig. 9-14. MEFV curve versus clinical evaluation in children with cystic fibrosis. *Ordinate:* MEF50% TLC expressed in units of TLC per second to eliminate effect of variation in lung size between patients. *Abscissa:* clinical score assessed independently by a pediatrician. The correlation is significant at the 1% level. Drawn and dashed lines: mean normal values ± SE.[55] From reference 54.

Figure 12-2, p. 298. These curves were recorded with the computer system of Figure 9-7. After isoproterenol inhalation, flow rates increase, while the slope of the effort-independent portion of the curve is unchanged. Post-isoproterenol flows are still abnormally low, suggesting significant irreversible airway obstruction (see also Chap. 12, p. 316).

In experiments with constrictor agents, the decrease in flow rates on MEFV and PEFV curves is related to the drug's concentration in the inhaled aerosol. In some subjects, adequate dose-response relations can be obtained from measurements of $FEV_{1.0}$ as well as of MEF40% and MEF40% (P) (Fig. 9-15*A*). In other subjects, the deep inspiration required for measurement of $FEV_{1.0}$ and MEF40% appears to abolish the constrictor effect; only the PEFV curve then provides a dose-related response of flow rates (Fig. 9-15*B*). This experience suggests that subtle effects of inhaled agents may be missed if one relies exclusively on forced expirations after a maximal inspiration. The sensitivity of PEFV curves to induced small-airway obstruction is also shown by the experiment of Figure 9-16 in which a healthy subject is exposed to flax dust:[8] MEF values on the PEFV curve decreased more than those on the MEFV curve, while the change in $FEV_{1.0}$ was minimal. In patients with bronchial asthma, PEFV curves are highly sensitive to the effect of bronchodilatation with isoproterenol.[6] In healthy persons, flow rates on PEFV curves increase significantly after administration of atropine,[52] demonstrating the existence of a normal degree of airway muscle tone in small airways. In other studies, PEFV curves have been used to demonstrate airway obstruction after

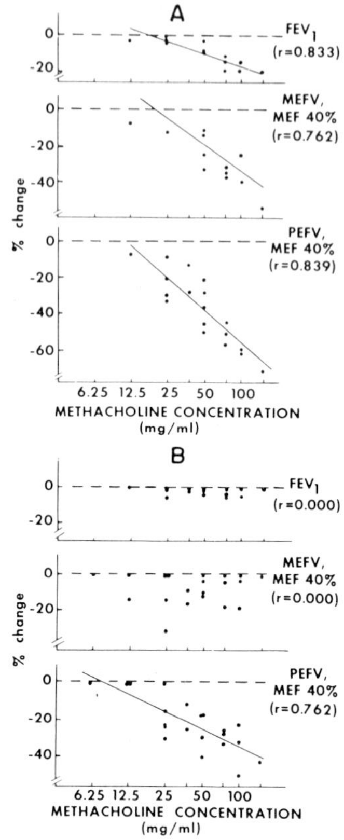

Fig. 9-15. Dose-response curves with methacholine aerosol inhalations. Each graph represents all data obtained from MEFV and PEFV curves in one subject. *Abscissa:* methacholine concentration in nebulized fluid. Duration of all inhalations—30 seconds. Subject *B* has no decrease of $FEV_{1.0}$ at any dose level, while flow decreases on the MEFV curve are erratic. Only MEF40% on the PEFV curve shows a dose-related decrease. In this subject, the drug effect is seen on the PEFV curve, but not consistently on the MEFV curve which was recorded immediately afterward. Thus, a single maximum inspiration often abolished the effect of the constrictor drug, at least temporarily. In subject *A*, the effect of the maximum inspiration was less and all three measurements show dose-related responses. As a percentage of control values, the PEFV curve showed the largest changes. Data contributed by Dr. C.A. Mitchell.[38]

inhalation of 1 ppm SO_2 in air (Chap. 12), after smoking one or two cigarettes,[57] and after 30 seconds' exposure to hairspray aerosols.[58]

Changes in flow rates on MEFV or PEFV curves do not reveal the cause of airway obstruction; they merely indicate its degree. In experiments with agents that alter smooth muscle tone acutely, this effect can explain the changes in airway caliber. In other instances, such as cigarette smoking, the nature of the obstruction is less clear since the biological effects of many pollutants on small airways have not been adequately studied. Inflammation of the mucosa and accumulation of secretions may play a role, while reduced elastic recoil must be considered in long-standing flow rate decreases. The evidence concerning the site of obstruction is likewise indirect. Such evidence rests in part on models of expiratory airflow, which indicate that small-airway caliber is a major determinant of maximum flow (p. 184); further evidence comes from concurring results of tests that measure other aspects of small-airway function, such as nitrogen clearance (Chap. 4), frequency-dependence of compliance (Chap. 7), and airway closing volume

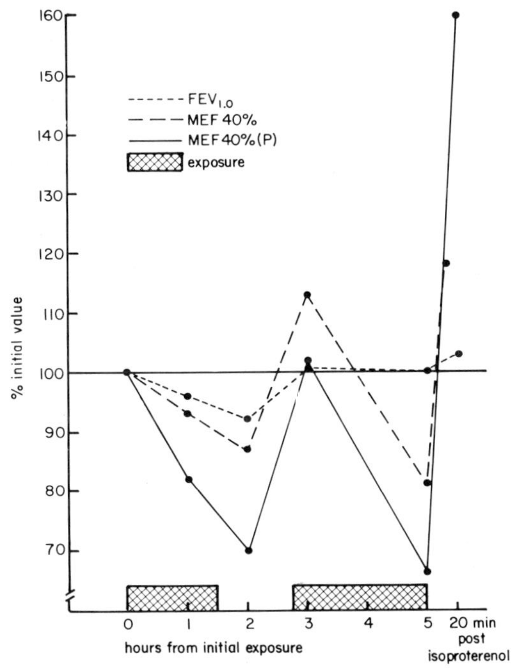

Fig. 9-16. Exposure to flax dust in a healthy subject. MEFV and PEFV curves as well as $FEV_{1.0}$ recorded with maneuver of Figure 9-9. *Ordinate:* percentage change from control values = 100%. The MEF measurements show constrictor responses to dust exposure, with recovery between exposures and, at the end of the experiment, after isoproterenol. See text for further comments. From reference 8.

(Chap. 4). For practical purposes, the PEFV curve has the advantage of being both simple to perform and highly sensitive to small changes in airway caliber.

SUMMARY

Maximum and partial expiratory flow-volume (MEFV and PEFV) curves describe maximum flows as a function of lung volume during forced expirations. Maximum expiratory flow rates are determined mainly by the flow resistance of peripheral airways and by lung elastic recoil; previous flows and inspired gas composition also affect flow rates. Lung size and age influence the shape and size of MEFV curves, and obstructive and restrictive lung disease produce abnormal curve patterns. To record MEFV curves, one uses a flowmeter to sense flow rate and integrating circuits to provide volume excursions. Data processing can be done on-line by computer. With similar equipment, PEFV curves can be recorded in reference to the point of maximum inspiration. Measurements of instantaneous flows at specified lung volumes (for nomenclature see Table 9-1) allow assessment of flow changes in comparison with normal values and with individual control data in acute experiments with inhaled agents. MEFV curves aid in diagnosis and management of asthma, bronchitis, cystic fibrosis, emphysema, and lung fibrosis. They are particularly suitable for detecting subclinical disease in industrial and community population groups, and for assessing effects of therapy on lung function in obstructive diseases of the airways. MEFV curves, and even more, PEFV curves, offer a highly sensitive, objective, and simple means of assessing small airway obstruction induced by smoking, dust, and air pollutants.

REFERENCES

1. Bargeton D, Florentin E, Menier R, Vardon G: Recording of second time derivative $\ddot{V}$ of displaced volume V in breathing. J Appl Physiol 34:259–262, 1973
2. Bouhuys A: Airways dynamics and bronchoactive agents in man, in Bouhuys A (ed): Airway Dynamics; Physiology and Pharmacology. Springfield, Charles C Thomas, 1970, pp 263–282
3. Bouhuys A: The clinical use of pneumotachography. Acta Med Scand 159:91–103, 1957
4. Bouhuys A: Recent applications of volume displacement body plethysmographs. Progr Respir Res 4:24–38, 1969
5. Bouhuys A, Gee JBL: Environmental lung disease, in: Harrison's Principles of Internal Medicine, ed 7. New York, McGraw-Hill, 1974, pp 1310–1320
6. Bouhuys A, Hunt VR, Kim BM, Zapletal A: Maximum expiratory flow rates in induced bronchoconstriction in man. J Clin Invest 48:1159–1168, 1969
7. Bouhuys A, Jonson B: Alveolar pressure, air flow rate and lung inflation. J Appl Physiol 22:1086–1100, 1967
8. Bouhuys A, Mitchell CA, Schilling RSF, Zuskin E: A physiological study of byssinosis in colonial America. Trans NY Acad Sci 35:537–546, 1973
9. Bouhuys A, van de Woestijne KP: Mechanical consequences of airway smooth muscle relaxation. J Appl Physiol 30: 670–676, 1971
10. Bouhuys A, van de Woestijne KP, with the technical assistance of Kane G, van Wayenburg J: Respiratory mechanics and dust exposure in byssinosis. J Clin Invest 49:106–118, 1970
11. Cherniack RM, Raber MB: Normal standards for ventilatory function using an

automated wedge spirometer. Am Rev Respir Dis 106:38–46, 1972
12. Clément J, van de Woestijne KP: Validity of simple physical models in interpreting maximal expiratory flow-volume curves. Respir Physiol 15:70–86, 1972
13. Da Silva AMT, Hamosh P: Effect of smoking a single cigarette on the "small airways." J Appl Physiol 34:361–365, 1973
14. Dayman H: Mechanics of airflow in health and in emphysema. J Clin Invest 30:1175–1190, 1951
15. Despas PJ, Leroux M, Macklem PT: Site of airway obstruction in asthma as determined by measuring maximal expiratory flow breathing air and a helium-oxygen mixture. J Clin Invest 51:3235–3243, 1972
16. DuBois AB, Botelho SY, Bedell GN, Marshall R, Comroe JH Jr: A rapid plethysmographic method for measuring thoracic gas volume: A comparison with a nitrogen washout method for measuring functional residual capacity in normal subjects. J Clin Invest 35:322–326, 1956
17. Finucane KE, Egan BA, Dawson SV: Linearity and frequency response of pneumotachographs. J Appl Physiol 32: 121–126, 1972
18. Fleisch A: Der Pneumotachograph; ein Apparat zur Geschwindigkeits registrierung der Atemluft. Pfluegers Arch 209: 713–722, 1925
19. Fry DL, Hyatt RE: Pulmonary Mechanics. A unified analysis of the relationship between pressure, volume and gasflow in the lungs of normal and diseased human subjects. Am J Med 29: 672–689, 1960
20. Grimby G, Stiksa J: Flow-volume curves and breathing patterns during exercise in patients with obstructive lung disease. Scand J Clin Lab Invest 25:303–313, 1970
21. Hankinson JL, Lapp NL: Time-pulse generator for flow-volume curves. J Appl Physiol 29:109–110, 1970
22. Hyatt RE: Dynamic lung volumes, in: Fenn WO, Rahn H (eds): Handbook of Physiology, Section 3: Respiration, vol II. Washington, D.C., American Physiological Society, 1965, pp 1381–1397
23. Hyatt RE, Black LF: The flow-volume curve: a current perspective. Am Rev Respir Dis 107:191–199, 1973
24. Hyatt RE, Schilder DP, Fry DL: Relationship between maximum expiratory flow and degree of lung inflation. J Appl Physiol 13:331–336, 1958
25. Ingram RH Jr, Schilder DP: Effect ot gas compression on pulmonary pressure, flow, and volume relationship. J Appl Physiol 21:1821–1826, 1966
26. Jordanoglou J, Pride NB: A comparison of maximum inspiratory and expiratory flow in health and in lung disease. Thorax 23:38–45, 1968
27. Knudson RJ, Mead J, Leith DE: Flow transients from the respiratory system. Fed Proc 27:227a, 1968
28. Lapp NL, Hyatt RE: Some factors affecting the relationship of maximal expiratory flow to lung volume in health and disease. Chest 51:475–481, 1967
29. Leuallen EC, Fowler WS: Maximal midexpiratory flow. Am Rev Tuberc Pulm Dis 72:783–800, 1955
30. Lloyd TC Jr, Wright GW: Evaluation of methods used in detecting changes of airway resistance in man. Am Rev Respir Dis 87:529–537, 1963
31. Lord GP, Gazioglu K, Kaltreider N: The maximum expiratory flow-volume in the evaluation of patients with lung disease. Am J Med 46:72–79, 1969
32. McCall CB, Hyatt RE, Noble FW, Fry DL: Harmonic content of certain respiratory flow phenomena of normal individuals. J Appl Physiol 10:215–218, 1957
33. McFadden ER Jr, DeGroot WJ: An assessment of closing volumes and maximum mid-expiratory flow rates as tests of small airway disease. Clin Res 21:667, 1973
34. McFadden ER Jr, Lyons HA: Serial studies of factors influencing airway dynamics during recovery from acute asthma attacks. J Appl Physiol 27:452–459, 1969
35. McFadden ER Jr, Newton-Howes J, Pride NB: Acute effects of inhaled isoproterenol on the mechanical characteristics of the lungs in normal man. J Clin Invest 49:779–790, 1970
36. Mead J, Turner JM, Macklem PT, Little JB: Significance of the relationship between lung recoil and maximum expiratory flow. J Appl Physiol 22:95–108, 1967
37. Mellins RB, Lord GP, Fishman AP:

Dynamic behavior of the lung in acute asthma. Med Thorac 24:81–98, 1967
37a. Miller RD, Hyatt RE: Obstructing lesions of the larynx and trachea: clinical and physiologic characteristics. Mayo Clin Proc 44:145–161, 1969
38. Mitchell CA, Piscitelli D, Bouhuys A: Interaction of humoral agents on airway smooth muscle responses (ASMR) in man. Physiologist 15:219, 1972
39. Motoyama EK, Goto H, Wu B, de Leuchtenberg N: Evidence of lower airway obstruction in children with heart disease. Ped Res 7:425, 1973.
40. Murtagh PS, Proctor DF, Permutt S, Kelly B, Evering S: Bronchial closure with mecholyl in excised dog lobes. J Appl Physiol 31:409–415, 1971
41. Overrath G, Konietzko N, Matthys H: Die diagnostische Aussagekraft des expiratorischen Flussvolumendiagramms. Pneumonologie 146:11–25, 1971
42. Park SS, Goldring IP, Shim CS, Williams MH Jr: Mechanical properties of the lung in experimental pulmonary emphysema. J Appl Physiol 26:738–744, 1969
43. Pascual RS, Mosher MB, Sikand RS, De Conti RC, Bouhuys A: Effect of bleomycin on pulmonary function in man. Am Rev Respir Dis 108:211–217, 1973
44. Peslin R, Mead J: Influence de l'histoire antérieure de débit sur la rélation débit expiratoire maximum/volume pulmonaire. Unpublished manuscript
45. Peslin R, Morinet-Lambert J, Duvivier C: Étude de la réponse en fréquence de pneumotachographes (Frequency response of pneumotachographs). Bull Physiopathol Respir (Nancy) 8:1363–1376, 1972
46. Peters JM, Mead J, van Ganse WF: A simple flow-volume device for measuring ventilatory function in the field. Am Rev Respir Dis 99:617–622, 1969
47. Schilder DP, Roberts A, Fry DL: Effect of gas density and viscosity on the maximal expiratory flow-volume relationship. J Clin Invest 42:1705–1713, 1963
48. Seely JE, Zuskin E, Bouhuys A: Cigarette smoking: Objective evidence for lung damage in teen-agers. Science 172: 741–743, 1971
49. Stubbs SE, Hyatt RE: Effect of increased lung recoil pressure on maximal expiratory flow in normal subjects. J Appl Physiol 32:325–331, 1972
50. Takishima T, Grimby G, Graham W, Knudson R, Macklem PT, Mead J: Flow-volume curves during quiet breathing, maximum voluntary ventilation, and forced vital capacities in patients with obstructive lung disease. Scand J Respir Dis 48:384–393, 1967
51. Takishima T, Takahashi K: "Closing volumes" and decreased maximum flow at low lung volumes in young subjects. J Appl Physiol 34:188–193, 1973
52. Vincent NJ, Knudson R, Leith DE, Macklem PT, Mead J: Factors influencing pulmonary resistance. J Appl Physiol 29:236–243, 1970
53. Virgulto J, Bouhuys A: Electronic circuits for recording of maximum expiratory flow-volume (MEFV) curves. J Appl Physiol 35:145–147, 1973
54. Zapletal A, Motoyama EK, Gibson LE, Bouhuys A: Pulmonary mechanics in asthma and cystic fibrosis. Pediatrics 48:64–72, 1971
55. Zapletal A, Motoyama EK, van de Woestijne KP, Hunt VR, Bouhuys A: Maximum expiratory flow-volume curves and airway conductance in children and adolescents. J Appl Physiol 26:308–316, 1969
56. Zuskin E, Lewis AJ, Bouhuys A: Inhibition of histamine-induced airway constriction by ascorbic acid. J Allergy Clin Immunol 51:218–226, 1973
57. Zuskin E, Mitchell CA, Bouhuys A: Interaction between effects of beta blockade and cigarette smoke on airways. J Appl Physiol 36:449–452, 1974
58. Zuskin E, Bouhuys A: Acute airway responses to hairspray preparations. N Engl J Med 290:660–663, 1974
59. Zamel N, Kass I, Fleischli GJ: Relative sensitivity of maximum expiratory flow-volume curves using spirometer versus body plethysmograph to detect mild airway obstruction. Am Rev Respir Dis 107:861–863, 1973

Chapter 10

Control of Breathing

The respiratory control system regulates a series of usually complementary but sometimes competitive or even incompatible activities. It must (1) maintain, through involuntary controls, a regular rhythmic breathing pattern; (2) adjust the tidal volume and the rate of breathing so that the minute volume of ventilation is sufficient to meet the demands for gas exchange in the lungs; and (3) adjust the breathing pattern so that it is consistent with other activities that use the same muscles, such as speech and the control of posture. Under most circumstances, breathing is controlled so well that the arterial partial pressures of oxygen and carbon dioxide remain constant within narrow limits.

Breathing is a motor act and its control resembles that of other movements. According to Luria, "The system is self-regulating: the brain judges the result of every action in relation to the basic plan and calls an end to the activity when it arrives at a successful completion of the program. This mechanism is equally applicable to elementary, involuntary forms of behavior, such as breathing and walking, and to complicated, voluntary ones such as reading, writing, decision-making and problem-solving." [76] The output of the breathing apparatus can be measured by recording respiratory muscle activity, lung volume changes, and arterial or alveolar gas tensions. In addition, many components of the control system have been studied in detail. However, we have as yet no adequate concept of how the control system fits all incoming signals together to determine the required motor output pattern. This chapter attempts a synthesis insofar as that is possible with our current knowledge. The following reviews offer more detailed discussions as well as access to the voluminous literature on the control of breathing: References 14, 17, 22, 26, 32, 34, 62, 69, 73, 85, 90, 104, 105, 116, 121, and 123.

ORGANIZATION OF THE CONTROL SYSTEM

Breathing is usually involuntarily controlled, but voluntary control is important for many special motor acts—such as speech (Chap. 11)—that use the respiratory bellows. The involuntary rhythmic breathing movements are initiated by networks of nerve cells in the brain stem ("brain stem centers" in Fig. 10-1). The autonomous activity of the brain stem centers is modified by nervous and chemical stimuli and is regulated in the framework of a complex control system that has three main functional components (Fig. 10-1).

Control of the Breathing Pattern (block 1 in Fig. 10-1)

The periodic motor output of the brain stem centers, which leads to regular rhythmic breathing, is conducted via bulbospinal neurons to the segments in the spinal cord. These segments contain the motoneurons for the diaphragm (phrenic nerves, 3rd to 5th cervical segments), the intercostal muscles (1st to 6th thoracic segments), and the abdominal muscles (7th to 12th thoracic and 1st

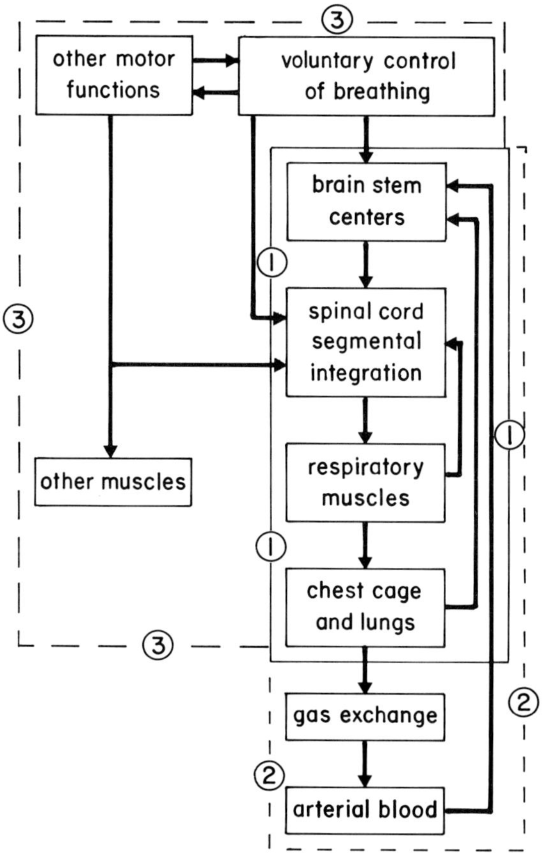

Fig. 10-1. Organization of respiratory control system. Blocks *1*, *2*, and *3* contain the elements concerned with the three main goals of the control system (see text). Brain stem centers are often called "respiratory centers." However, additional integrative control centers for breathing are located in the spinal cord. Together with the brain stem centers they comprise the main central nervous system networks for involuntary control of breathing. In the text the term "centers" refers to the brain stem centers unless specified otherwise.

lumbar segments). At the segmental level, the actions of these individual muscles are coordinated by neuronal networks that receive, in addition to commands from the brain stem centers, signals from the muscle spindles in the respiratory muscles which indicate the state of muscle contraction. Integration of these and possibly other signals at the segmental level results in precise timing and frequency of impulses to each muscle's motor units. The result of respiratory muscle contraction—increase or decrease of the volume of the chest cage and, hence, of the lungs—is monitored by the brain stem centers, which receive information on lung volume from receptors in the lungs via vagal afferent fibers, and from receptors in the chest wall via spinal afferents.

Control of Ventilation (block 2 in Fig. 10-1)

The motor output of the control system (the ventilatory drive) must be adjusted to meet the metabolic demands for gas exchange. For this adjustment, the centers use information on the arterial partial pressures of O_2 and CO_2 and on the H^+ ion concentrations in arterial blood, information provided by chemoreceptor cells near the centers themselves as well as in strategic sites in major arteries (carotid body, aorta). Appropriate modification of the motor output requires processing, storage, and integration of this information with other signals received by the centers. In this way, the ventilation of the lungs, per unit time, is regulated to maintain arterial O_2 and CO_2 tensions constant within narrow limits under most physiological conditions.

Integrative Control of Breathing (block 3 in Fig. 10-1)

The control of breathing must be integrated with the control of other motor functions using the same muscles: posture, speech, singing, swallowing, laughing. There may be neural connections which subserve voluntary control over the brain stem centers (corticobulbar fibers), but most voluntary commands to the respiratory muscles are probably conducted directly to spinal integration centers via corticospinal neurons. To a large extent, integration of breathing with other motor acts may also take place at segmental levels in the spinal cord.

THE BRAIN STEM CENTERS

The brain stem centers contain intricate networks of neurons that maintain coordinated rhythmic breathing even in the absence of afferent inputs. When the connection between the brain stem and the rest of the brain is severed (transection *1* in Fig. 10-2), normal breathing resumes after the animal recovers from the operation. When the pons is separated from the medulla oblongata (transection *4* in Fig. 10-2), breathing often becomes irregular. However, even in the absence of connections with rostral parts of the brain stem and of cranial nerve afferents, the medulla can generate a rhythmic respiratory drive (see review in ref. 85). When the medulla is sectioned a few millimeters lower (transection *5*), breathing stops. Thus, centers crucial for rhythmic breathing appear to be situated between transections *4* and *5* in the upper part of the medulla.

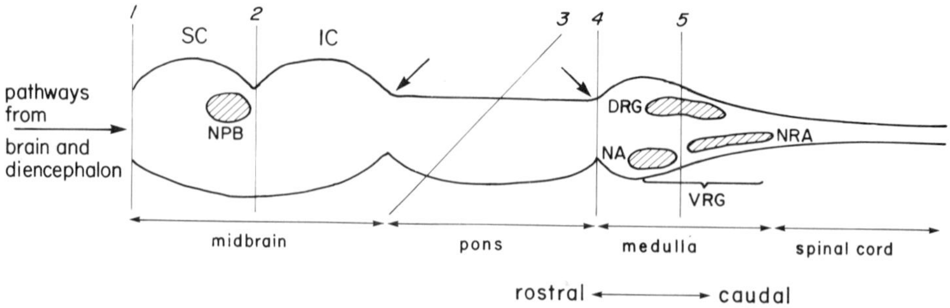

Fig. 10-2. Schematic diagram of brain stem structures, with levels of transections discussed in text. IC and SC = inferior and superior colliculus, respectively. Between arrows: floor of the 4th ventricle. NPB = nucleus parabrachialis (= pneumotaxic center). Respiratory neurons in medulla (after Mitchell and Berger [85]): DRG = dorsal respiratory group, near nucleus tractus solitarius; VRG = ventral respiratory group, with neurons in nucleus ambiguus (NA) and in nucleus retroambigualis (NRA). The diagram represents a sagittal section lateral to the midline of the brain stem.

Until recently most physiologists thought that inspiratory and expiratory centers in the medulla, although capable of functioning automatically, depend on connections to other brain stem centers for the generation of a regular respiratory rhythm. This "classic" view is shown schematically in Figure 10-3. After transection *3* (see also Fig. 10-2), combined with vagotomy, respiratory arrest occurs in an inspiratory position (apneusis). Thus, the lower part of the pons appears to contain a center (apneustic center) which, when isolated from higher centers and from vagal afferents, promotes inspiration and inhibits expiration. After transection *1*, breathing usually remains normal. Thus, when the apneustic center is connected to the midbrain, the action of the apneustic center is inhibited and breathing is rhythmic, even when the vagi have been cut. When the vagi are intact after transection *3*, apneusis does not occur either. Hence, both vagal afferents and stimuli from a center in the midbrain (pneumotaxic center) affect the function of the apneustic center; apneusis occurs only when both sources of stimuli have been removed.

Recently, through improved neurophysiological and histological methods, we have learned a great deal about the location of the inspiratory and expiratory neurons in the medulla, and about their connection to respiratory muscle motoneurons. A crucial assumption in the classic view was that the medullary centers could not maintain regular rhythmic breathing on their own. However, this is now known not to be true.[85] As a result, recent studies have emphasized the role of the medullary centers in the involuntary control of breathing, and the role of the pneumotaxic and apneustic centers is being reassessed (see below).

Cellular action potentials synchronous with breathing can be recorded from different sites in the pons and medulla.[21] By combining such recordings with antidromic (i.e., from the axon to the cell body of a neuron) stimulation of spinal cord or peripheral motor nerve fibers, one can trace the connections of central neurons, which show electrical activity (depolarization or hyperpolarization; spikes) in some relation to the breathing cycle.

The two main groups of respiratory neurons in the medulla are the dorsal and ventral respiratory groups (DRG and VRG; Fig. 10-2). The dorsal group,

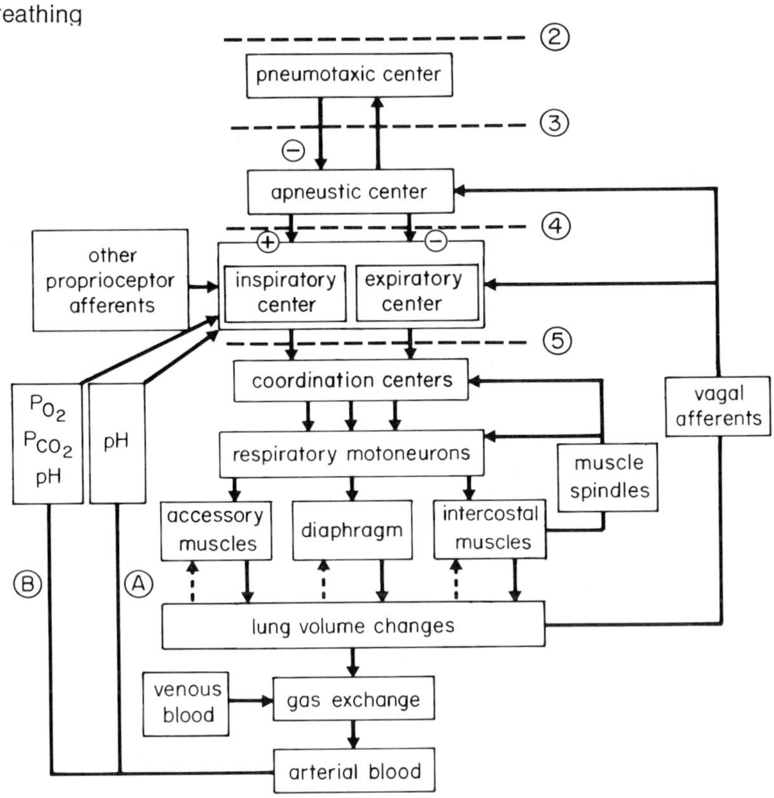

Fig. 10-3. Main functional components of the control system and the breathing apparatus. Dashed lines 3, 4, and 5 indicate the corresponding transections in Figure 10-2. Facilitatory (+) and inhibitory (−) effects in the brain stem shown where appropriate. Dashed arrows indicate mechanical effect of lung volume changes on muscles (p. 239). *A*: central chemoreceptors; *B*: peripheral chemoreceptors. The "classic" view of the brain stem centers, as shown in this diagram, is no longer accepted but has not yet been replaced by a comprehensive alternative model. See text for discussion.

near the nucleus of the tractus solitarius, contains neurons that discharge just before and during inspiration (as determined from recordings of phrenic nerve activity). Most of these inspiratory neurons have their axons in bulbospinal fiber bundles;[7] i.e., they are connected to segmental integration centers in the spinal cord. The ventral group, in the nucleus ambiguus and nucleus retroambigualis, contains approximately equal numbers of inspiratory and expiratory neurons.[86] Of the inspiratory neurons, about 60 percent have bulbospinal connections.[7] Most of the remaining inspiratory neurons appear to have short axons within the medulla since they cannot be stimulated antidromically from peripheral sites.[7] These "propriobulbar" neurons occur rarely in the dorsal group. They fire, as a group, earlier than inspiratory neurons with bulbospinal connections, which suggests that the propriobulbar neurons may play a role in the early stage of activation of the other inspiratory neurons. The activation patterns of the inspiratory neurons (and the inhibition of expiratory neurons; see below) correspond closely with the pattern of phrenic nerve discharge. The similarity of firing patterns, and of changes in resting potentials, in the inspiratory neurons of the ventral group led Mitchell and

Herbert[87] to conclude that these neurons are activated by already highly synchronized input signals. Hence, they believe that the inspiratory neurons in the VRG are not themselves the source of regularly recurring inspiratory stimuli—the rhythm must be generated elsewhere in the medulla or pons.

Neurons that discharge during expiration and are inhibited during inspiration have been found only in the ventral group, intermingled with inspiratory neurons.[7] These neurons hyperpolarize during inspiration and depolarize, often with bursts of spikes, during expiration.[86] About one-third of the expiratory neurons have bulbospinal connections, 45 percent are propriobulbar neurons, and the remainder are expiratory laryngeal neurons.[7] The activity of medullary expiratory neurons can be inhibited easily by even slight activation of inspiratory neurons. For instance, slight stimulation of the cat's nasopharynx with a thin wire elicits a brief burst of activity in inspiratory neurons in the medulla (sniff reflex); this results in marked and sometimes prolonged inhibition of expiratory neurons.[4] Conversely, inspiratory neurons are not inhibited when expiratory neurons are activated during expiration.[81]

The sniff reflex experiments showed [4] that inspiratory neurons in the dorsal group were the first to be activated, even after weak stimuli, whereas VRG inspiratory neurons required stronger stimuli and responded later. Some of the DRG inspiratory neurons are activated by stimulation of the vagus or by inflation of the lungs.[38] For these reasons, Mitchell and Berger [85] suggest that the DRG may be an initial integration center for the Hering-Breuer as well as the sniff reflex, and perhaps for other reflexes as well. They believe that the DRG itself, or closely associated neurons, may act as the medullary respiratory rhythm generator.

Nevertheless, how the rhythm of breathing is established is far from clear. It could be due to inherent automaticity of individual nerve cells in or near the medulla (pacemaker cells), or it may result from interconnections between nerve cells in a network. There is no evidence for the existence of pacemaker cells in the brain stem, but it is difficult to be sure of their absence since the cells cannot be studied in isolation.[85] In neural networks, an oscillating output may be maintained by time delays in neural connections.[82] Different models of neural networks have been proposed,[85] and in all of these models reciprocal inhibition between discharging neurons is a key feature in explaining rhythmicity. Indirect support for the existence of central neural networks comes from experiments with active and passive hyperventilation in cats.[37] When their ventilatory drive is actively increased (by stimulating the carotid body nerve), ventilation continues after the stimulation ceases. Presumably, internal feedback loops with time delays enable the centers to keep firing after the stimulus stops. With passive hyperventilation (by a respirator) the centers are not activated, so breathing stops because of lack of appropriate stimuli when the artificial ventilation ceases.[37] It is likely that a similar mechanism prevents apnea after active voluntary hyperventilation in man.[119]

How the pneumotaxic and apneustic centers relate to the medullary centers remains unclear. Apneusis (after transection *3*; Fig. 10-2) is not a permanent state,[111] so promotion of inspiration by a center in the lower pons may be less crucial in the normal regulation of breathing than used to be thought. The pneumotaxic centers, now known to be located in the nucleus parabrachialis and associated structures, may modulate the rhythmic centers in the medulla.[7a] Some investigators believe that it can generate an oscillating discharge pattern on its own, essential to drive the medullary centers. Others think the pneumotaxic centers may not be essential for rhythmic breathing.[85]

CONTROL OF THE BREATHING PATTERN

Mechanical Factors

To inspire and expire a tidal volume requires inspiratory and expiratory muscle activity, adapted to the lung volume and to the chest cage configuration. The recoil forces of the chest and lungs determine how much force is needed, and in which direction. For instance, inspiring a small tidal volume from FRC requires only inspiratory muscle activity; expiration is mainly passive, through elastic recoil. At higher lung volumes, the same tidal volume requires more inspiratory force to counteract the increased recoil force of the lungs and chest (Figs. 7-1, 7-8). At lung volumes below FRC, expiration always requires active muscle force. During breathing against positive pressure, inspiration may be passive (since inspiratory force is supplied), while expiration must be active. The respiratory motoneuron output must be adapted to meet these varying demands. Hence, the relation between muscle force and tidal volume is not constant.

In addition, the relation between the nervous stimuli that reach the muscles and the force developed depends on the initial length of the muscles. For the same degree of stimulation, muscles develop more force when they are stretched. Thus, to develop a similar inspiratory force, the inspiratory muscles require more stimulation when they are shortened (at high lung volumes).

The regulation of the division of labor between inspiratory and expiratory muscles is not clear but may require vagal afferent signals.[9] In cats, pressure breathing leads to contraction of abdominal muscles, which provide added expiratory force to overcome the load. This response is abolished by vagotomy, even when breathing is stimulated by CO_2.[8] However, responses to pressure breathing in man are probably more complex (see below).

Because of the complex relations between motoneuron output, muscle force, and tidal volume, the latter is a reliable measure of total motoneuron output only when the mechanical conditions are constant. Additional information on motoneuron output can be obtained from recordings of phrenic nerve discharge and of intercostal muscle electromyograms, which reflect important components of the motor drive but do not indicate its integral. Thus, none of these measurements provides a full picture of the output of the controlling system.

Proprioceptive Control by Muscle Afferents

The respiratory muscles contain two kinds of proprioceptive receptors—muscle spindles and tendon receptors—which sense their state of contraction. These sensors can initiate reflex changes in muscle tension via coordinating centers in the spinal cord. The nerve fibers from the sensors (γ-afferents) reach the spinal cord via the dorsal roots (Fig. 10-4). When these roots are cut, the electrical activity

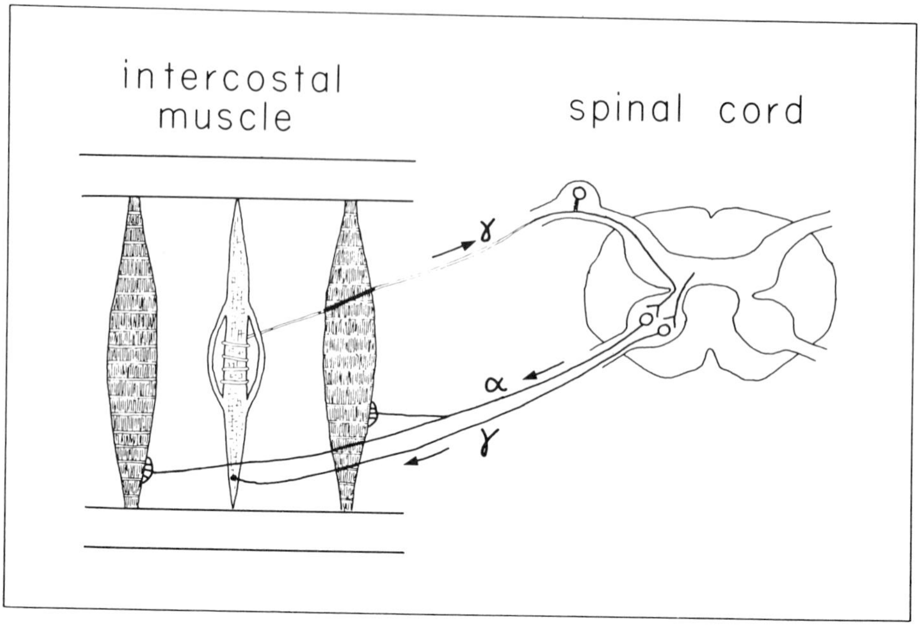

Fig. 10-4. Schematic diagram of respiratory muscle, with a muscle spindle, and its main neural connections with the spinal cord. γ-afferent fibers to the spinal cord and α- and γ-efferent fibers to the muscle fibers and the spindles, respectively, are shown. The γ-afferent fibers have their cell bodies in the dorsal root ganglion and synapse with α-motoneurons in the spinal cord (interneurons not shown). The termination of a motor pathway descending from higher centers is also shown.

in the external intercostal muscles decreases, in man [91] as well as in adult cats.[77] Thus, inputs from the γ-afferents affect inspiratory muscle activity.

Muscle spindles and tendon receptors influence muscle contraction in opposite directions. Stretching the intercostal muscles (which contain many spindles) increases muscle force (facilitation), while stretching the diaphragm (which contains mainly tendon receptors) inhibits its contraction.[31] The motor control of the intercostal muscles differs from that of the diaphragm; they also influence each other via mechanical and nervous linkages. Movement of the rib cage exerts force on the diaphragm, which is attached to it. More indirectly, movements of the rib cage affect the position of the diaphragm via changes in pleural pressure, and vice versa (see p. 271). In addition, contraction of intercostal muscles influences the diaphragm via nervous reflexes. In cats, contraction of the diaphragm can reinforce itself via an intercostal-to-phrenic nerve reflex, elicited by the pull of the diaphragm on the chest cage.[29] While this reflex may help to coordinate posture control and straining maneuvers,[30, 31] its role in breathing per se is uncertain.

Although the proprioceptive control system appears particularly well suited for rapid adaptations of muscle forces to changing demands, its importance in the control of breathing is not clear. Section of dorsal roots in man causes only temporary respiratory muscle paralysis.[91] When sudden loads (e.g., positive pressure at the mouth) are imposed on the breathing apparatus, proprioceptive stimuli elicit a "load-compensating reflex," which alters muscle activity appropriately. However, this response lasts so briefly that it can hardly affect ventilation.[92] In addition, responses to loading in man are influenced by anticipation of its effects and by learning in successive experiments.[49, 93, 114] Furthermore, changes in lung volume due to positive mouth pressures can explain at least some responses mechanically (via changes in elastance) without the need to invoke nervous control mechanisms.[45, 83]

Thus, the physiological function of proprioceptive muscle control in the control of breathing is not established. Since the muscles, chest cage, and lungs form a slow-responding mechanical system, which receives its motor input from fast-traveling nerve signals, afferent signals from sensors in the muscles would seem to be indispensable for control. Yet, perhaps the afferent signals have a less direct function, since their control function does not appear to influence ventilation under conditions (loading) in which it would seem most needed. The linkage of a fast nervous system to a slow-responding mechanical system is reminiscent of the linkage of a high-speed computer to a slow output device, such as a teletype. If the computer gave its output at its own rate to the teletype, only a fraction of the information would be recorded. In computer technology this problem is solved by buffers and flags. That is, the computer stores its information temporarily in a memory unit (buffer) and waits for a signal (a flag), indicating that the teletype is ready to produce an output signal. Thus, information is transferred sequentially at a discontinuous rate that the teletype can handle. If the analogy has any value, the muscle afferents may function as flags that signal the state of the muscles to the coordination centers. Such a function would not necessarily affect the motor output but merely facilitate its transmission to the muscles.

Proprioceptive Control by Vagal Afferents

More than 100 years ago, Hering and Breuer[104] proposed that inspiration is self-limiting because lung inflation stimulates receptors in lung tissue (stretch receptors) which, via vagal afferent fibers, lead to cessation of inspiration. This concept was based on the finding that intact animals stop breathing when their airway is closed after the lungs have been inflated. With the vagi cut, they attempt to inspire against the closed airway. Thus, vagal afferents appear to inhibit inspiration.

In a recent, more detailed concept of vagal control,[20] the ventilatory drive of the respiratory centers sets the rate of inspiratory muscle contraction and hence inspiratory flow rate (the slope of lines *1*, *2*, and *3* in Fig. 10-5). This drive terminates after a time interval set by the centers (about 1.7 seconds in Fig. 10-5). However, this interval limits inspiration only when the ventilatory drive is minimal and inspiration therefore is slow (*3* in Fig. 10-5). The greater the ventilatory drive (*1* and *2*), the sooner inspiration ends (i.e., earlier in *1* than in *2*). After vagotomy, inspiration lasts equally long in all three instances, presumably when the respiratory centers stop firing of their own accord. It is likely that the hyperbolic relation between inspired volume (V_I) and the duration of inspiration, represented by curve *BC* in Figure 10-5, is related to firing of vagal afferent fibers from the lungs.

Vagal afferent signals from the lungs do not alter the centers' ventilatory drive[39] but influence the combination of tidal volume and breathing rate chosen for a given minute ventilation. After vagotomy in cats, tidal volume increases and

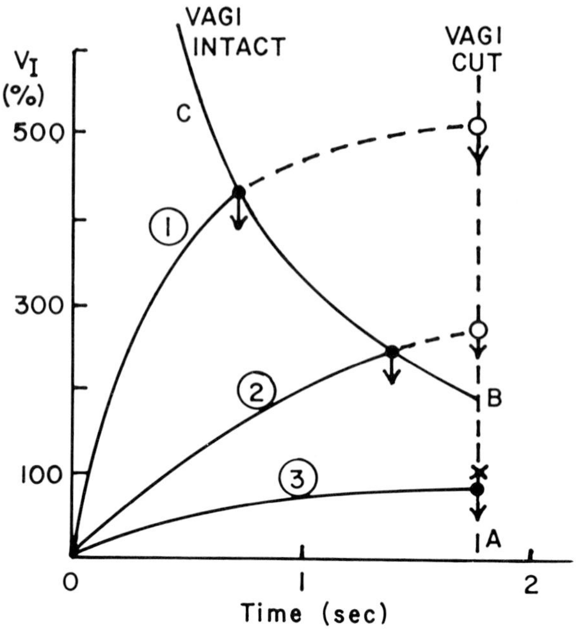

Fig. 10-5. Effect of vagotomy on relation between inspired volume (V_I; tidal volume during quiet breathing = 100%) and duration of inspiration (time). Lines *1, 2,* and *3* represent three inspirations with different ventilatory drives, before (*drawn lines*) and after (*drawn + dashed lines*) vagotomy. The slope of these lines indicates inspiratory flow rate. The arrows indicate the end of inspiration in each instance, before and after vagotomy. Clark and Euler [20] place the normal tidal volume level (*X*) in the range *AB*. As discussed in the text, it may lie close to *B*. A comparison of lines *1* and *2* shows how vagal control amplifies the effect of increased ventilatory drive. Flow rate in *1* is about three times larger than in *2*; since inspiration lasts only half as long, tidal volume is about twice as large in *1* as in *2*. Because the rate has doubled, ventilation increases about fourfold. After vagotomy, rate is low and fixed; both tidal volume and ventilation are twice as large in *1* as in *2*. After reference 20.

rate decreases, while minute ventilation remains constant.[9] Conditions that normally affect breathing rate (e.g., breathing of CO_2-enriched air, airway obstruction) do not do so after vagotomy. In intact humans, too, breathing rate usually increases when tidal volume increases (with V_T up to about half the VC[58]). Hence, large inspirations are brief, in accordance with the hyperbolic relation between V_I and time in Figure 10-5.

In man at rest, vagal block does not affect the breathing pattern.[55] On the other hand, vagal afferent signals have been recorded in man at FRC, and these signals increase at larger lung volumes.[53, 56] Also, breathing rate increases as soon as tidal volume increases when the vagi are intact.[58] During normal breathing in man the control system appears to operate close to point *B* in Figure 10-5. As long as inspiration ends close to point *B* on the hyperbolic curve *BC*, vagal block would have little effect on the breathing pattern; yet, detectable afferent firing might occur. When ventilatory drive increases, the inspiratory point moves up the hyperbolic curve, and the breathing rate increases because of vagal inhibition.

Thus, the principle of self-limited inspiration proposed by Hering and Breuer seems to be well established as an important mechanism that limits lung volume changes during breathing.[9] Even though the consequences of the vagal afferent activity on ventilation are imperceptible during quiet breathing, this activity appears to be largely responsible for the increase in rate when tidal volume increases, during exercise, hypercapnia and hypoxia.[20, 100, 101, 109]

Hering and Breuer also proposed that expiration is self-limiting, due to receptors which respond to decreases in lung volume (deflation receptors). Yet, there is no evidence for a role of deflation reflexes in the control of breathing patterns,[65] and it is not known at precisely which lung volume, presumably below FRC, they are activated. Deflation reflexes may be important under abnormal conditions where inspiratory efforts counteract collapse of peripheral lung units, as in pneumothorax or guinea pig anaphylaxis.[64, 65]

The concept of vagal control over tidal volume and rate appears to conflict with mechanical theories suggesting that the breathing rate is adjusted to optimal values in terms of the work or force of breathing (Chap. 7, p. 164). The mechanisms which accomplish this goal are not clear, and since the minima are far from critical, the fact that work and force are close to optimal may be just a useful but fortuitous consequence of the total system design. In fact, it has been suggested that minimal work would require a square wave inspiratory flow pattern and an exponentially decaying expiratory flow pattern,[125] while apneustic breathing at a constant minute ventilation causes a higher Pa_{O_2} and a lower Pa_{CO_2} than a sinusoid breathing pattern (Chap. 5, p. 87). None of these patterns occurs in man at rest or during moderate hyperventilation. The vagal control represents a more precise mechanism of rate control that may have developed independently or may have become adapted to the mechanical system design.[20]

Synthesis

The breathing pattern reflects mechanical conditions of the lungs and chest as well as the ventilatory drive provided by the respiratory centers in the medulla and pons, modified by afferent inputs from vagal nerve fibers which signal changes in lung volume. Coordination of the respiratory muscle action may involve vagal afferent stimuli at the level of the centers as well as proprioceptive input from the muscles at the spinal level. Two types of sensors in the muscles provide afferent information to the spinal cord centers, and the muscles' proprioceptive control system can adjust muscle action to changes in loads and in other mechanical conditions. However, the physiological function of this system remains elusive. The role of vagal control is better established. Vagal afferents from stretch receptors in the lungs inhibit inspiration during lung inflation (Hering-Breuer reflex) and determine the end point of inspiration when tidal volume is increased during breathing. This rate control of the vagal nerve afferents amplifies the chemical control of ventilation. When an increase in chemical stimuli enhances the inspiratory drive, tidal volume increases. At the same time, vagal control leads to a rate increase (Fig. 10-5), which multiplies the effect of the increased respiratory drive on minute ventilation. Hence, the centers controlling ventilatory drive need only vary the rate of inspiratory drive in order to increase or decrease minute ventilation.[20]

CONTROL OF VENTILATION

The cells in the medullary respiratory centers can increase the ventilatory drive by firing more frequently, by increasing the number of firing cells, or both. Inspiratory drive is usually the only output, expiration being passive. The inspiratory drive is modulated by many different inputs into the centers, including inputs from (1) central chemoreceptor cells sensitive to H^+ concentration; (2) peripheral chemoreceptors sensitive to P_{O_2}, P_{CO_2}, and H^+ concentration in arterial blood; (3) higher centers in the midbrain; and (4) cerebral centers: (a) voluntary stimuli, as during breath holding or voluntary hyperventilation; and (b) in the context of other motor acts, including complex reflex events like posture control and swallowing, as well as learned patterns of motor behavior such as speech and singing (Chap. 11).

Central Chemoreceptors

The central chemoreceptors are located near the ventrolateral surface of the medulla, about 0.1 to 0.2 mm below the surface, and relatively far from the medullary respiratory centers. Stimulation of central chemoreceptor cells depends on the composition of the brain's extracellular fluid (ECF), specifically its pH.[73, 88, 98] In turn, the pH near the receptor cells depends on the local P_{CO_2} and HCO_3^- ion concentration, since other buffer systems are probably not important. Hence, the pH of brain ECF is determined by the Henderson-Hasselbalch equation (Chap. 6). At any given HCO_3^- concentration, the relation between pH and P_{CO_2} is fixed. The P_{CO_2} of brain ECF depends on the P_{CO_2} of blood perfusing the medulla, on local CO_2 production, and on tissue blood flow. CO_2 can also diffuse into the tissue from the cerebrospinal fluid (CSF) (Fig. 10-6). The concentration of HCO_3^- in brain ECF is largely determined by its concentration in the CSF bathing the medulla, since HCO_3^- does not easily pass the blood-brain barrier. When the HCO_3^- concentration and P_{CO_2} of CSF are kept constant, CO_2 breathing can still cause large ventilation increases, acting via increased blood P_{CO_2}.[98] However, sudden changes in CSF composition alter ventilation very rapidly—after 3 sec when CSF P_{CO_2} is raised and after 8 sec when CSF (HCO_3^-) is increased.[88] Hence, the central chemoreceptor cells appear to be easily accessible to CO_2 and HCO_3^- diffusing into brain tissue from CSF; they must be superficially located.

The central chemoreceptor cells are connected to respiratory neurons in the medulla or pons in order to signal local tissue pH changes which lead to increased or decreased ventilation, but these connections have not yet been traced. It used to be thought that the respiratory neurons themselves were sensitive to changes in P_{CO_2} and/or pH, but this is no longer accepted. In fact, the respiratory neurons closest to the ventrolateral surface of the medulla are hyperpolarized, not activated, by increases of P_{CO_2}.[86] These respiratory neurons (of the VRG, Fig. 10-2) are probably not directly connected with the central chemoreceptors.[86]

The fact that the pH near the central chemoreceptors is influenced both by CSF and blood pH and P_{CO_2}, and by HCO_3 concentrations in the CSF, becomes important when the acid-base status of CSF differs from that of blood. The blood-brain barrier is easily permeable to CO_2 but not to bicarbonate, lactic acid, and other fixed acids. Hence, CSF P_{CO_2} follows the P_{CO_2} changes in arterial blood

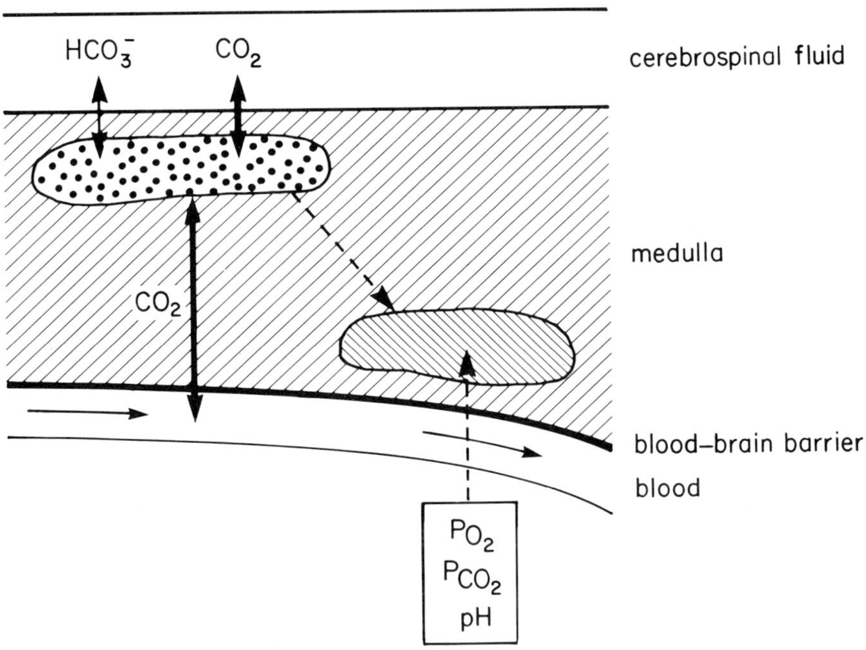

Fig. 10-6. The pH near the central chemoreceptors (*stippled area*) is affected by (*1*) diffusion of CO_2 from the bloodstream and the CSF and (*2*) diffusion of bicarbonate from CSF. CO_2 diffuses more rapidly (*heavy arrows*) than HCO_3^- (*light arrows*). Neural connections between central chemoreceptors and central respiratory neurons (*dark hatching*) and between peripheral chemoreceptors (*block below*) and central respiratory neurons are indicated by dashed arrows.

while levels of CSF bicarbonate and thus CSF pH may differ appreciably from those of blood. This explains why a similar degree of acidosis affects ventilation differently when it is caused by CO_2 breathing than when it is caused by lactic acid accumulation, as during heavy exercise. In the case of CO_2, CSF P_{CO_2} increases rapidly, and hence CSF pH decreases. Consequently, the tissue pH near the central chemoreceptors is decreased because of a low pH in blood as well as in CSF. In the case of lactic acid, no primary change in CSF pH occurs since this ion does not penetrate the blood-brain barrier. However, the resulting decrease in blood pH stimulates ventilation via the peripheral chemoreceptors (see below)—arterial P_{CO_2} decreases, followed rapidly by a decrease of CSF P_{CO_2}. Hence, CSF pH increases, and this partially offsets the decrease of ECF pH near the chemoreceptor cells brought about by the lowering of blood pH. Thus, for the same change of blood pH, CO_2 is a more effective stimulus to breathing than other acids.

Peripheral Chemoreceptors

Peripheral chemoreceptors are located in the carotid bodies, near the bifurcation of the common carotid artery and near the arch of the aorta (aortic bodies). The carotid bodies weigh only 1–2.5 mg and have a disproportionately large blood flow (1–2 liters/min/100 gm tissue at 130 mm Hg pressure [78]). Hence, their O_2 consumption is negligible compared to the amount of O_2 flowing through them, and their cells may be exposed to close to arterial P_{O_2} values. The chemoreceptor cells of the carotid and aortic bodies discharge in response to a decrease in arterial P_{O_2} and an increase in arterial P_{CO_2}. The carotid bodies also respond to a decrease in arterial pH; the aortic bodies do not.[111a] The stimuli from these cells reach the central nervous system via the glossopharyngeal nerve (from the carotid bodies) and via the vagus nerve (from the aortic bodies), and may first reach the respiratory neurons of the dorsal group.[85] The resulting change in the centers' ventilatory drive ordinarily activates inspiratory, but not expiratory, muscles.[8] Stimulation of chemoreceptor cells also changes heart rate and vascular tone. Peripheral chemoreceptor cells at other sites [22] probably do not play as important a role as the carotid and aortic bodies. At least in human adults, the hypoxia response is chiefly mediated through the carotid bodies, since bilateral resection of the carotid bodies [59, 75] and denervation of the carotid body [122] abolish or greatly reduce the hypoxia response. Blockade of the vagal and glossopharyngeal nerves in man has the same effect.[54]

Although arterial P_{O_2} is usually the main determinant of carotid body stimulation, this is not so when blood flow through the carotid bodies is reduced, as in severe *hemorrhagic shock.* Tissue P_{O_2} in the bodies may then decrease, even though Pa_{O_2} may be normal; in addition, tissue pH in the bodies may decrease as acid metabolites accumulate. Hence, carotid body stimulation may increase ventilation in patients with shock even though their Pa_{O_2} is normal. In *anemia,* on the other hand, cardiac output and hence carotid body blood flow are high, and arterial P_{O_2} is normal; no stimulation of the carotid bodies occurs. In *CO poisoning,* arterial P_{O_2} and carotid body blood flow are also normal. Yet, chemoreceptor stimulation may occur because CO affects the shape and position of the Hb dissociation curve (see Fig. 6-9, p. 116); this may decrease the local P_{O_2} in the chemoreceptor tissues even if Pa_{O_2} is unchanged.[84]

The mechanism of chemoreceptor cell sensitivity probably involves a good deal more than a direct effect of low P_{O_2} on afferent nerve endings. Recent electron microscopic studies suggest that glossopharyngeal nerve endings can conduct impulses in two directions—toward the nerve as well as toward the glomus cells of the carotid body on which they end.[79] The presence of these "reciprocal synapses" suggests that nerve endings and glomus cells work closely together, but the exact mechanism is not yet clear. It may be that hypoxia (and also hypercapnia) stimulates the afferent nerve endings directly, with the glomus cells functioning as an interconnected network of neuron-like cells which modulate the sensitivity of the afferents.[79] Or, it might be that hypoxia acts on the glomus cells, altering the rate of chemotransmitter secretion [40] by glomus cells and thus stimulating afferent nerve fibers indirectly. In this hypothesis,[96] acetylcholine secretion from the nerve endings would modulate chemotransmitter secretion by glomus cells. Both hypotheses thus include a feedback mechanism that regulates the chemoreceptive function; the reciprocal synapses are a likely substrate for this feedback mechanism.

Ventilatory Responses to CO_2

Carbon dioxide affects ventilation via the central as well as via the peripheral chemoreceptors. Its effect on the peripheral chemoreceptors is direct and rapid,

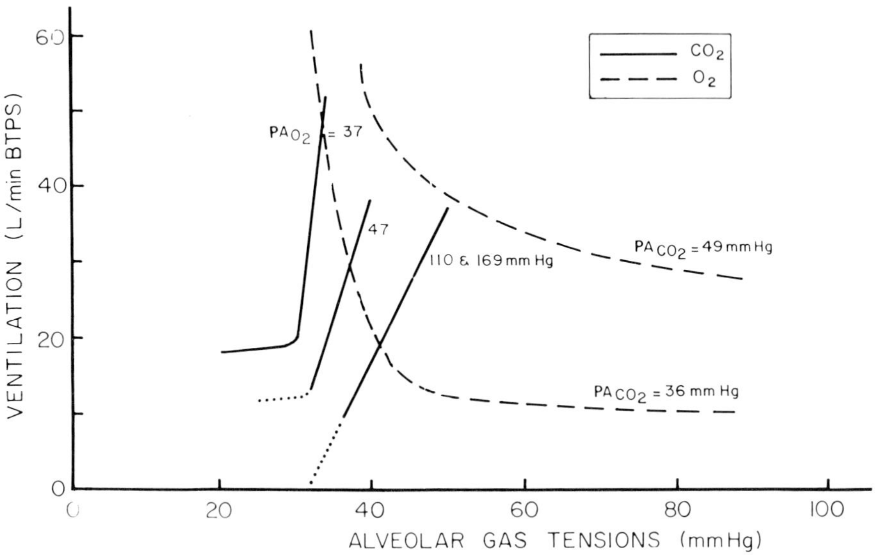

Fig. 10-7. Ventilatory responses to CO_2 at constant PA_{O_2} (*drawn lines*) and to O_2 at constant PA_{CO_2} (*dashed lines*). Data for CO_2 responses from reference 94 and for O_2 responses from reference 74.

but it contributes only a small portion of the total ventilatory drive. The indirect (via changes in tissue pH, see p. 244) effect of CO_2 on the central chemoreceptors is slower, but in dogs it provides about 80 percent of the total ventilatory drive.[6]

When healthy persons breathe 3–7 percent CO_2 in air, tidal volume, breathing rate, and minute ventilation increase. Graphs of minute ventilation versus arterial or alveolar P_{CO_2} (Fig. 10-7) describe the sensitivity of the control system to CO_2, but their interpretation is complex. In principle, the slope of the curve ($\Delta\dot{V}_E/\Delta P_{CO_2}$) reflects the "gain" or sensitivity of the CO_2 controller, but the curves are often alinear and determination of their slopes is inaccurate.[36] In addition, ventilatory response may be affected by mechanical factors. For instance, during pressure breathing in cats, minute ventilation responds less to CO_2, while phrenic motoneuron activity increases as usual.[8] The decreased compliance of the lungs and chest due to the increased lung volume prevents ventilation from increasing in response to increased motoneuron output. An analogous condition occurs in patients with severe airway obstruction (p. 257).

At near-normal alveolar gas tensions, ventilation responds to a small increase in CO_2 tension (Fig. 10-7). When the arterial P_{CO_2} is decreased by hyperventilation, minute ventilation is temporarily reduced and often stops briefly (apnea).[3] During breathing of CO_2-enriched air, arterial P_{CO_2} increases, but less than it would if ventilation did not increase too. Hence, the difference between arterial and inspired P_{CO_2} decreases, with the arterial P_{CO_2} always remaining the higher one. At high inspired CO_2 pressures, the narcotic effect of CO_2 reduces ventilation and causes rapid retention of CO_2 in blood and tissues. The centers' sensitivity to CO_2 may depend on impulses from higher centers. In patients with bilateral cerebral lesions, CO_2 responses were often increased,[103] suggesting that stimuli from the brain normally inhibit the CO_2 response (cf. also reference 120).

Ventilatory Responses to Hypoxia

When one breathes room air, the chemoreceptors are active and they increase their activity when the inspired P_{O_2} is decreased. Inspiration of a single breath of pure oxygen leads to temporary reduction of minute ventilation (Fig. 10-8), suggesting that hypoxic drive contributes to ventilation during room-air breathing. With prior breathing of a hypoxic gas mixture, the O_2 breath reduces ventilation more, reflecting an increased hypoxic drive in hypoxia. At near-normal alveolar gas tensions, small changes in alveolar P_{O_2} affect ventilation much less than changes in alveolar P_{CO_2} (Fig. 10-7). The ventilatory responses to hypoxia lead to secondary changes in arterial P_{CO_2}. Since the controlling system is very sensitive to CO_2, the response to hypoxia per se can only be studied adequately when Pa_{CO_2} is kept constant (see next section).

Athletes respond less to hypoxia and to CO_2 than do untrained healthy persons; both hypoxic and hypercapnic responses correlate negatively with the maximum working capacity.[16] Whether these diminished ventilatory responses are related to chemoreceptor function or to differences in central processing of chemoreceptor information is not known.

Interaction Between CO_2 and O_2 Stimuli

By carefully manipulating inspired gas concentrations, one can keep alveolar and arterial P_{O_2} tensions constant while changing P_{CO_2}, and vice versa. This procedure yields graphs of minute ventilation versus P_{CO_2} at constant P_{O_2}, and of minute ventilation versus P_{O_2} at constant P_{CO_2} (Fig. 10-7). Clearly, the level of alveolar P_{O_2} influences the response to CO_2-tension changes, and vice versa.[74, 94] At low values of P_{O_2}, the response to CO_2 is alinear; there appears to be a threshold below which P_{CO_2} changes do not affect ventilation. Above the threshold, ventila-

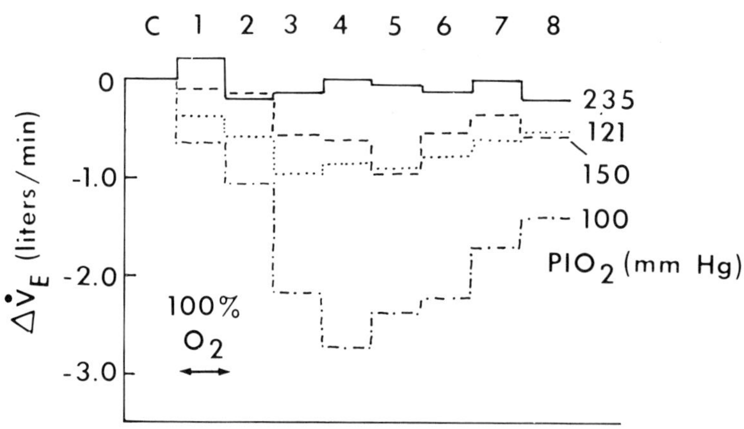

Fig. 10-8. Changes in minute ventilation ($\Delta\dot{V}_E$, *ordinate*) induced by a single breath of 100 percent O_2 (breath 1) in subjects who breathed different O_2 mixtures (O_2 partial pressures at right) during the control period (*C*) and during breaths 2–8. Average data from 3 subjects of Dejours et al., J Physiol (Paris) 49:115–119, 1957. Inspired O_2 tensions calculated assuming that atmospheric pressure was 760 mm Hg (altitude, 50 meters).

tion increases steeply with increased P_{CO_2}, more so than when the alveolar P_{O_2} is normal or increased. Conversely, at near-normal alveolar P_{CO_2}, large decreases of P_{O_2} are required before ventilation increases markedly. At a higher alveolar P_{CO_2}, lesser degrees of hypoxia elicit a response, and the sensitivity to P_{O_2} changes in the range between 50 and 80 mm Hg appears to increase. The mechanism of the interaction between CO_2 and hypoxic stimuli is not known. At least in part, interaction takes place in the carotid bodies,[44] but the cellular events involved in the interaction have not been identified.

Physiological Events Involving the Control of Ventilation

In this section the foregoing discussions of the components of the ventilatory control system are applied to conditions during breath holding, exercise, and sojourn at high altitude.

Breath holding. Man can voluntarily suspend breathing for periods of less than a minute to over 10 minutes, depending on his motivation, his initial lung volume, and his alveolar gas tensions at the beginning of breath holding. Both the CO_2 stimulus and the hypoxic stimulus influence the "breaking point" at which the subject can no longer resist the urge to breathe. After someone quietly breathes room air, he commonly reaches the breaking point when PA_{CO_2} is about 50 mm Hg and PA_{O_2} about 70 mm Hg.[62] Breath holding can be prolonged (1) by first hyperventilating, (2) by first inspiring a breath of 100 percent O_2, and (3) maximally by first hyperventilating while inspiring 100 percent O_2. When P_{O_2} is high, alveolar P_{CO_2} determines the breaking point and vice versa, when P_{CO_2} is low, alveolar P_{O_2} is the limiting factor. At the end of a voluntary breath hold, breathing a gas low in O_2 and high in CO_2 can enable the subject to hold his breath again, even though alveolar gas composition has not improved.[48] This suggests that chest movements play a role in determining the end point of breath holding.

Exercise. Ventilation may increase from its resting value of about 5 liters/min to 60 liters/min or more during exercise. This adaptation to the increased demand for oxygen and to the need to excrete more CO_2 is so effective that arterial P_{O_2} need not decrease even during maximum work, while arterial P_{CO_2} need not increase.

Ventilation increases upon the onset of exercise (Fig. 10-9)[34, 35] so rapidly that flow rate increases during the phase of the breath in which work begins.[60] This immediate response must be due to nervous stimuli, since it occurs too rapidly to be explained by blood-borne chemical stimuli. Since ventilation also increases when the limbs are passively exercised, these nervous stimuli to breathing may be elicited by proprioceptors in the limb muscles or joints,[23, 34] which sense muscular contraction, particularly the rate of movement.[2] For instance, passive stretching of a leg muscle increases phrenic nerve discharge in dogs.[63] However, ventilation increases more during active than during passive exercise, and, in addition, the initial response may be too rapid to be explained by afferent neural stimuli.[99] Hence, the increased neurogenic ventilatory drive at the start of exercise may originate centrally, as a set of impulses from the brain to the respiratory centers,

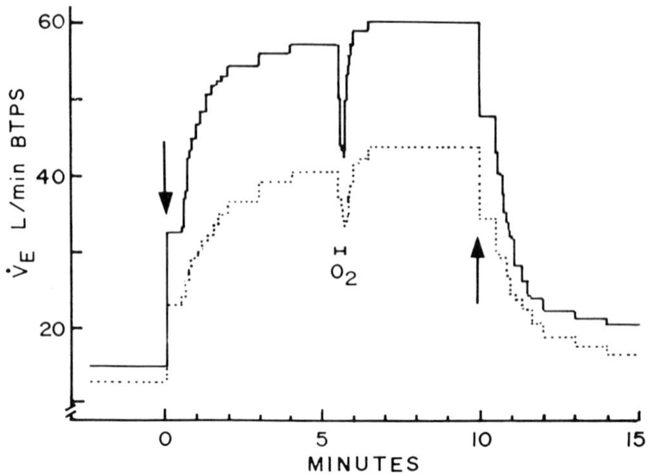

Fig. 10-9. Mean ventilatory responses to exercise in lowlanders (*solid line*) and highlanders (*dotted line*) at 3660 meters (12,300 ft) altitude. Arrows indicate beginning and end of work (load: 120 watts). Both the initial and steady-state responses are less in highlanders than in lowlanders. Three inspirations of 100 percent O_2 were given in the sixth minute of exercise. The ensuing decrease of $\dot{V}_E$ indicates the contribution of hypoxic drive to ventilation before and after the O_2 breaths. The hypoxic drive is less in the highlanders than in the lowlanders. Modified from reference 71.

concomitant with motor impulses to the exercising muscles. The abrupt increase in ventilatory drive might be a learned response rather than part of a feedback control system.[5, 61]

After its rapid initial increase, ventilation increases further, slowly, before it levels off during the steady state of exercise. The neurogenic drive (see above) continues to provide a large fraction of the total ventilatory drive during this phase.[27, 34] When one suddenly stops exercising, there is a rapid initial decline of ventilation, followed by a slow decrease (Fig. 10-9). This recovery pattern is similar to that after cessation of active hyperventilation in cats.[37] It may reflect the gradual decline of activity in central neuronal networks (see p. 238). Another part of the ventilatory drive during exercise is provided by the peripheral chemoreceptors: a few breaths of 100 percent O_2, taken during exercise, abruptly reduce ventilation (Fig. 10-9).

Since arterial P_{CO_2} is often unchanged during transition from rest to work, and usually decreases during heavy work, CO_2 stimuli were long thought to be unimportant in increasing ventilation during exercise.[43] However, the relation between P_{CO_2} and ventilation may be obscured by other stimuli, in particular the increased neurogenic drive when work begins. When these other stimuli are kept constant (as when changing from light to heavier exercise in unanesthetized dogs, increasing treadmill grade, and keeping rate of leg movements constant), the relation between changes in P_{CO_2} and ventilation is similar to that obtained with CO_2 inhalation.[2] Under these conditions, changes in P_{CO_2} during exercise can account for the ventilatory increase. During heavy exercise, arterial pH decreases because of accumulation of lactic and pyruvic acid in blood. Carotid body stimulation by increased blood acidity then provides additional ventilatory drive, which lowers the arterial P_{CO_2}.

High altitude. When a sea-level resident first arrives at high altitude, his ventilation at rest and during work increases in response to the acute hypoxia. Without hyperventilation, P_{CO_2} would remain constant and the alveolar point would be situated at 1″ in Figure 10-10. Due to hyperventilation, P_{CO_2} decreases, and P_{O_2} increases about 6 mm Hg (to point 1′, at 4600 meters = 15,000 feet). The gain in alveolar P_{O_2} continues when ventilation increases further during continued stay at altitude (arrows in Fig. 10-10). Thus, acclimatization results in increases in alveolar P_{O_2} at the expense of increased ventilation and decreased alveolar P_{CO_2}.

Acclimatization of sea-level residents ("lowlanders") involves increased sensitivity and a decreased threshold to CO_2, which occur within 3 days after arrival at altitude (4540 meters [66]). Responses to hypoxia remain unchanged during the first 11 days at this altitude.[66] The increased CO_2 sensitivity may in part be related to a decreased HCO_3^- concentration in the brain extracellular fluid (ECF). In this view, immediately after arrival at altitude alveolar P_{CO_2}, and concurrently CSF P_{CO_2}, decrease because of the hypoxic drive via the arterial chemoreceptors.[13] The decreased CSF P_{CO_2} leads to an increase in ECF pH, which inhibits the ventila-

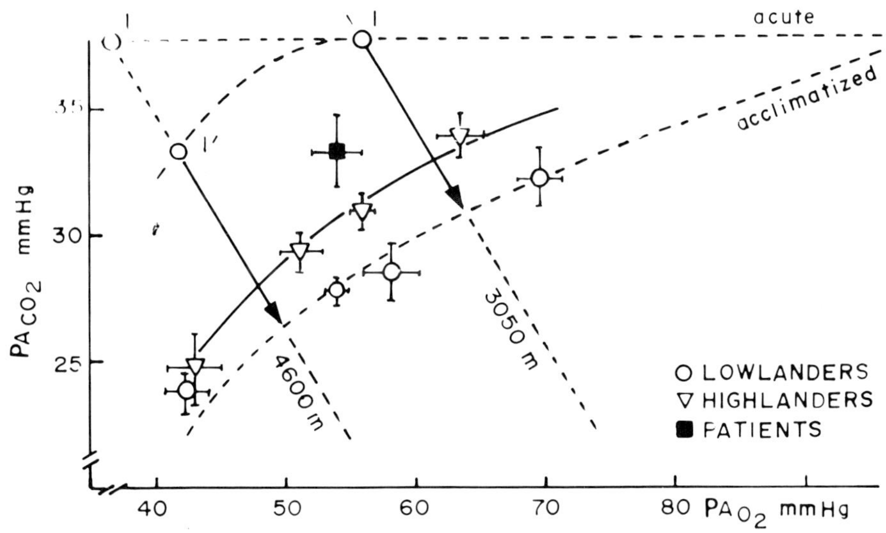

Fig. 10-10. O_2-CO_2 diagram (see Chap. 5) with *R* lines for two altitudes (3050 meters = 10,000 feet; 4600 meters = 15,000 feet). Inspired P_{O_2} = 100 and 80 mm Hg, respectively (note that the ordinate has been interrupted so that the *R* lines do not intersect the abscissa at the PI_{O_2} value). Line labeled "acute" shows changes in alveolar gas tensions during an acute transfer from sea level to altitude (alveolar point 1 at 3050 meters; point 1′ at 4600 meters). Point 1″ is the alveolar point that would occur at 4600 meters without hyperventilation. Arrows indicate changes in alveolar gas during acclimatization. In highlanders, especially those with airway obstruction (see p. 257), PA_{O_2} is lower and PA_{CO_2} higher than in acclimatized lowlanders. The point for the patients is an average of 9 patients (mean age 52 years). Bars indicate 2 SE for PA_{O_2} and PA_{CO_2}. Modified from reference 70.

tory drive. Gradually, CSF bicarbonate concentration is adjusted to the low P_{CO_2}, and ECF pH decreases. Thus, the initial inhibitory effect of the high ECF pH on ventilatory drive is removed, and ventilation increases further.[115] How the ECF HCO_3^- concentration decreases is not known; in severe hypoxia, formation of lactic acid in the brain might be involved. However, recent studies [47] have questioned the validity of this concept of altitude acclimatization. Forster et al. found that CSF pH remained slightly elevated in humans acclimatizing to 4300 meters altitude; hence, compensation of ECF pH by decreases in HCO_3^- appeared to be incomplete. Complete compensation may occur only in high-altitude natives.[10]

The increased ventilation of lowlanders at altitude improves their oxygenation at the expense of increased work of breathing. Native highlanders ventilate less at the same oxygen uptake than recently acclimatized lowlanders.[68] Since they utilize a smaller portion of their ventilatory capacity for the same work, they are less dyspneic than lowlanders. However, their reduced ventilatory response leads to lower alveolar O_2 tensions (Fig. 10-10). In one study, PA_{O_2} averaged 56 mm Hg in highlanders and 61 mm Hg in acclimatized lowlanders at similar work loads.[71] Highlanders may tolerate hypoxia better than acclimatized lowlanders, and can therefore work harder, but the mechanisms of this tolerance are ill understood. Short-term acclimatization to altitude (weeks or months) does not lead to an adaptation that equals that of native highlanders.

Native highlanders have a smaller ventilatory response to hypoxia than acclimatized lowlanders (Fig. 10-9). This "blunted hypoxic drive" occurs in persons native to altitudes of 2900 meters and higher, and in persons of widely varying ethnic origins, living in the Andes, in Colorado, and in the Himalayas.[46, 68, 117] Animals native to high altitude (yaks, heifers, and sheep in the Himalayas; dogs and llamas in the Andes) have a normal response to hypoxia.[15, 67, 70] The decreased hypoxic response may explain why highlanders ventilate less and have a lower PA_{O_2} and a higher PA_{CO_2} than acclimatized lowlanders (Fig. 10-10).

The blunted hypoxic response of highlanders has been attributed to failure of the peripheral chemoreceptors, which might also account for the slower response of highlanders to CO_2.[72, 124] However, in cats, development of the blunted hypoxic response appears to require intact connections between the brain stem and higher brain centers. In these animals, a blunted hypoxic response can be evoked during stays of up to 4 months in a low-pressure chamber (atmosphere equivalent to 5500 meters = 18,000 feet altitude).[120] Experiments with decerebration or removal of the cerebral cortex in cats suggest that cortical centers inhibit the response to hypoxia at altitude, while centers in the diencephalon facilitate it.[120]

Synthesis. Central chemoreceptor cells in the medulla respond to H^+-ions with increased chemoreceptor drive, leading to increased ventilation. The local pH near these cells is determined by the composition of blood and of CSF. Peripheral chemoreceptor cells in carotid bodies and aortic wall respond to decreased arterial P_{O_2} and pH and to increased arterial P_{CO_2}, leading to afferent nervous stimuli, which increase ventilatory drive. The relations between increased ventilatory drive induced by central and peripheral chemoreceptor stimuli on the one hand, and lung ventilation on the other hand, are complicated by (1) the mechanical properties of muscles, chest wall, and lungs and (2) interaction between CO_2 and hypoxic stimuli. The breaking point of *breath holding* may be determined by the CO_2 and by hypoxic stimuli. The increased ventilation during *exercise* is elicited by (1) rapid-acting neurogenic stimuli from muscle or joint receptors in the limbs or from brain centers, or both; (2) responses to increased P_{CO_2}, which can be detected when other stimuli are kept constant; and (3) responses to decreased arterial pH during heavy exercise. At *high altitude,* the hypoxic stimulus increases ventilation in newly arrived lowlanders; further hyperventilation results from increased CO_2 sensitivity, perhaps a result of changes in the pH of brain extracellular fluid. Native highlanders ventilate less and respond less to hypoxia than acclimatized lowlanders.

INTEGRATIVE CONTROL OF BREATHING

"The course of events in the organism forms a network, with circular or net-like connections between several chains of events. . . . the existence of such networks provides the general conditions for regulation of an event."[108] Thus, in 1921 Rohrer introduced the principle of the control of breathing as a regulatory system involving positive and negative feedback ("Hin- und Rückkoppelung von Teilvorgängen"). In recent years, mathematical models have been used extensively to describe quantitatively how feedback loops can regulate the output of the controller (i.e., the ventilatory drive of the respiratory centers) so that the controlled quantities (arterial gas tensions) remain close to constant.[19, 107]

In addition, breathing movements must be coordinated with other motor functions using the same muscles, which necessitates nervous connections between respiratory and other motor centers. For instance, pathways from the cerebellum to the phrenic nerve center may provide a means for integrating diaphragmatic contraction in the control of posture.[30] In the cerebral cortex, an area close to Broca's speech center may help integrate speech and breathing (Chap. 11). Electrical stimulation of the motor area in the cortex causes individual muscles to contract but does not lead to coordinated breathing movements. Voluntary changes in coordinated breathing probably involve indirect (extrapyramidal) pathways from the cerebral cortex to the spinal cord, with coordination occurring at a subcortical level.

The integration of breathing with the control of speech, singing, and wind-instrument playing (Chap. 11) poses special problems, as for the trumpet player who marches in a band, especially uphill! Marching bands generally prefer brass instruments, which require higher flow rates than most woodwinds and are therefore more compatible with exercise requirements. Integrative control of breathing during these activities has its limits; for instance, it is impossible to speak normally during heavy exercise, since the flow rate requirements for the two activities differ too much. The integration between swallowing and breathing has been discussed in Chapter 2. In several animals, heat loss through the respiratory system helps regulate body temperature. When placed in a hot environment, they hyperventilate, thus increasing heat loss through the respiratory passages. An increase in body temperature in cats leads to an increased ventilatory drive of the respiratory centers.[39] In unanesthetized goats, breathing rate increased from about 40 breaths per minute to 270 breaths per minute during thermal polypnea, with an increase in rectal temperature of only 1° C.[57] This response was accompanied by a decrease of arterial P_{CO_2} from 39 to 25 mm Hg. Dogs, too, depend to a large extent on respiratory heat elimination for their body temperature control. In conscious, trained dogs, arterial P_{CO_2} decreases by 4–7 mm Hg during exercise on a treadmill.[1] Apparently, the thermoregulatory process requires goats and dogs to ventilate in excess of their requirements for gas exchange.

Thus, the needs of other regulatory processes sometimes appear to take precedence over ventilation control for purposes of gas exchange. In man, too, the ventilatory control system does not always ideally fulfill its task of keeping blood gas tensions within normal limits. During exercise, ventilation can be altered by the ventilatory load even though the oxygen uptake is constant.[89] When the breathing apparatus is unloaded by breathing a light gas (He-O_2; see also Chap. 8), ventilation increases for the same oxygen uptake, and P_{CO_2} decreases from 35 to 30 mm Hg. During the same work, with the subject breathing room air, P_{CO_2} remained constant at 35 mm Hg. The control system seems to set the level of ventilation in accordance with expected requirements and fails to adjust the ventilatory drive under the unusual condition of a decreased ventilatory load. There are apparently no stimuli that inform the control system of the altered load. But also under conditions where powerful stimuli increase the ventilatory drive, blood gas tensions are not always kept constant. During heavy exercise, arterial P_{CO_2} may decrease to 30 mm Hg or less when O_2 uptake is more than 3 liters/min,[12, 34] due primarily to the metabolic acidosis of exercise. Hyperventilation may occur in part because the inspiratory muscles participate in the work itself, for instance, by moving and stabilizing the shoulder girdle.

One might therefore say that the control system is imperfect. But maybe it is better to say that nature has avoided "over-engineering" the controls; short periods of slight or moderate hyperventilation are well tolerated. And the possibility that physiologists would one day try to trick the system by having people breathe helium-oxygen may have been overlooked at the Creation—or dismissed as of no real consequence.

DEVELOPMENT OF THE CONTROL OF BREATHING

Breathing begins before birth—as early as 13 weeks' gestation in human fetuses.[28] Fetal breathing movements are rapid and irregular, with diurnal variations in amplitude.[28, 80] They are accompanied by slight but measurable to-and-fro movements of fluid in the trachea. In some respects the fetal respiratory control system behaves as it does after birth; e.g., hypercapnia increases fetal breathing in lambs. In other respects it does not; e.g., mild fetal hypoxemia does not stimulate but may stop fetal breathing.[28] If breathing begins in utero, the initiation of air breathing after birth may be a less dramatic event—as far as the control system is concerned—than used to be thought. Apparently, the newborn enters the atmosphere well prepared. But the control system does not yet function optimally and develops further during the first stages of postnatal development.

Initiation of Breathing

The fluid which fills the lungs in utero is expelled during delivery (Chap. 1). Some air may enter the infant's lungs as his chest and lungs recoil to a resting position immediately after his chest has passed through the birth canal. However, forceful inspiratory maneuvers are needed to expand the lungs during the first few breaths and to keep them inflated (see p. 165, Chap. 7). Some studies suggest that the ventilatory drive required to produce this force is largely initiated by changes in the newborn's blood gas tensions, i.e., an increase in P_{CO_2} and a decrease in P_{O_2}. For instance, in fetal lambs delivered by caesarean section, the circulation can be maintained by cross-perfusion. If the arterial blood gases are controlled at close to normal levels in such animals, they do not begin to breathe.[97] Lowering P_{O_2} or increasing P_{CO_2} in their arterial blood, or both, invariably triggers breathing, while clamping the cord does not. The low P_{O_2} and high P_{CO_2} stimuli interact much as they do in adults (p. 248). But in human infants breathing often starts before the cord is clamped, and the relative insensitivity and slow response of the peripheral chemoreceptors suggest that other stimuli (temperature, tactile stimuli) may be more important than changes in blood gases in the initiation of breathing in man.[80, 110]

Several elements of the respiratory control system function at birth. Newborn infants decrease their ventilation when breathing 100 percent O_2 during 8–15 seconds, or during 5 breaths,[24, 106] suggesting that the peripheral chemoreceptors are tonically active, as they are in adults (p. 248). In newborn animals, ventilatory responses to hypoxia are not sustained more than a few minutes, although the carotid nerve afferents keep firing.[112] Thus, exhaustion of immature central or effector neurons[113] rather than immaturity of receptors or afferent fibers may be involved. In the highly immature newborn opossum, responses to CO_2 and hypoxia occur in 5-day-old animals (weighing 350 mg; age from conception 18 days).[42] In 15–20-day-old opossums, interaction between CO_2 and hypoxic stimuli occurs as described on p. 248. In newborn infants an inflation reflex can be elicited, presumably through activation of stretch receptors in lungs; this reflex disappears after a few days.[25] Newborn infants are highly sensitive to CO_2 during the first weeks of life.[118] The importance of the Hering-Breuer reflex to newborn infants is discussed in the next section.

In spite of the presence of functional vagal afferents and chemoreceptors for CO_2 and hypoxia, rhythmic control of breathing is not fully developed at birth. In particular, higher integrative control appears to be lacking. For instance, the human newborn swallows air and inspires air into the lungs at the same time;[11] he must learn to integrate swallowing and breathing as they occur in the adult (see Chap. 2). It has even been suggested that the first few breaths are in fact modified swallows, similar to the breathing maneuvers of frogs.[11]

Early Development of Control Mechanisms

In human infants during the first weeks of life, responses to CO_2 decrease[118] while responses of tidal volume to 100 percent oxygen (5 breaths) increase.[24] The roles of vagal afferents and of proprioceptive control also appear to change during development.

Vagal afferents. The newborn's most important need is to maintain lung inflation. In particular, insufficient development of lung surfactant (Chap. 1, p. 9) may lead to alveolar collapse in premature newborns. Thus, it is not surprising that ventilatory responses to changes in lung volume are well developed at birth, even in the highly immature opossum.[41] These responses differ, at least in opossums, from those in adults and include gasping and prolonged inspirations. In some immature animals, vagal input is critical for the control of breathing. Newborn kittens survive decerebration only if the vagi are intact—they stop breathing and die when the vagi are cut. The mature (21 days) decerebrated rabbit develops increased inspiratory force when the trachea is occluded, even after the vagi have been cut. The immature newborn rabbit, also decerebrated, shows this response only when the vagi are intact.[112] Thus, input from vagal afferents appears to be critical for maintaining breathing in these immature animals, and this may be related to their prime need to maintain lung inflation. The adult animal's lungs are mechanically more stable and hence less susceptible to collapse. For adults, vagal afferent input appears to be less critical during quiet breathing as well as during exercise, and deflation reflexes play a role only under pathological conditions with lung collapse.[65] In newborn, especially premature, human infants the Hering-Breuer reflex is strong and acts to increase the rate of breathing. In turn, the high breathing rate keeps lung volume at a level well above residual volume.[95]

Proprioceptive control. In comparison with vagal input, proprioceptive input from the respiratory muscles appears to be relatively unimportant for the young animal. In the mature cat (28 days), sectioning 7 adjacent dorsal roots on both sides decreases EMG activity in external intercostal muscles. In the newborn kitten, the same muscles show unchanged activity after the same dorsal root section.[112] Hence, proprioceptive control of the respiratory muscles functions in the mature cat but not in the newborn kitten. Integration of the control of breathing with proprioceptive muscle control [31, 39] may be essential for integrating breathing with other motor acts (walking, running, posture control). But while this integration is essential for the mature animal, it is less important for the newborn whose motor abilities are immature.

CLINICAL APPLICATIONS

While breathing-control disorders as separate clinical entities are relatively rare, many pharmacological substances affect the central control mechanisms, and depression of breathing by anesthetics and other drugs is a common clinical problem.[69] Decreased ventilation as a result of structural damage to the central nervous system usually occurs together with other signs of neurological disorders. In clinical practice, depressed ventilatory control is usually detected only when it leads to overt ventilatory failure, requiring artificial ventilation.

Decreased ventilation caused by failure of control mechanisms must be distinguished from that caused by parenchymal lung disease and airway obstruction. Since lung disease and failure of control may coexist, this is not always easy. A patient with decreased minute ventilation, reduced vital capacity, and forceful chest movements during breathing usually has severe airway obstruction. In case of doubt, one can use esophageal pressure recordings (Chap. 7) to distinguish between lack of respiratory drive and ventilatory failure due to lung disease. When the respiratory drive and the respiratory muscles are intact, pleural-pressure swings during the breathing cycle are usually normal or increased, reflecting adequate forces applied to the lungs. In patients with respiratory muscle paralysis or insufficient ventilatory drive, the inadequate force is reflected by decreased pleural-pressure swings. Electromyography of respiratory muscles, using surface or needle electrodes for the intercostal and abdominal muscles and an intraesophageal electrode for the diaphragm,[17] may be used to record individual muscle function. In patients with normal lungs and depressed ventilatory drive, measurements of ventilation at rest, during voluntary breathing maneuvers (VC; hyperpnea), exercise, or inspiration of CO_2, low oxygen mixtures and 100 percent O_2 can yield information on the control system. Single-breath tests with 100 percent O_2, during a period of breathing 13 percent O_2, can indicate the presence of a hypoxic ventilatory drive.[33] Vital capacity breaths of 5 percent or 15 percent CO_2 in N_2 or O_2, with subsequent measurement of ventilation, also permit assessment of chemoreceptor drive.[50] However, these tests have been insufficiently standardized, and the variability of normal responses is large. Nevertheless, in selected patients and in the context of other diagnostic information, they may help to determine the role of ventilatory control mechanisms in ventilatory failure.

Ventilatory Control in Airway Obstruction

In patients with severe chronic airway obstruction, responses of ventilation to low P_{O_2} or increased P_{CO_2} are often less than in normal persons. Ventilatory drive may be inappropriately strong (Chap. 8, p. 196), but the increased work of breathing leads to insufficient ventilation even though the forces applied by the respiratory muscles are normal or increased. The hypercapnia which sometimes occurs during O_2 breathing in these patients has been attributed to lack of central response to CO_2. Thus, ventilation would be driven largely by the hypoxic drive from the peripheral chemoreceptors, and administration of oxygen would abolish this input. However, increased airway resistance at the mouth, combined with an added dead space, causes a similar response to O_2 in healthy subjects, suggesting that hypercapnia in patients may also be explained on the basis of the increased work of breathing[18] (see also p. 165). Although the responses to CO_2 and O_2 in patients with obstruction are low in absolute terms (measured in liters per minute), they equal those of normal persons when measured as a fraction of the maximum voluntary ventilation.[52] Thus, both patients and healthy persons use a similar proportion of their ventilatory capacity when responding to similar CO_2 and hypoxic stimuli. In patients with airway obstruction and ventilatory failure, relief of obstruction is obviously the more important treatment goal, for when this is achieved, the response to ventilatory stimuli improves.

At altitude, even a person with moderate airway obstruction may have severe dyspnea, polycythemia, and hypercapnia[70] (Fig. 10-10). In part, his higher P_{CO_2} and lower P_{O_2}, in comparison with a healthy highlander, may be caused by relative lack of ventilatory response to low P_{O_2} and high P_{CO_2}.[72]

During sleep, ventilatory drive is normally reduced, resulting in increases in arterial P_{CO_2} from 2–10 mm Hg. Similar increases occur in patients with airway obstruction and are accompanied by decreases in arterial P_{O_2} (avg. 7.4 mm Hg[102]).

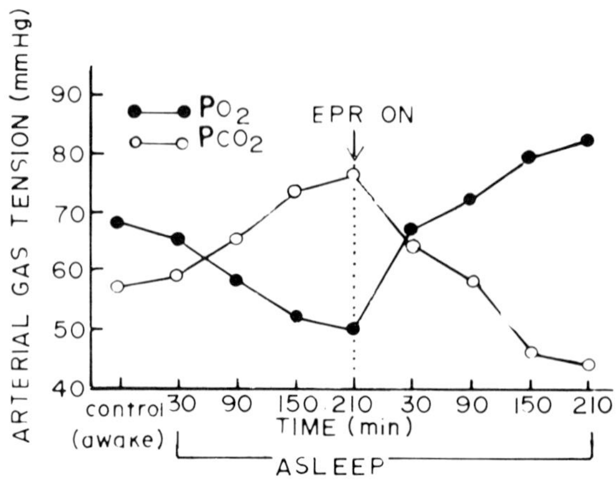

Fig. 10-11. Normalization of blood gas tensions by electrophrenic respiration (EPR) in a patient with encephalitis. During sleep, PA_{O_2} decreased and PA_{CO_2} increased, until EPR was initiated. From reference 51.

These changes are, however, not much greater than those in healthy sleepers. When ventilation is depressed and cardiac output is normal, the average $\dot{V}_A/\dot{Q}$ ratio decreases. Since recumbency by itself leads to decreased $\dot{V}_A/\dot{Q}$ ratios in parts of the lungs (p. 93; Chap. 5), one might expect that during sleep, patients with severe airway obstruction and a nonuniform distribution of $\dot{V}_A/\dot{Q}$ would have appreciable decreases in P_{O_2} combined with some increases in P_{CO_2}, according to the shape of the $\dot{V}_A/\dot{Q}$ lines (Fig. 5-6, p. 89). In fact, the distribution of $\dot{V}_A/\dot{Q}$ ratios in these patients may already be large due to the disease itself, and the incremental distribution abnormality due to sleep may be difficult to detect.

Central Hypoventilation

Reduced ventilatory drive in the presence of normal lung and respiratory muscle function occurs in patients with neurological disease, e.g., encephalitis or brain stem lesions. Some patients with insufficient ventilatory drive are thought to be "lazy breathers." Rohrer described two physicians who thought that they had temporarily lost ventilatory control during a severe illness, "so that only the conscious will to continue to breathe had brought them through this critical condition."[108] Such observations have been made in other patients who lack central ventilatory drive and may require admonitions to breathe. They often ventilate normally during the day but develop ventilatory failure during sleep. They may need artificial ventilation every night to prevent hypoxemia and CO_2 retention. In recent years, unilateral stimulation of the phrenic nerve (electrophrenic respiration) has been used successfully to supplement the inspiratory drive and to normalize gas exchange in these patients[51] (Fig. 10-11). Since at least some patients with central hypoventilation appear to have a localized neurological defect with few symptoms other than failure of ventilatory drive, one wonders whether the plasticity of the brain would permit re-education through a conditioning approach, perhaps using rhythmic sensory stimulation.

Cheyne-Stokes Breathing [19]

Cheyne-Stokes breathing is a pattern of waxing and waning breathing, in which periods with large tidal volumes alternate with apnea or minimal breathing lasting 15–60 seconds. An oscillating output can occur in any control system involving feedback (Rohrer, 1921 [108]), for instance, when the temporal relation between the feedback and the output signal is disrupted, or when the system is insufficiently damped. The oscillating ventilatory drive in Cheyne-Stokes breathing is promoted by time delays in the feedback signals, for instance, prolongation of the circulation time. In disease of the central nervous system, where inhibitory impulses from higher centers are removed, the CO_2 controller may become less stable, or its response may be so depressed that the alinear O_2 controller takes over. This promotes output oscillations, since O_2 stores in the body are small and the O_2 controller is therefore less damped and inherently less stable than the CO_2 controller.

SUMMARY

A complex nervous control system—with humoral as well as nervous inputs—regulates the rhythmic pattern of breathing, adjusts ventilation to match the needs for gas exchange, and coordinates breathing with other motor activities. Respiratory centers in the brain stem initiate the nervous ventilatory drive; coordinating centers in the spinal cord ensure appropriate dosage and timing of nervous impulses to participating muscles. Respiratory muscle force depends on muscle length and hence on lung volume. Muscle force, along with the mechanical state of the chest and lungs (lung volume, airway caliber, airway pressure), determines the tidal volume which results from a given level of ventilatory drive.

The respiratory centers in the brain stem receive feedback information concerning the output of the control system from (1) proprioceptive muscle afferents, (2) vagal afferents from the lungs, (3) central chemoreceptors sensitive to the level of H^+ ions in brain extracellular fluid, and (4) peripheral chemoreceptors (in carotid and aortic bodies), which respond to decreases in arterial P_{O_2} and pH and to increases of arterial P_{CO_2}. CO_2 and O_2 stimuli interact in their effect on ventilation. The physiological importance of the control system becomes clear from experiments on breath holding in man, and from studies on responses to exercise and high-altitude hypoxia in man and animals.

Integration of breathing with other motor acts (speech, swallowing, thermal polypnea in animals, postural control) requires nervous connections between nerve centers subserving breathing and those subserving other motor activities. Under some conditions, the requirements of other motor acts appear to prevail over the main goal of the breathing apparatus, i.e., to keep arterial blood gas levels constant within narrow limits.

The respiratory control system functions at birth but undergoes further development during maturation. In newborn animals, vagal afferents from the lungs are essential to maintain breathing, while proprioceptive muscle control is as yet undeveloped.

In assessing disease states with ventilatory failure, one must differentiate between (1) lack of ventilatory drive (due to drugs or central nervous system damage), (2) respiratory muscle paralysis, and (3) inability to ventilate the lungs because of lung disease in spite of adequate ventilatory drive and muscle force. Central hypoventilation, often a result of brain stem lesions, can now be treated by implanting an electrode that stimulates the phrenic nerve and supplements the efferent motor stimuli to the diaphragm.

REFERENCES

1. Bainton CR, Mitchell RA: Effect of skin cooling on exercise ventilation in the awake dog. J Appl Physiol 30: 370–377, 1971
2. Bainton CR: Effect of speed vs. grade and shivering on ventilation in dogs during active exercise. J Appl Physiol 33:778–787, 1972
3. Bainton CR, Mitchell RA: Posthyperventilation apnea in awake man. J Appl Physiol 21:411–415, 1966
4. Batsel HL, Lines AJ Jr: Bulbar respiratory neurons participating in the sniff reflex in the cat. Exp Neurol 39: 469–481, 1973
5. Beaver WL, Wasserman K: Tidal volume and respiratory rate changes at start and end of exercise. J Appl Physiol 29:872–876, 1970
6. Berger AJ, Krasney JA, Dutton RE: Respiratory recovery from CO_2 breathing in intact and chemodenervated awake dogs. J Appl Physiol 35:35–41, 1973
7. Bianchi AL: Modalités de décharge et propriétés anatomo-fonctionnelles des neurones respiratoires bulbaires. J Physiol (Paris) 68:555–587, 1974

7a. Bertrand F, Hugelin A, Vibert JF: A stereologic model of pneumotaxic oscillator based on spatial and temporal distributions of neuronal bursts. J Neurophysiol 37:91–107, 1974

8. Bishop B, Bachofen H: Comparison of neural control of diaphragm and abdominal muscle activities in the cat. J Appl Physiol 32:798–805, 1972
9. Bishop B, Bachofen H: Vagal control of ventilation and respiratory muscles during elevated pressures in the cat. J Appl Physiol 32:103–112, 1972
10. Blayo MC, Marc-Vergnes JP, Pocidalo JJ: P_{CO_2} and P_{O_2} of cisternal cerebrospinal fluid in high altitude natives. Respir Physiol 19:298–311, 1973
11. Bosma JF, Truby HM, Lind J: Studies of neonatal transition: Correlated cineradiographic and visual-acoustic observations. Acta Paediatr Scand [Suppl] 163:93–109, 1965
12. Bouhuys A, Pool J, Binkhorst RA, van Leeuwen P: Metabolic acidosis of exercise in healthy males. J Appl Physiol 21:1040–1046, 1966
13. Bouverot P, Candas V, Libert JP: Role of the arterial chemoreceptors in ventilatory adaptation to hypoxia of awake dogs and rabbits. Respir Physiol 17: 209–219, 1973
14. Brooks McC, Kao FF, Lloyd BB (eds): Cerebrospinal Fluid and the Regulation of Ventilation. Oxford, Blackwell Scientific Publications, 1965
15. Brooks JG, Tenney SM: Ventilatory response of llama to hypoxia at sea level and high altitude. Respir Physiol 5:269–278, 1968
16. Byrne-Quinn E, Weil JV, Sodal IE, Filley GF, Grover RF: Ventilatory control in the athlete. J Appl Physiol 30:91–98, 1971
17. Campbell EJM, Agostoni E, Newsom Davis J (eds): The Respiratory Muscles; Mechanics and Neural Control, ed 2. Philadelphia, WB Saunders Co, 1970
18. Cherniack RM, Chodirker WB: Hypercapnia with relief of hypoxia in normal individuals with increased work of breathing. J Appl Physiol 33:189–192, 1972
19. Cherniack NS, Longobardo GS: Cheyne-Stokes breathing: An instability in physiologic control. N Engl J Med 288:952–957, 1973
20. Clark FJ, von Euler C: On the regulation of depth and rate of breathing. J Physiol (Lond) 222:267–295, 1972
21. Cohen MI: How respiratory rhythm originates: evidence from discharge patterns of brain stem respiratory neurones, in Porter R (ed): Breathing:

Hering-Breuer Centenary Symposium. Ciba Found Symp, London, J & A Churchill, 1970, pp 125–150
22. Comroe JH Jr: The peripheral chemoreceptors, in Fenn WO, Rahn H (eds): Handbook of Physiology, Section 3: Respiration, vol I. Washington, D.C., American Physiological Society, 1964, pp 557–583
23. Comroe JH Jr, Schmidt CF: Reflexes from the limbs as a factor in the hyperpnea of muscular exercise. Am J Physiol 138:536–547, 1943
24. Crance JP, Becquart P, Bouverot P, Arnould P: Réponses ventilatoires du nouveau-né au test oxygène. J Physiol (Paris) 63:32A, 1971
25. Cross KW, Klaus M, Tooley WH, Weisser K: The response of the newborn baby to inflation of the lungs. J Physiol (Lond) 151:551–565, 1960
26. Cunningham DJC, Lloyd BB (eds): The Regulation of Human Respiration. Philadelphia, FA Davis Company, 1963
27. D'Angelo E, Torelli G: Neural stimuli increasing respiration during different types of exercise. J Appl Physiol 30: 116–121, 1971
28. Dawes GS: Breathing before birth in animals and man—an essay in developmental medicine. N Engl J Med 290: 557–559, 1974
29. Decima EE, von Euler C: Excitability of phrenic motoneurones to afferent input from lower intercostal nerves in the spinal cat. Acta Physiol Scand 75: 580–591, 1969
30. Decima EE, von Euler C: Intercostal and cerebellar influences on efferent phrenic activity in the decerebrate cat. Acta Physiol Scand 76:148–158, 1969
31. Decima EE, von Euler C, Thoden U: Intercostal-to-phrenic reflexes in the spinal cat. Acta Physiol Scand 75: 568–579, 1969
32. Dejours P: Chemoreflexes in breathing. Physiol Rev 42:335–358, 1962
33. Dejours P: Control of respiration by arterial chemoreceptors, in: Regulation of Respiration. Ann NY Acad Sci 109: 682–695, 1963
34. Dejours P: Control of respiration in muscular exercise, in Fenn WO, Rahn H (eds): Handbook of Physiology, Section 3: Respiration, vol I. Washington, D.C., American Physiological Society, 1964, pp 631–648
35. Dejours P: The regulation of breathing during muscular exercise in man. A neurohumoral theory, in Cunningham DJC, Lloyd BB (eds): The Regulation of Human Respiration. Philadelphia, FA Davis Company, 1963, pp 535–547
36. Dejours P, Puccinelli R, Armand J, Dicharry M: Concept and measurement of ventilatory sensitivity to carbon dioxide. J Appl Physiol 20:890–897, 1965
37. Eldridge FL: Central neural respiratory stimulatory effect of active respiration. J Appl Physiol 37:723–735, 1974
38. Euler, C von, Hayward JN, Marttila I, Wyman RJ: Respiratory neurones of the ventrolateral nucleus of the solitary tract of cat: Vagal input, spinal connections and morphological identification. Brain Res 61:1–22, 1973
39. Euler C von, Herrero F, Wexler I: Control mechanisms determining rate and depth of respiratory movements. Respir Physiol 10:93–108, 1970
40. Eyzaguirre C, Koyano H: Origin of sensory discharges in carotid body chemoreceptors. Cold Spring Harbor Symp Quant Biol 30:227–231, 1965
41. Farber JP: Development of pulmonary reflexes and pattern of breathing in the Virginia Opossum. Respir Physiol 14: 278–286, 1972
42. Farber JP, Hultgren HN, Tenney SM: Development of the chemical control of breathing in the Virginia Opossum. Respir Physiol 14:267–277, 1972
43. Fenn WO: Introductory remarks, in Nahas GG (ed): Regulation of Respiration. Ann NY Acad Sci 109:415–417, 1963
44. Fitzgerald RS, Parks DC: Effect of hypoxia on carotid chemoreceptor response to carbon dioxide in cats. Respir Physiol 12:218–229, 1971
45. Flenley DC, Pengelly LD, Milic-Emili J: Immediate effects of positive-pressure breathing on the ventilatory response to CO_2. J Appl Physiol 30: 7–11, 1971
46. Forster HV, Dempsey JA, Birnbaum ML, Reddan WG, Thoden J, Grover RF, Rankin J: Effect of chronic exposure to hypoxia on ventilatory response to CO_2 and hypoxia. J Appl Physiol 31:586–592, 1971
47. Forster HV, Dempsey JA, Chosy LW:

Incomplete compensation of CSF [H^+] in man during acclimatization to high altitude (4,300 m). J Appl Physiol 38:1067–1072, 1975
48. Fowler WS: Breaking point of breath-holding. J Appl Physiol 6:539–545, 1954
49. Freedman S, Weinstein SA: Effects of external elastic and threshold loading on breathing in man. J Appl Physiol 20:469–472, 1965
50. Gabel RA, Kronenberg RS, Severinghaus JW: Vital capacity breaths of 5% or 15% CO_2 in N_2 or O_2 to test carotid chemosensitivity. Respir Physiol 17:195–208, 1973
51. Glenn WWL, Holcomb WG, Gee JBL, Rath R: Central hypoventilation; long-term ventilatory assistance by radiofrequency electrophrenic respiration. Ann Surg 172:755–773, 1970
52. Godfrey S, Edwards RHT, Copland GM, Gross PL: Chemosensitivity in normal subjects, athletes, and patients with chronic airways obstruction. J Appl Physiol 30:193–199, 1971
53. Guz A, Noble MIM, Eisele JH, Trenchard D: The role of vagal inflation reflexes in man and other animals, in Porter R (ed): Breathing: Hering-Breuer Centenary Symposium. Ciba Found Symp, London, J & A Churchill, 1970, pp 17–40
54. Guz A, Noble MIM, Widdicombe JG, Trenchard D, Mushin WW: Peripheral chemoreceptor block in man. Respir Physiol 1:38–40, 1966
55. Guz A, Noble MIM, Widdicombe JG, Trenchard D, Mushin WW: The effect of bilateral block of vagus and glossopharyngeal nerves on the ventilatory response to CO_2 of conscious man. Respir Physiol 1:206–210, 1966
56. Guz A, Trenchard DW: Pulmonary stretch receptor activity in man. A comparison with dog and cat. J Physiol (Lond) 213:329–343, 1971
57. Heisey SR, Adams T, Hofman W, Riegle G: Thermally induced respiratory responses of the unanesthetized goat. Respir Physiol 11:145–151, 1971
58. Hey EN, Lloyd BB, Cunningham DJC, Jukes MGM, Bolton DPG: Effects of various respiratory stimuli on the depth and frequency of breathing in man. Respir Physiol 1:193–205, 1966
59. Holton P, Wood JB: The effects of bilateral removal of the carotid bodies and denervation of the carotid sinuses in two human subjects. J Physiol (Lond) 181:365–378, 1965
60. Ingemann Jensen J, Vejby-Christensen H, Petersen ES: Ventilatory response to work initiated at various times during the respiratory cycle. J Appl Physiol 33:744–750, 1972
61. Ingemann Jensen J, Vejby-Christensen H, Petersen ES: Ventilation in man at onset of work employing different standardized starting orders. Respir Physiol 13:209–220, 1971
62. Kellogg RH: Central chemical regulation of respiration, in Fenn WO, Rahn H (eds): Handbook of Physiology, Section 3: Respiration, vol I. Washington, D.C., American Physiological Society, 1964, pp 507–534
63. Kindermann W, Pleschka K: Phrenic nerve response to passive muscle stretch at different arterial CO_2 tensions. Respir Physiol 17:227–237, 1973
64. Koller EA, Ferrer P: Discharge patterns of the lung stretch receptors and activation of deflation fibers in anaphylactic bronchial asthma. Respir Physiol 17:113–126, 1973
65. Koller EA, Ferrer P: Studies on the role of the lung deflation reflex. Respir Physiol 10:172–183, 1970
66. Lahiri S: Dynamic aspects of regulation of ventilation in man during acclimatization to high altitude. Respir Physiol 16:245–258, 1972
67. Lahiri S: Unattenuated ventilatory hypoxic drive in ovine and bovine species native to high altitude. J Appl Physiol 32:95–102, 1972
68. Lahiri S, Milledge JS, Sørensen SC: Ventilation in man during exercise at high altitude. J Appl Physiol 32:766–769, 1972
69. Lambertsen CJ: Effects of drugs and hormones on the respiratory response to carbon dioxide, in Fenn WO, Rahn H (eds): Handbook of Physiology, Section 3: Respiration, vol I: Washington, D.C., American Physiological Society, 1964, pp 545–555
70. Lefrançois R, Gautier H, Pasquis P: Ventilatory oxygen drive in acute and chronic hypoxia. Respir Physiol 4: 217–228, 1968
71. Lefrançois R, Gautier H, Pasquis P, Vargas E: Factors controlling respira-

tion during muscular exercise at altitude. Fed Proc 28:1296–1300, 1969
72. Lefrançois R, Gautier H, Pasquis P, Cevaer AM, Hellot MF, Leroy J: Chemoreflex ventilatory response to CO_2 in man at low and high altitudes. Respir Physiol 14:296–306, 1972
73. Leusen I: Regulation of cerebrospinal fluid composition with reference to breathing. Physiol Rev 52:1–56, 1972
74. Loeschcke HH, Gertz KH: Einfluss des O_2-Druckes in der Einatmungsluft auf die Atemtätigkeit des Menschen, geprüft unter Konstanthaltung des alveolaren CO_2-Druckes. Pflueger's Arch 267: 460–477, 1958
75. Lugliani R, Whipp BJ, Seard C, Wasserman K: Effect of bilateral carotid-body resection on ventilatory control at rest and during exercise in man. N Engl J Med 285:1105–1111, 1971
76. Luria AR: Functional organization of the brain. Sci Am 222:66–78, 1970
77. Lynne-Davies P, Couture J, Pengelly LD, Milic-Emili J: Immediate ventilatory response to added inspiratory elastic loads in cats. J Appl Physiol 30: 512–516, 1971
78. McCloskey DI, Torrance RW: Autoregulation of blood flow in the carotid body. Respir Physiol 13:23–35, 1971
79. McDonald DM, Mitchell RA: The innervation of glomus cells, ganglion cells and blood vessels in the rat carotid body: a quantitative ultrastructural analysis. J Neurocytol 4:177–230, 1975
80. Merlet-Bénichou C: Mouvements respiratoires chez le foetus et installation de la respiration à la naissance. Bull Physiopathol Respir 9:1365–1387, 1973
81. Merrill EG: Finding a respiratory function for the medullary respiratory neurons, in Bellairs R, Merrill EG (eds): Essays on the Nervous System. Oxford, Clarendon Press, 1974, pp 451–486
82. Merton PA: Discussion, in Porter R (ed): Breathing: Hering-Breuer Centenary Symposium. Ciba Found Symp, London, J & A Churchill, 1970, pp 156–157
83. Milic-Emili J, Pengelly LD: Ventilatory effects of mechanical loading, in Campbell EJM, Agostoni E, Newsom Davis J (eds): The Respiratory Muscles; Mechanics and Neural Control, ed 2. Philadelphia, WB Saunders Company, 1970, pp 271–290
84. Mills E, Edwards MW Jr: Stimulation of aortic and carotid chemoreceptors during carbon monoxide inhalation. J Appl Physiol 25:494–502, 1968
85. Mitchell RA, Berger AJ: Neural regulation of respiration. Am Rev Respir Dis 111:206–224, 1975
86. Mitchell RA, Herbert DA: The effect of carbon dioxide on the membrane potential of medullary respiratory neurons. Brain Res 75:345–349, 1974
87. Mitchell RA, Herbert DA: Synchronized high frequency synaptic potentials in medullary respiratory neurons. Brain Res 75:350–355, 1974
88. Mitchell RA, Loeschcke HH, Massion WH, Severinghaus JW: Respiratory responses mediated through superficial chemosensitive areas on the medulla. J Appl Physiol 18:523–533, 1963
89. Murphy TM, Clark WH, Buckingham IPB, Young WA: Respiratory gas exchange in exercise during helium-oxygen breathing. J Appl Physiol 26:303–307, 1969
90. Nahas GG (ed): Regulation of respiration. Ann NY Acad Sci 109: 411–948, 1963
91. Nathan PW, Sears TA: Effects of posterior root section on the activity of some muscles in man. J Neurol Neurosurg Psychiatry 23:10–22, 1960
92. Newsom Davis J: Spinal control, in Campbell EJM, Agostoni E, Newsom Davis J (eds): The Respiratory Muscles; Mechanics and Neural Control, ed 2. Philadelphia, WB Saunders Company, 1970, pp 205–233
93. Newsom Davis J, Sears TA: The proprioceptive reflex control of the intercostal muscles during their voluntary activation. J Physiol (Lond) 209:711–738, 1970
94. Nielsen M, Smith H: Studies on the regulation of respiration in acute hypoxia. Acta Physiol Scand 24:293–313, 1951
95. Olinsky A, Bryan MH, Bryan AC: Influence of lung inflation on respiratory control in neonates. J Appl Physiol 36:426–429, 1974
96. Osborne MP, Butler PJ: New theory for receptor mechanisms of carotid body chemoreceptors. Nature 254: 701–703, 1975

97. Pagtakhan RD, Faridy EE, Chernick V: Interaction between P_{O_2} and P_{CO_2} in the initiation of respiration of fetal sheep. J Appl Physiol 30:382–387, 1971
98. Pappenheimer JR, Fencl V, Heisey SR, Held D: Role of cerebral fluids in control of respiration as studied in unanesthetized goats. Am J Physiol 208: 436–450, 1965
99. Paulev P-E: Cardiac rate and ventilatory volume rate reactions to a muscle contraction in man. J Appl Physiol 34:578–583, 1973
100. Phillipson EA, Hickey RF, Bainton CR, Nadel JA: Effect of vagal blockade on regulation of breathing in conscious dogs. J Appl Physiol 29:475–479, 1970
101. Phillipson EA, Murphy E: Vagal control of respiratory rate and depth independent of lung inflation in conscious dogs. Fed Proc 32:355 (abstract), 1973
102. Pierce AK, Jarrett CE, Werkle G Jr, Miller WF: Respiratory function during sleep in patients with chronic obstructive lung disease. J Clin Invest 45:631–636, 1966
103. Plum F: Neurological integration of behavioural and metabolic control of breathing, in Porter R (ed): Breathing: Hering-Breuer Centenary Symposium. Ciba Found Symp, London, J & A Churchill, 1970, pp 159–175
104. Porter R (ed): Breathing: Hering-Breuer Centenary Symposium. Ciba Found Symp, London, J & A Churchill, 1970
105. Porter R, Knight J (eds): High Altitude Physiology: Cardiac and Respiratory Aspects. Edinburgh, Churchill Livingstone, 1971
106. Reinstorff D, Fenner A: Ventilatory response to hyperoxia in premature and newborn infants during the first three days of life. Respir Physiol 15:159–165, 1972
107. Reynolds WJ, Milhorn HT Jr, Holloman GH Jr: Transient ventilatory response to graded hypercapnia in man. J Appl Physiol 33:47–54, 1972
108. Rohrer F: Die Regulation der Atmung. Schweiz Med Wochenschr 4: 73–79, 1921
109. Rosenstein R, McCarthy LE, Borison HL: Constancy of the relationship between respiratory frequency and tidal volume with respect to alveolar carbon dioxide and oxygen in decerebrate cats. Fed Proc 32:356a, 1973
110. Rudolph AM, Heymann MA: Fetal and neonatal circulation and respiration. Annu Rev Physiol 36:187–207, 1974
111. St. John WM, Glasser RL, King RA: Rhythmic respiration in awake vagotomized cats with chronic pneumotaxic area lesions. Respir Physiol 15:233–244, 1972
111a. Sampson SR, Hainsworth R: Responses of the aortic body chemoreceptors of the cat to physiological stimuli. Am J Physiol 222:953–958, 1972
112. Schwieler GH: Some aspects of respiratory regulation during the postnatal development in cats and rabbits. Life Sci [II] 6:1803–1810, 1967
113. Schwieler GH, Douglas JS, Bouhuys A: Postnatal development of autonomic efferent innervation in the rabbit. Am J Physiol 219:391–397, 1970
114. Sears TA: Breathing: a sensori-motor act. Sci Basis Med 7:129–147, 1971
115. Severinghaus JW, Mitchell RA, Richardson BW, Singer MM: Respiratory control at high altitude suggesting active transport regulation of CSF pH. J Appl Physiol 18:1155–1166, 1963
116. Sørensen SC: The chemical control of ventilation. Acta Physiol Scand [Suppl] 361: 1–72, 1971
117. Sørensen SC, Severinghaus JW: Irreversible respiratory insensitivity to acute hypoxia in man born at high altitude. J Appl Physiol 25:217–220, 1968
118. Stahlman M: Respiratory regulation in the newborn, in Nahas GG (ed): Regulation of Respiration. Ann NY Acad Sci 109:882–891, 1963
119. Tawadrous FD, Eldridge FL: Posthyperventilation breathing patterns after active hyperventilation in man. J. Appl Physiol 37:353–356, 1974
120. Tenney SM, Scotto P, Ou LC, Bartlett D Jr, Remmers JE: Suprapontine influences on hypoxic ventilatory control, in Porter R, Knight J (eds): Ciba Found Symp on High Altitude Physiology: Cardiac and Respiratory Aspects. Edinburgh, Churchill Livingstone, 1971, pp 89–102
121. Torrance RW (ed): Arterial Chemo-

receptors. Oxford, Blackwell Scientific Publications, 1968

122. Wade JG, Larson CP Jr, Hickey RF, Ehrenfeld WK, Severinghaus JW: Effect of carotid endarterectomy on carotid chemoreceptor and baroreceptor function in man. N Engl J Med 282: 823–829, 1970

123. Wang SC, Ngai SH: General organization of central respiratory mechanisms, in Fenn WO, Rahn H (eds): Handbook of Physiology, Section 3: Respiration, vol 1. Washington, D.C., American Physiological Society, 1964, pp 487–505

124. Weil JV, Byrne-Quinn E, Sodal IE, Filley GF, Grover RF: Acquired attenuation of chemoreceptor function in chronically hypoxic man at high altitude. J Clin Invest 50:186–195, 1971

125. Yamashiro SM, Grodins FS: Optimal regulation of respiratory airflow. J Appl Physiol 30:597–602, 1971

Chapter 11

Voluntary Breathing Acts: Speech, Singing, and Wind-Instrument Playing

Man's breathing apparatus is essential to his ability to speak. Although other animals can communicate through voice sounds, only man can speak at a rate that exceeds the flicker fusion frequency of the eye.[44] Man's speaking facility is made possible by a detailed coding system. Only human speech sounds have the characteristics that allow coding as well as decoding; hence, human language requires human speech.[44] Individual speech sounds do not stand alone, but rather derive meaning from a context of phonemes, syllables, words, and sentences. The respiratory bellows provide the power, with a pressurized stream of air, for the vocal apparatus. Man's upper airways include a number of specialized organs for speech —a larynx for voicing sounds, a mobile pharynx for varying those sounds, and the soft palate, tongue, and lips, which further alter the resonant properties of the supravocal tract and help form consonants (e.g., /p/ with the lips; /k/ with the soft palate).

These adaptations of the supravocal tract and the larynx for speech also allow other forms of human communication. Singing and wind-instrument playing use the respiratory tract to express a wide range of emotions in a highly organized fashion. In contrast with the songbird's small, species-specific repertoires,[48] man's music covers the total range of his religious, historical, and cultural experience. As in speech, individual sounds in music derive their meaning from a context of phrases, movements, and compositions.

In this chapter I discuss the respiratory aspects of speech, singing, and wind-instrument performance. These include the generation of pressure and airflow and the coordination of muscular events; breathing patterns and control mechanisms are discussed also. Some attention is given to the relationship between respiratory and speech disorders and to the development of speech and language. Detailed discussions of the physiology of the larynx and of phonetic and linguistic aspects of speech are available elsewhere.[15, 28, 30, 39, 44, 53, 55]

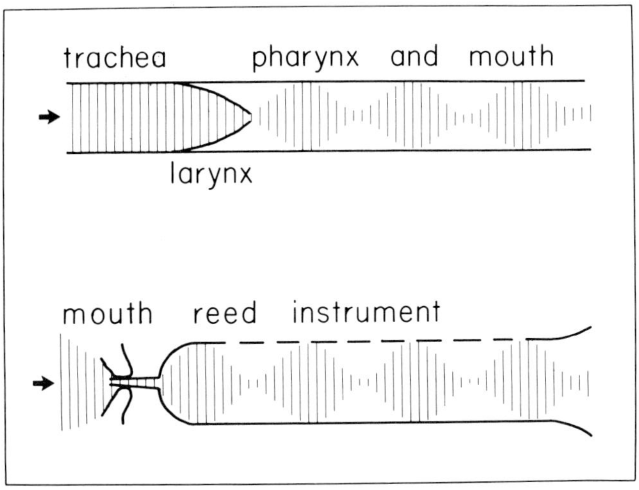

Fig. 11-1. Generation of sound waves in the larynx and in a reed instrument. From reference 5.

RESPIRATORY MECHANICS

Generation of Sound

Sound waves are produced when (1) mechanical systems—such as the strings of violins, the membranes of drums, and the vocal folds of the human glottis—create vibrations in the surrounding air, or (2) an airstream in a fixed mechanical system is disturbed, as in the flute and the organ pipe.

During speech and singing, the vocal folds in the larynx transform a pressurized stream of air from the lungs into a series of air pulses (Fig. 11-1). This process (phonation) generates the fundamental frequency of the voice. The supravocal tract then lets energy through at certain multiples of this frequency (harmonics), while other frequencies are damped. The resonance of the supravocal tract determines which sounds pass through with minimum loss. The characteristics vary with the tract's length and shape. The frequencies at which energy maxima occur (the formants) are characteristic for each speech sound, vowel or consonant. Vowels are voiced sounds produced while the supravocal tract assumes a fixed shape and is open to the atmosphere. Consonants involve either constriction or abrupt changes in the shape of the supravocal tract; consonants may be voiced (e.g., /m/, /b/) or unvoiced (e.g., /p/, /s/).

In brass instruments, the human lips form a vibrating reed; in most woodwinds, the instrument's mouthpiece contains a reed. In both instances, the player's expiration creates an air column which causes the reed to vibrate. Flutes have no reeds and belong to the class of "aerodynamic whistles"[13]—the tone is formed by blowing an airstream across a hole in the mouthpiece. In all wind instruments, the horn functions as a resonance chamber; its length and thus its resonating frequency can be altered. The vibrations set up in the horn in turn determine the vibrating frequency of the reed. The reed and the horn are interdependent and the horn "enslaves the reed" (Benade, in discussion of reference 6). In wind instruments the fundamental frequency of the reed corresponds to one tone at that frequency, with its harmonics. The human voice is much more versatile. Since the glottis is only loosely coupled with the supravocal tract,[27] we can speak or sing different vowels by altering the configuration of the supravocal tract, independent of the glottal fundamental.

Voice Input and Output

The flow rate and the pressure head of the expiratory airstream during speech or singing are the input characteristics of the vocal apparatus. Its output can be measured with acoustical methods (sound pressure, frequency spectrogram, i.e., a recording of dominating voice frequencies versus time).

Driving Pressure

During speech and singing, the pressure drop across the glottis or supravocal tract provides the driving pressure for sound generation. During phonation, the principal pressure drop occurs across the phonating glottis, since the supravocal tract is open to the atmosphere. During articulated speech, the site of the main pressure drop shifts, depending on the speech sounds. For instance, explosive consonants like /p/ are preceded by increased pressure on the alveolar side of an occlusion in the upper airway. In any case, the pressure difference between the subglottal area and the atmosphere is the total pressure drop across the vocal apparatus.

Although tracheal puncture provides a safe, direct measurement of subglottal pressure (Ps), many persons find this method unacceptable. Indirect measurements of Ps, such as those derived from esophageal pressure measurements (Fig. 7-6), are therefore preferred. By recording the lung static recoil curve separately, one can measure Ps as the horizontal distance between the esophageal pressure points on a pressure-volume curve and the static recoil curve (Fig. 11-2). Although this method ignores the pressure drop contributed by lower-airway resistance, this is usually minimal compared to the pressure drop across the vocal apparatus.[9] Comparisons with the direct (tracheal puncture) method, during speech, have validated the esophageal pressure method.[42] Another indirect measurement of Ps is based on the compression of alveolar gas which results from increased alveolar pressure (Palv). This method, which requires a body plethysmograph to record the chest volume changes due to gas compression,[33] eliminates the need for an esophageal balloon and may also respond faster to rapid pressure changes than the esophageal pressure method.

During wind-instrument playing, driving pressures can be measured directly by inserting an air-filled balloon[4] or a miniature pressure transducer[59] into the mouth. The indirect methods discussed above can also be used. Since the pressure drop across the lips or reed is usually much larger than other pressure drops in the airways, one may assume that mouth pressure, Pm, equals Palv.

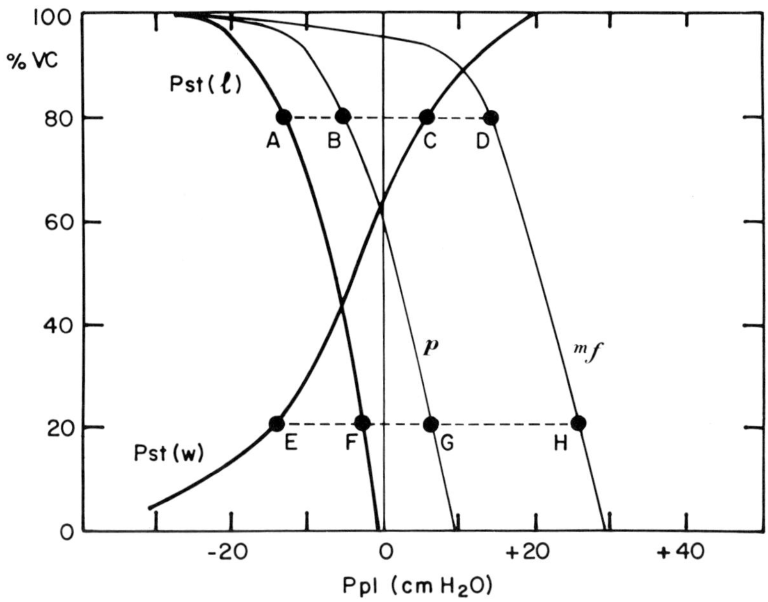

Fig. 11-2. Pressure-volume diagram of the lungs and chest. Pst(*l*) = static recoil curve of the lungs. Pst(w) = static recoil curve of chest wall. Lines marked *p* and *mf* show pressure-volume curves during singing of a soft (*p*) and a louder (*mf*) tone. AB = FG = subglottic pressure for soft tone. AD = FH = subglottic pressure for louder tone. Pmus shown at 80% and 20% VC. At 80% VC, Pmus is negative (inspiratory) for the soft tone (BC) and positive for the louder tone (CD). At 20% VC, Pmus is positive for both tones (EG and EH, respectively). Modified from reference 8.

Generation of Driving Pressures

The pressures needed to drive the vocal apparatus or a horn result from (1) the elastic recoil forces of the lungs and the chest cage, (2) active contraction of expiratory muscles, and (3) relaxation of inspiratory muscles. The analysis of recoil and muscular pressures [Pst(*l*), Pst(w), and Pmus] in Chapter 7 (pp.159 and Fig. 7-7) helps explain the complex mechanical problem faced by speakers, singers, and wind musicians. For example, to maintain a constant sung tone throughout the vital capacity, the singer must maintain a constant subglottic pressure even though his lung and chest recoil forces change as lung volume decreases. An analogy with the bow of a violin may be useful. The length of the bow limits the duration of a tone on the violin; similarly, the vital capacity limits the duration of tones during singing. But the violinist can hold the bow against the strings at any point, while the singer must continuously work with or against the elastic forces of the lungs and chest. "Imagine the difficulties a violinist would have sustaining a steady tone with strings attached to his bow!"[51]

The contributions of elastic and muscular forces are analyzed quantitatively in Figure 11-2, which is similar to Figure 7-7. The graph shows pressure-volume curves recorded while the subject sang two constant tones and relates these to the Pst(*l*) and Pst(w) curves. The subject inspired to TLC, initiated the tone, and

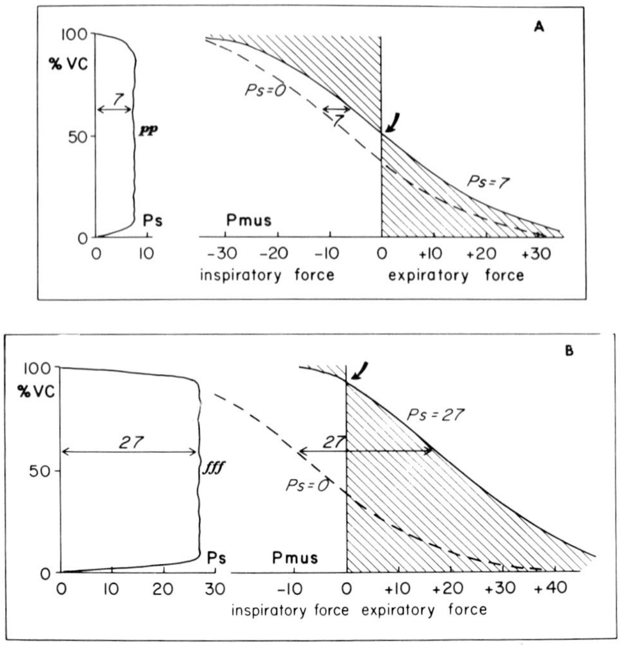

Fig. 11-3. Inspiratory and expiratory force (*right-hand graphs*) during singing of tones at constant subglottic pressures, Ps (*left-hand graphs*), as a function of lung volume (ordinate). Dashed lines represent forces required to hold the breath at all lung volumes (Ps = 0). Drawn lines labeled Ps = 7 (*A*) and Ps = 27 (*B*) represent net muscle force during singing. At curved arrows, net muscle force is zero. From reference 51.

maintained it at constant pitch and loudness throughout the VC. The first part of each curve reflects the compression of alveolar gas required to increase alveolar (=subglottic) pressure. Both curves lie to the right of the Pst (*l*) curve, indicating that Palv is positive throughout, and they run at equal horizontal distances from the Pst(*l*) curve. Thus, subglottic pressure was maintained constant once the proper level to produce the tone had been reached. The curve for the soft tone (*p*) runs to the left of the Pst(w) curve until lung volume reaches about 60 percent of the VC. In this portion of the curve, Pmus is negative; i.e., the subject exerts a net inspiratory muscle force. Below 60 percent VC, Pmus becomes positive —the subject now exerts net expiratory muscle force to sustain the tone at equal loudness. The louder tone (*mf*) required net expiratory force almost immediately after the tone was initiated. The legend of Figure 11-2 indicates how to read the numerical values of Ps and Pmus from the graph. Each curve intersects with the Pst(w) curve; at this point Pmus = 0.

By plotting Pmus versus lung volume (Fig. 11–3), one can visualize the direction and degree of muscular effort. In general, inspiratory muscles maintain low subglottic pressures at high lung volumes, while higher subglottic pressures, at lower lung volumes, require contraction of the expiratory muscles. Hence, near

TLC, to maintain a low subglottic pressure in *A*, the inspiratory muscles must literally "brake" the expiratory flow. As the tone continues, inspiratory effort gradually relaxes in order to keep Ps constant. At about 50 percent VC, net muscle force is zero, since the elastic recoil of the lungs and chest exactly balance one another at the required subglottic pressure level (+7 cm H_2O). Lower lung volumes require increasing net expiratory force to maintain the tone. A louder tone requires expiratory muscle action at high lung volumes; the inspiratory muscle brake is then only necessary near TLC (*B*). At 90 percent VC, the combined chest and lung recoil force provides the required subglottic pressure (+27 cm H_2O). At all lower volumes expiratory force is used. Higher subglottic pressures (or mouth pressures, in the case of wind instruments) require expiratory muscle force as soon as the tone is initiated.

Pmus indicates the net inspiratory or expiratory muscle force that results from different combinations of inspiratory and expiratory muscle effort. For instance, when Pmus = 0, all respiratory muscles may be relaxed, or the contractions of the inspiratory and expiratory muscles (agonists and antagonists) may just balance one another. An electromyogram (EMG—a recording of electrical activity in individual muscles) indicates which participating muscles are contracted. The EMG therefore complements the information provided by the pressure-volume diagram: while the former indicates which muscles are active, the latter shows the net forces developed by muscle contraction. During speech, EMG recordings indicate inspiratory muscle activity (external intercostal muscles) at high lung volumes.[23] As lung volume decreases, inspiratory muscle activity decreases, while that of the expiratory muscles (internal intercostals) increases.[57] Even though considerable inspiratory force is required to produce soft tones at high lung volumes (Fig. 11-3*A*), EMG recordings suggest that the strongest inspiratory muscle, the diaphragm, does not contribute to this force. The diaphragm remains electrically silent, while the external intercostal muscles show marked EMG activity. The diaphragm's inactivity probably results from its lack of muscle spindles (see p. 240). Fortunately, since the mechanical interaction between the intrapleural and intra-abdominal pressures regulates the position of the diaphragm (see next section), contraction of the diaphragm is not needed to regulate subglottic pressure.

Intra-abdominal Pressure

When man is upright, the weight of the abdominal organs contributes to the mechanical control of intrapleural pressures.[9] The elasticity of the external abdominal wall provides the primary support for the viscera. The diaphragm is subject to an upward pull exerted by the negative intrapleural pressure. Hence, lung elastic recoil tends to pull the diaphragm and the abdominal viscera upward. This tendency is counteracted by the weight of the abdominal viscera, an opposing force which is greater the larger the hydrostatic pressure gradient in the abdominal cavity. Hence, the opposing force increases with elevation of the diaphragm. A person who begins to sing a soft tone near TLC expands the rib cage by contracting inspiratory muscles and relaxing the abdominal muscles. Although the negative intrapleural pressure pulls the diaphragm upward, this force is checked by the weight of the abdominal contents, which tends to pull it downward. In this way, the weight of the abdominal viscera replaces active contraction of the diaphragm with a passive inspiratory force and makes possible the production of soft sung tones at high lung volumes while the diaphragm remains relaxed. Analysis of intra-abdominal (intragastric) and intrapleural pressures suggested that this maneuver required an elevated rib cage and relaxed abdominal muscles.[9] Direct measurements of rib cage and abdominal wall displacements during singing have confirmed this conclusion.[37]

Airflow Rate

The driving pressure and the resistance of the vocal apparatus together determine the expiratory airflow rate during speech and singing. With wind instruments, mouth pressure and the resistance of the opening between the lips or in the reed determine flow. Since sound is produced by alternately closing and opening the vocal folds or the reed, or by periodic occlusions at other sites during articulated speech, instantaneous flow rate varies as a function of these rapid changes in the glottis, supravocal tract, or mouthpiece. During stable events (singing of constant tones), the mean expiratory flow rate remains approximately constant and can be measured from the slope of a recording of lung volume versus time, with the subject seated in a body plethysmograph.[9] This method is not suitable when flows are more variable, as during articulated speech. Instantaneous flow rates can then be measured with face masks incorporating a wire mesh flowmeter screen [33, 36] (p. 211). When correctly designed, these masks impede articulation only minimally. Flow measurements are best interpreted in relation to simultaneous driving pressure and sound output measurements (see below).

Lung Volume

Lung volume changes during production of speech or other sounds reflect alveolar gas compression and expiratory airflow rates. Sounds can be produced at all lung volume levels within the constraints of the pressure-volume diagram (see below). Thus, lung volume recordings are chiefly of indirect interest—they allow construction of pressure-volume diagrams (Fig. 11-2), visualization of breathing patterns (Fig. 11-9), and measurement of total ventilation during speech (Fig. 11-12). Their slopes also indicate inspiratory and expiratory flow rates. When the subject is seated in a body plethysmograph with his head out and a seal around the neck, lung volumes during speech, singing, and wind-instrument playing can be recorded and studied without attaching measuring devices to the subject's mouth.[6, 9] These recordings reflect alveolar gas compression as well as expiratory airflow and thus can help relate lung recoil pressures to pressures during sound production. Since the latter pressures may vary from near-static values to maximum expiratory pressures, alveolar gas compression varies considerably, a fact not reflected in volume recordings made with instruments connected to the mouth (Chap. 9, p. 212).

Relations Between Driving Pressure, Airflow Rate, and Sound Level

Singing. Simultaneous measurements of airflow, subglottic pressure, and sound levels during singing of tones of constant pitch and loudness are plotted as a function of lung volume in Figure 11-4. One subject (DFP) is trained and the

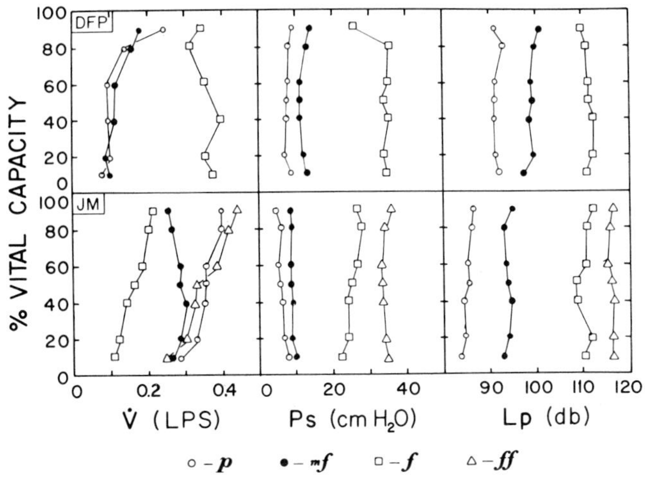

Fig. 11-4. Airflow rate ($\dot{V}$, *left graphs*), subglottic pressure (Ps, *middle graphs*), and sound level (Lp, *right graphs*) in a trained amateur singer (DFP, *upper row of graphs*) and in an inexperienced and untrained singer (JM, *lower row of graphs*). All data are plotted versus lung volume in percent of vital capacity. Symbols indicate different sound levels for the same tone (B♭3) in both subjects. Lung volume measured with body plethysmograph, $\dot{V}$ from slope of volume recording, Ps with esophageal balloon (as in Fig. 11-2), and sound level with microphone in front of the mouth. From reference 8.

other (JM) untrained in singing. In both subjects, sound level increases with increasing subglottic pressures. The latter vary within narrow limits during each tone; flow rates vary more and often decrease with lung volume, especially in JM. Moreover, the relation between flow rate and sound level differs between the subjects. The trained singer (DFP) uses minimal flow rates when he sings softly; flow increases when he sings louder tones. JM, on the other hand, uses high flow rates for the softest tone; with increasing sound level, flow rate decreases, except at the highest sound level, where higher flows again appear. This difference between the two singers is clearer in Figure 11-5, in which subglottic pressures and flow rates are plotted against one another. Each data point represents a tone sung at constant pitch and loudness; the symbols indicate tones of different pitch. The trained singer (*A*) increases flow as well as pressure when he sings a tone louder; the untrained singer (*B*) usually decreases flow while increasing pressure for tones of increasing loudness.

Differences in the pressure-flow behavior of the two subjects in Figure 11-5 suggest differences in the mechanical efficiency of the phonating glottis. With louder tones, the untrained singer's mechanical efficiency increases much more than that of the trained singer. The two sets of lines in Figure 11-5 illustrate this phenomenon. One set of diagonal straight lines indicates equal values of the product Ps · $\dot{V}$, which is the power spent in producing the constant tones (see Fig. 8-21, p. 198). At right angles with these lines are the lines of equal resistance,

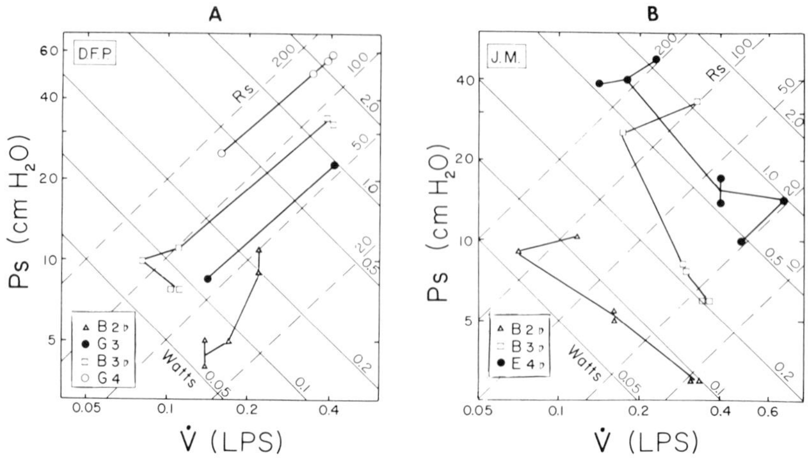

Fig. 11-5. Subglottic pressure (Ps, *ordinate*) and flow rates ($\dot{V}$, *abscissa*) for different tones in a trained (*A*) and an untrained (*B*) singer. The lines connect points at different sound levels for each tone. Ps increases with sound level in both graphs. Drawn diagonal lines are lines of equal power (= Ps · $\dot{V}$) in watts. Dashed diagonal lines indicate equal values of the equivalent dc resistance of the glottis (Rs). From reference 8.

i.e., the ratio Ps/$\dot{V}$, which represents the equivalent dc resistance values of the phonating glottis. The trained singer (*A*) spends increasing amounts of power, up to more than 2 watts, when he increases loudness. Except for the tone with the lowest pitch, the dc resistance of his glottis remains nearly constant. The untrained singer, on the other hand, sings softly with high flow rates; as he sings louder, flow decreases while Ps increases, and the product Ps · $\dot{V}$ remains nearly constant except for the loudest tones. Hence, this subject produces louder tones while spending the same power; i.e., the mechanical efficiency of his glottis increases with loudness. At the same time, the equivalent dc resistance of his glottis increases about tenfold. Other studies have shown that experienced singers, too, may increase the mechanical efficiency of their glottides when singing louder, but to a lesser extent than untrained singers.[12]

Analysis of the harmonic contents of tones produced by the inexperienced and the trained singers of Figures 11-4 and 11-5 [8] helps explain the differences in mechanical efficiency. The frequency spectra of the trained singer suggest that the air pulses through his glottis have a similar waveform for soft and loud tones (Fig. 11-6). The untrained subject's louder tones are richer in high frequencies (i.e., they are harsher sounds), and the glottal air pulse becomes more peaked as loudness increases. When subject JM sings softly, a substantial portion of the central airstream through the glottis does not participate in sound production. Apparently, the vocal folds do not close at any time during the cycle. Thus, there is a constant expired airstream through the glottis, or a "dc air leak." When JM sings louder tones, the dc leak decreases and disappears. Then all of the airstream participates in sound production, which explains why the mechanical efficiency of sound production increases so dramatically. The trained subject DFP may have a small dc leak when he sings softly, but there is no marked change in

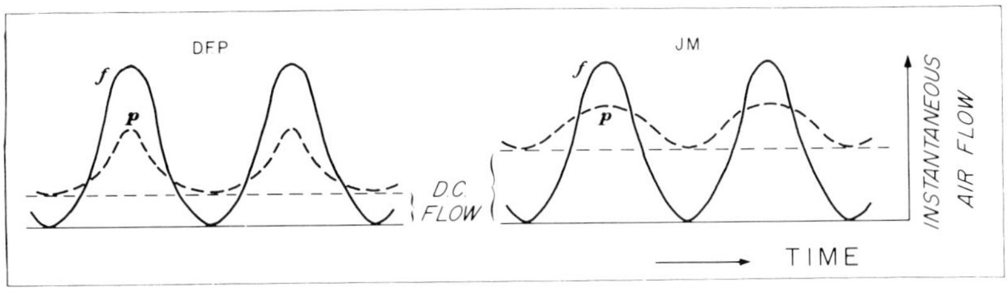

Fig. 11-6. Schematic representation of glottal waveforms (instantaneous airflow rate versus time) in subjects DFP (trained) and JM (untrained). *Dashed lines:* soft tones (*p*). DC flow: constant airstream through glottis, larger in JM than in DFP. *Solid lines:* loud tones (*f*). From reference 8.

waveform as he increases loudness. Figures 11-5 and 11-6 suggest that there are important differences in the control of vocal fold vibrations in trained and untrained singers. The untrained singer is apparently unable to adduct the vocal folds completely, or nearly so, when he sings softly. This results in a "breathy" character of these soft tones.

Speaking. While tones sung at constant pitch and loudness help demonstrate the mechanical events during phonation and speech, they have no linguistic meaning and display few of the complexities of articulated speech. The combination of consonants and vowels in phonemes, the elementary building blocks of speech, causes complex changes in pressure and flow which are often out of phase with one another. In Figure 11-7, subglottal pressure is high and flow rate low when the vowel /a/ is spoken. The high mechanical efficiency of the phonating glottis leads to a high sound-output level. In contrast, one produces the consonant /h/ with the nonphonating glottis wide open. Since there is little resistance in the supravocal tract, subglottal pressure is low and flow rate is high. In spite of the high flows, little sound is produced. Thus, the relation between sound output, on the one hand, and pressures and flows, on the other hand, is much more complex during speech than during singing of constant tones.

Figure 11-7 shows that the speaker exerts rapid, precise control over the glottis and supravocal tract. Each time the glottis narrows for vowel production, the vocal folds vibrate at exactly the same pitch as they did during the previous vowel (as when saying ha-ha-ha). High-speed movies indicate that the folds actually begin to vibrate, at nearly the correct pitch, even before the glottal chink is fully closed, while the folds still "flutter in the wind." [36] As a consequence, it is difficult to decide where the consonant ends and the vowel begins.

When short-lasting sounds are spoken at approximately constant loudness, subglottic pressures vary only slightly (see Figs. 3 to 5 in Lieberman [42]). In contrast, flow rates vary considerably, and different phonemes have characteristic flow rate patterns.[36] Phonemes with voiceless consonants (Fig. 11-7) are associated with high flow rates (/hah/ , /pap/), while phonemes with voiced consonants generally have low flows (/zaz/, /vav/). As a result, speech material that includes many high-flow phonemes requires larger amounts of expired air than material with many low-flow phonemes.[10, 60]

Thus, variations in flow rate are a prominent respiratory feature in articulated

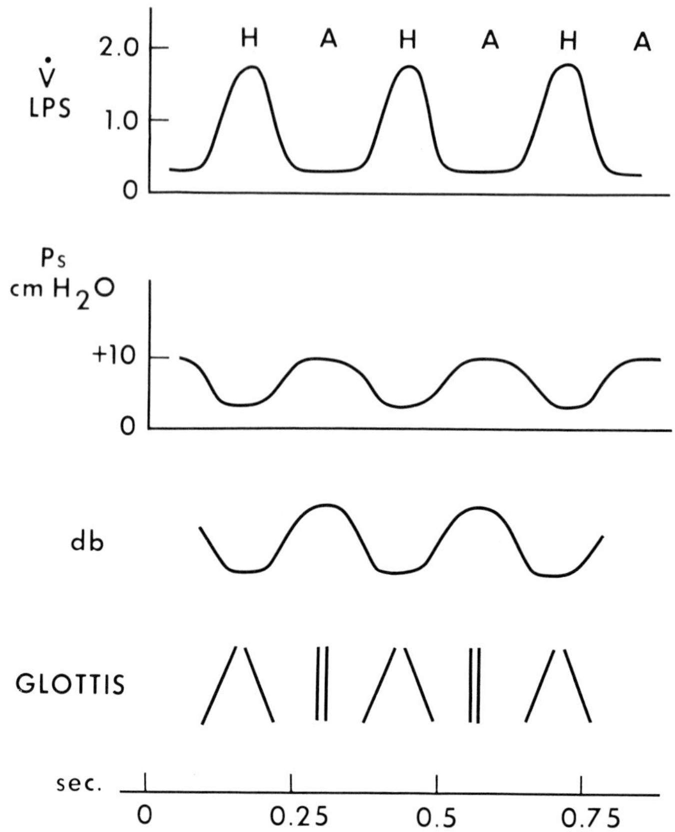

Fig. 11-7. Schematic diagram of flow rate, subglottic pressure, and sound level during utterance ha-ha-ha. See text for discussion. Modified from reference 3.

speech; different classes of speech sounds have distinct flow rate patterns. Variations in flow rate, at constant subglottic pressure, reflect the resistance of the glottis and supravocal tract, and therefore depend upon the neuromuscular control of these organs. Subglottic pressure usually increases with loudness, as in singing and during stress of syllables.[38, 42] Consequently, one must integrate control of respiratory muscles (which control subglottal pressure) and laryngeal and articulatory muscles (which control the syllable). In some languages, e.g., in Swedish, stress has linguistic significance; precise coordination between respiratory and laryngeal muscles then assumes special importance.

The interaction between subglottal pressure and laryngeal control therefore largely determines the pitch, loudness, and quality of voiced speech sounds. One can study this interaction with excised human larynges,[52, 58] in which vocal-fold tension and subglottal pressure can be controlled independently. At constant vocal-fold tension, pitch rises with increased subglottic pressure. Thus, if one increases subglottic pressure in order to produce a louder tone, vocal-fold tension must be adjusted to maintain a constant pitch. To sing a tone progressively louder or softer while maintaining constant pitch, singers must learn this fine control of

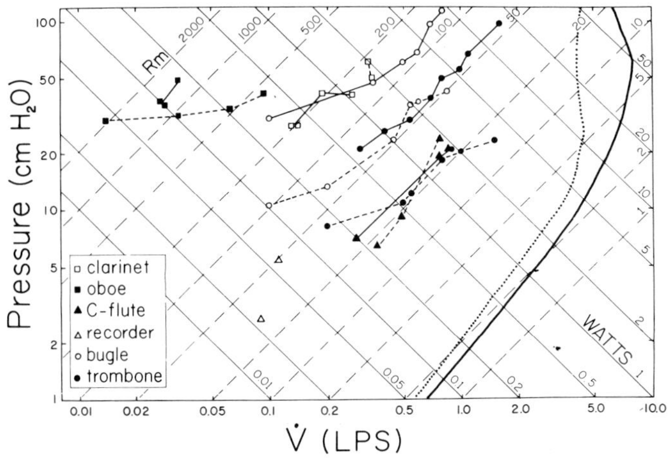

Fig. 11-8. Pressure-flow data for different wind instruments, with broken lines indicating a low tone and solid lines a high tone on each instrument. The solid and the dotted curves at the right are isovolume pressure-flow curves at two different lung volumes during expiration in a healthy subject. Drawn diagonal lines indicate power input values (as in Fig. 11-5); dashed diagonal lines indicate equivalent dc resistance values across lips and instrument (Rm = mouth pressure/flow rate). From reference 6.

respiratory and laryngeal muscles. Public speakers also need this control to express emotional content (e.g., in reading poetry) or simply to avoid monotony by varying pitch, loudness, and voice quality.

Wind-instrument playing. The requirements for mouth pressures and flow rates on wind instruments vary with the type of instrument and with pitch and loudness (Fig. 11-8). In some instruments, such as the oboe, the vibrating reed has a high resistance, and tone production (Fig. 11-1) requires relatively high pressures at low flow rates. In others, both pressure and flow are small (e.g., the recorder). For brass instruments and flutes, pressure and flow rise with increasing loudness, while resistance across the opening between the lips remains close to constant. High tones on brass generally require higher pressures than low tones. A brass player's power input (Pm · $\dot{V}$) may reach up to about 20 watts, compared with up to 2 watts in singers (Fig. 11-5*A*). Measurements of sound level, pressure, and flow indicate that the singing voice and wind instruments have similar levels of efficiency in converting airflow pulses into sound waves, i.e., up to about 1 percent.[7, 8]

BREATHING PATTERNS

For all types of sound production, breathing patterns are determined by (1) the pressure and flow requirements of the sound output and (2) the ventilatory requirements for gas exchange.

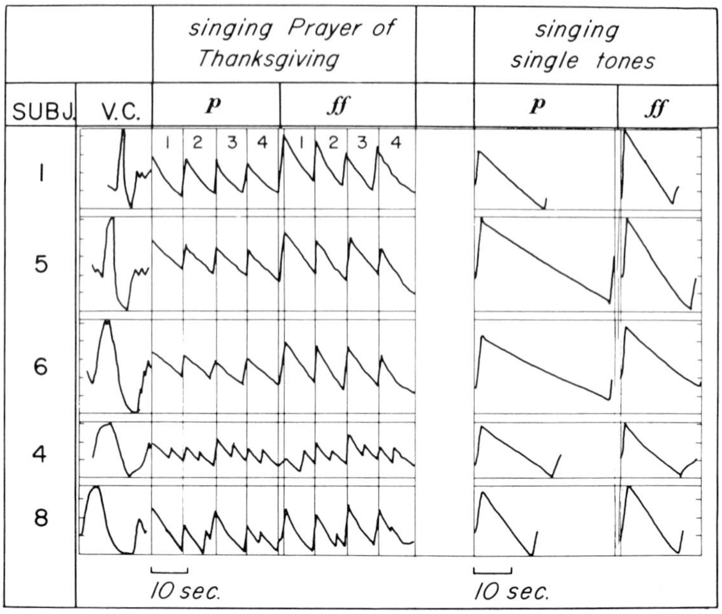

Fig. 11-9. Good-quality (subjects 1, 5, 6) and poor-quality (subjects 4, 8) volume recordings during singing of a song ("Prayer of Thanksgiving"). At left, vital capacity recording with volume scale in liters. At right, volume traces during singing of constant tones by the same subjects. The steeper their slopes, the higher the rate of flow during the tone. See text for discussion. From reference 8.

Singing

Breathing movements during singing consist of rapid inspirations followed by prolonged expirations (Fig. 11-9). The exact pattern adopted for the same song varies among individuals and may be related to singing proficiency.[9] Presumably, good phrasing (i.e., no inspirations in midphrase) and using most of the vital capacity without expiring to near RV are desirable from a standpoint of breathing economy. The three subjects in Figure 11-9, who had good-quality volume traces by such standards, increased total expired volume when a song was rendered loud (ff) rather than soft (p). These subjects also increased flow rates when singing tones louder. On the other hand, singers with poor-quality volume traces used high rates for single soft tones. These subjects appeared to behave like the untrained singer of Figure 11-5, in that they used excessive flow rates for soft tones. The breathing pattern adopted by trained singers depends greatly on the composition. Prolonged phrases, especially those sung forte, often require using nearly the full vital capacity (see Fig. 3 in Bouhuys et al.[9]).

Speaking

When one reads aloud, increasing voice volume calls for larger lung volume excursions; airflow rates may increase or remain the same.[9] Expiration often continues until lung volume decreases below functional residual capacity. As with singing, phrasing depends on the speech content and purpose; good public speakers use phrasing in conjunction with other mechanisms to achieve maximum impact. For one to read poetry, and perhaps even to write it, breath control is especially important. The American poet Charles Olson regarded poetry lines as elements shaped, in part, by the pattern of the poet's breath: "The line comes (I swear it) from the breath, from the breathing of the man who writes, at the moment that he writes . . . for only he, the man who writes, can declare, at every moment, the line, its metric and its ending—where its breathings shall come to termination."[41] When an experienced reader seated in a body plethysmograph read Olson's poetry, his volume recordings indeed showed that the breathing pattern helped to structure and define the lines and phrases, to clarify the intent of the poet, and to improve rhythm.[41]

Wind-Instrument Playing

The breathing pattern during wind-instrument playing resembles that during speech and singing—rapid inspirations are followed by prolonged expirations (see Figs. 2 and 3 in reference 4). The length of the expiration varies with the composition. By specifying when the player may inspire, many composers control their performers' breathing patterns. Since composers usually do not take into account ventilatory constraints, experienced instrumentalists should tell them whether their specifications can be met in practice.

Wind-instrument players often use nearly the full vital capacity and close to maximum expiratory pressures (Fig. 11-10). During prolonged expiration, alveolar

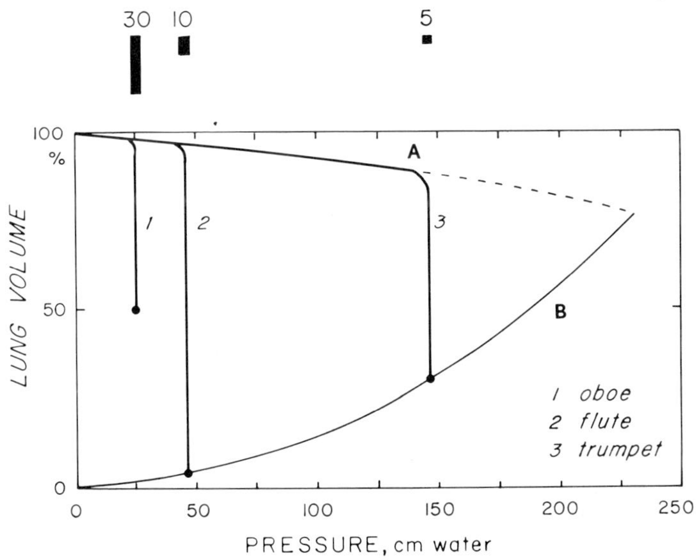

Fig. 11-10. Maximum expiratory pressure-volume diagram; lung volume in percentage VC. Curve *B* (beginning at lung volume 0) represents highest expiratory pressures at any lung volume. Lines 1, 2, and 3 represent pressure-volume events when playing single tones on different instruments (duration of each tone, in seconds, indicated above diagram). Continuous and dashed line *A* beginning at lung volume 100 percent represents pressure-volume events when air in the lungs is compressed by expiratory effort while no air leaves the lungs. Modified from reference 5.

CO_2 tension rises, with an additional increment caused by the elevated alveolar pressures. Thus, more than the singer or speaker, the horn player faces mechanical as well as gas-exchange constraints. The restrictions imposed by the instrument sometimes lead to special breathing patterns. For instance, typical flow rates for the oboe range from 50 to 150 ml/sec, far less than is needed to meet ventilatory requirements. Therefore, the player learns to perform additional quick expirations and inspirations between phrases (Fig. 11-12). In addition, some oboe players learn to breathe through their noses while continuing to produce tones. Apparently, they keep mouth pressure elevated by closing the oral cavity with the tongue, the epiglottis, and/or the soft palate.[4] Oriental snake charmers and players of the zurnah, a shawnlike instrument used in Turkey, reportedly also use this technique.[2]

RESPIRATORY CONSTRAINTS

The vital capacity determines the maximum volume that can be expired for a prolonged utterance or musical phrase. If driving pressures and flow rates are low, one may use nearly the full VC. However, a high pressure or flow, or both, prevents use of the full VC. Although the size of the vital capacity is presumably unrelated to musical aptitude, a performer with large VC may have a selective advantage. Brass players have larger than predicted vital capacities,[4] a fact more apt to reflect initial selection than training. Although some wind-instrument teachers recommend special breathing exercises to increase VC in their students, there is no evidence that the exercises are effective.

Maximum expiratory pressure. Figure 11-10 shows pressure-volume curves during playing of single tones on wind instruments, and these are compared with maximum expiratory pressures (p. 164; Fig. 7-9). Since the flute tone requires a mouth pressure of 50 cm H_2O, a value that can be maintained over most of the VC, the player can use nearly the full VC. Trumpet players, however, use much higher pressures for playing high and loud tones. Part of the VC is spent in compressing alveolar gas from 100 percent VC to about 90 percent VC. The resulting pressure level can be maintained from about 90 to about 30 percent of VC (Fig. 7-9). Below 30 percent VC, the trumpet player can no longer maintain the required pressure because it exceeds the maximum expiratory pressure at lower lung volumes. Hence, the player can effectively use only about half the VC for high or loud tones. Maximum expiratory pressures depend on age and sex,[17] but even young children (7–10 years) are able to produce pressures higher than 100 cm H_2O over about half the VC. Since only the high and loud tones require such high pressures on brass, children can play these instruments quite well. Maximum expiratory pressures decrease slightly with age.[17] Although, theoretically, this decrease could limit the older brass performer, superior musical skill may compensate for the loss.

Maximum expiratory flow rates. During speech and singing, average expiratory flow rates rarely exceed 0.5 liters/sec. While healthy subjects can maintain flows of this order over nearly the full VC (Chap. 9), patients with severe airway obstruction may have difficulty (see Fig. 9-6). Such patients often break speech

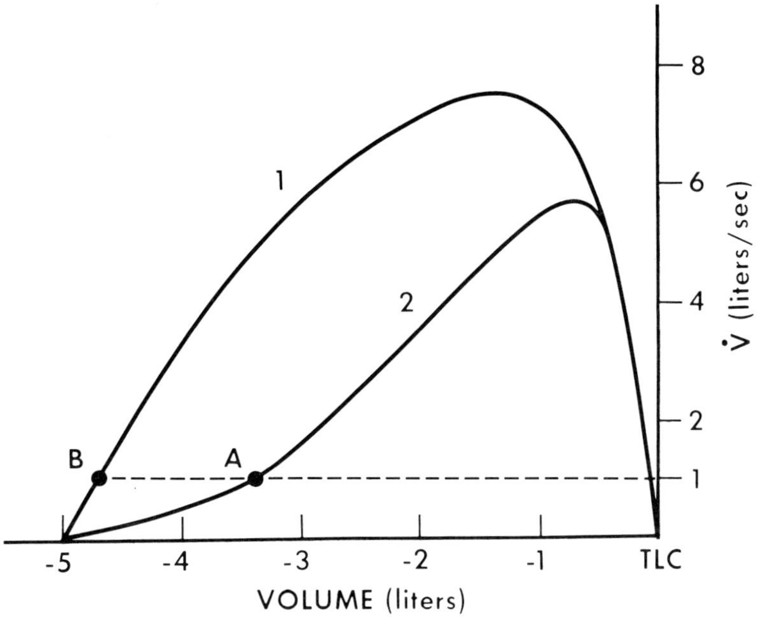

Fig. 11-11. Typical MEFV curves of young (*1*) and old (*2*) wind-instrument players. Dashed line indicates flow of 1 liter/sec required for tone. See text for discussion.

phrases frequently, probably because they can maintain the required flow rate only at higher lung volumes. Gas-exchange limitations may also contribute to the halting speech of dyspneic patients.

Older brass-instrument players frequently complain that they "run out of breath" sooner than they used to. This complaint may reflect flow limitations, as illustrated in Figure 11-11. Brass players frequently use flow rates of 1–2 liters/sec (Fig. 11-8). The player with MEFV curve *1* can maintain a flow of 1 liter/sec over nearly the full VC; this flow is maximal at point B, which is near RV. The player with MEFV curve *2*, on the other hand, can sustain a 1 liter/sec flow for only 3.4 seconds (i.e., not at volumes less than at A), while player *1* can play this tone for 4.7 seconds, i.e., 38 percent longer. Curves *1* and *2* typify MEFV curves of younger and older men, respectively (compare Fig. 9-12, p. 221). They might also represent MEFV curves for nonsmoking and smoking players of similar age (compare Fig. 12-5, p. 311). Since many wind players smoke heavily,[2, 4] smoking as well as age may reduce performance by decreasing maximum flows at low lung volumes.

Breath-holding time. The oboe player often uses flow rates as low as 50 ml/sec. To expire to a full VC of 5 liters at this flow would take 100 seconds, much longer than most people can hold their breath. Therefore, the oboe player usually plays over only a portion of the VC before inspiring again, or he performs a rapid expiration followed by a deep inspiration (Figs. 11-10 and 11-12). The need for gas exchange restricts his performance.

Hyperventilation. High flow rates at low pressures are used for low tones on brass instruments, e.g., the bass tuba.[4] During prolonged passages with such tones, these players may complain of dizziness, presumably caused by hyperventilation.

Circulatory limitations. High alveolar pressures impede the flow of venous blood to the heart and cause arterial blood pressure to drop.[25] Because of diminished cerebral blood supply, this drop in pressure may lead to dizziness and fainting. Since the coronary blood supply might also decrease, strenuous brass performance may pose risks for older players. The effects of hyperventilation and of high pressures may potentiate one another with respect to symptoms of dizziness during playing (Campbell, in discussion of reference 6).

CONTROL OF BREATHING

To speak, sing, or play a horn requires fine control over respiratory, laryngeal, pharyngeal, oral, and facial muscles. Even a simple act like singing a tone of constant pitch and loudness requires continuous, precise adjustments of inspiratory and expiratory muscle contraction (Fig. 11-3). At the same time, these muscles must be used to control ventilation for gas exchange (Chap. 10). For adequate performance, all participating muscles must contract to the correct degree, at the right time, and in proper sequence. Hence, the central nervous system must not only coordinate these elaborate sets of motor impulses, but also integrate them with those required for other motor acts involving the same muscles (breathing, swallowing, facial expression, posture). These sets of instructions and their mutual coordination develop during a process of trial and error. The learning process is guided by regular progress reports, or feedback information, from the moving structures as well as auditory and sometimes visual cues. We shall first discuss the sources of feedback information and, next, a concept of the integrated control system.

Sources of Feedback

The child learning to speak and the student of voice or wind instruments both require *auditory feedback* from their own sounds and those made by others. Birds do not learn to sing if they grow up in isolation.[48] When the initial learning process is complete, auditory feedback becomes less essential. Human speech begins to deteriorate markedly only over a year after the onset of nerve deafness,[19] and adult birds, when deafened, maintain normal song performance.[48] Additional sources of feedback include afferent signals from *muscle spindles* [11, 57] and from *sensory receptors* in laryngeal joints [35] and in the supravocal tract.

Muscle spindles indicate the relative state of muscle contraction. This information is integrated in the spinal cord, with impulses which travel down from higher centers in the brain and brainstem—together these assure the proper degree of muscle contraction. Muscle spindles are numerous in the intercostal muscles, the most important muscles in regulating subglottic pressure. The diaphragm, which has few muscle spindles, performs no active role during speech or singing (see p. 271). Perhaps surprisingly, the laryngeal muscles, which adjust the vocal-fold tension needed to control voice pitch precisely, contain no muscle spindles. In the cat, sensory receptors in the cricothyroid joint can signal changes in joint position to the central nervous system, resulting in efferent motor signals to intrinsic laryngeal muscles.[35] Since the relative positions of the thyroid and cricoid cartilages affect the length of the vocal folds and hence their tension, feedback from the cricothyroid sensory receptors may influence pitch control. Whether these particular receptors are present in man is not known. But the paucity of suitable laryngeal receptors suggests that auditory feedback is more important than other feedback sources for pitch control. Lastly, superficial sensory receptors along the supravocal tract, including the lips, probably help control articulation and wind-instrument performance.

Central Control Mechanisms

Although many nerve centers and pathways contribute to speech control,[24] its organization remains a mystery. Human language is one of the most highly organized outputs of the brain. However, since language is the main tool for studying the brain, no one has found a way to study how the brain controls speech.[62] Nevertheless, some general concepts of brain function can be derived from the study of language and other precise motor acts such as writing.[21, 30, 40]

Motor acts are often thought to result from a sequence of reflex events, involving efferent motor signals to the muscles and afferent signals to the central nervous system from muscles and other structures, which modify the efferent signals. However, many skilled motor acts preclude this explanation, since they are performed too rapidly to allow time for nerve conduction of afferent signals and processing of feedback information.[40] To sing a tone at nearly correct pitch, or to speak a word intelligibly, one has no time to conduct a complex series of reflex maneuvers (Fig. 11-7). Rather, one must perform such skilled motor acts according to preprogrammed instructions. The advance programming, or learning, also permits these acts to be performed in sequence. Thus, to speak even a single phoneme, the barest rudiment of human language, requires a predetermined, precisely quantitated and sequenced set of motor signals to the muscles; the impulses required to make the initial sound depend on the subsequent sounds within the phoneme.

Lashley [40] has emphasized that most skilled motor tasks require an "organized temporal order" for their execution. Individual parts of a set of events must occur in a prescribed sequence; they are part of a preprogrammed set of motor impulses. The instructions for each phoneme form a sort of subroutine for larger programs; phonemes are structured into syllables and words, and words into sentences and messages. The programming of human speech and language involves linguistic formulation as well as coordination of motor control per se.[30] Similarly, in music the performer develops a set of motor instructions that reflects the hierarchical and rhythmic order of notes, chords, measures, themes, parts, movements, and symphonies. Forty phonemes are used in English, incorporating only nine distinctive features.[14] Hence, a small number of basic instructions is enough to build up the elaborate structure of human language. Simpler organized sounds produced by animals may differ from human language mainly in the absence of higher levels of organization. In the katydid, the motor output for singing is emitted by a neuronal pacemaker that fires at the singing frequency; transmitting signals to the forewing muscles involves only a few neuronal elements.[34] Like human speech the purring of cats also involves coordination of vocal and respiratory muscles. Since purring persists even after afferent nerves from lungs and muscles have been cut, the alternating contractions of laryngeal muscles and diaphragm which cause purring must originate centrally. Thus, purring seems to be a good example of a stereotyped, programmed motor act.[56]

Even though programmed instructions may largely determine speech events, feedback information is also important. Feedback contributes to the ongoing assessment of performance, by detecting errors and modifying motor instructions. Feedback is particularly important for timing speech events and adjusting speech volume in relation to ambient noise levels.[30] When a subject's speech output is fed back to his ears via a delaying electronic circuit, speech is disrupted, primarily because of difficulties in articulation.[30] When loud random noise masks the sound of a wind instrument to the player's ear, he can usually remain on pitch, probably because he still receives tactile sensory input from his lips. However, ambient noise can make it impossible to produce a constant tone on the recorder, played through a tube inserted in the mouth, because the player receives neither auditory nor tactile information about tone production (personal observation).

The concepts of speech and language discussed in this section have practical importance not only in speech therapy, but also in efforts to synthesize speech artificially ("talking computers" [29]) and to understand and improve learning processes in children and music students.

Learning to Speak

The human infant learns to speak in response to speech sounds from those around him. Children born deaf do not develop speech without considerable special training. Although human language includes several added levels of complexities, the principles involved in human learning may be similar to those in songbird's learning.[48, 49] Young birds pick up selected auditory cues from their environment. Since they learn only their own song, and not those of other species, their brains must have some genetically determined pattern or template, which guides the selection process. Training may increase this template's precision, enabling the bird to improve vocalization, guided by auditory feedback from its own song and from others of the same species. This feedback information in turn further increases the template's precision.

Deaf-mute children lack appropriate control over breathing when they attempt to speak.[61] Yet, they have no trouble performing other coordinated acts, such as masticating and swallowing, which use the same muscle groups. Hence, since the children's lower coordination centers appear to function well, their speech defects must reflect a lack of central organization, rather than a lack of muscle coordination. The child that learns to speak develops a steadily increasing number of programmed sets of motor instruction, as well as the ability to organize these into an infinitely varying set of larger speech structures (words, sentences, messages). The early acquisition of speech apparently has a lasting effect on speech habits, and this often interferes with later acquisition of a new language. This is remarkable since man retains the capacity to learn many other skilled motor acts throughout his life. Perhaps the very early development of speech leads to fixed habits that inhibit the development of new patterns.

Integration With Ventilatory Control

The airflow requirements for speech must be reconciled with the ventilatory requirements for gas exchange. When one breathes room air at rest, ventilation per minute increases slightly during speech. The increase is greater when the speech material includes many high-flow consonants such as the /h/.[10] Significant hypocapnia has been observed in one study.[20] When ventilatory demands are increased, as during exercise or breathing of 3 percent CO_2, minute ventilation increases even though speech requires lower flows. Under these conditions, speech usually decreases the average minute ventilation (e.g., from an average of 18.9 to 16.0 liters/min during exercise; personal observation). Similarly, the speaker breathing 3 percent CO_2 in air has a minute ventilation which is less than the minute ventilation at rest during CO_2 breathing.[10] Thus, the speaker appears to achieve a compromise between ventilatory and speech demands on flow rates. How can he increase minute ventilation while maintaining flows compatible with intelligible speech? Figure 11-12 shows the solution to this problem schematically. Suppose that minute ventilation at rest is 7.5 liters/min, and the breathing rate is 15 breaths per minute. During speech, breathing rate declines to 12 breaths per

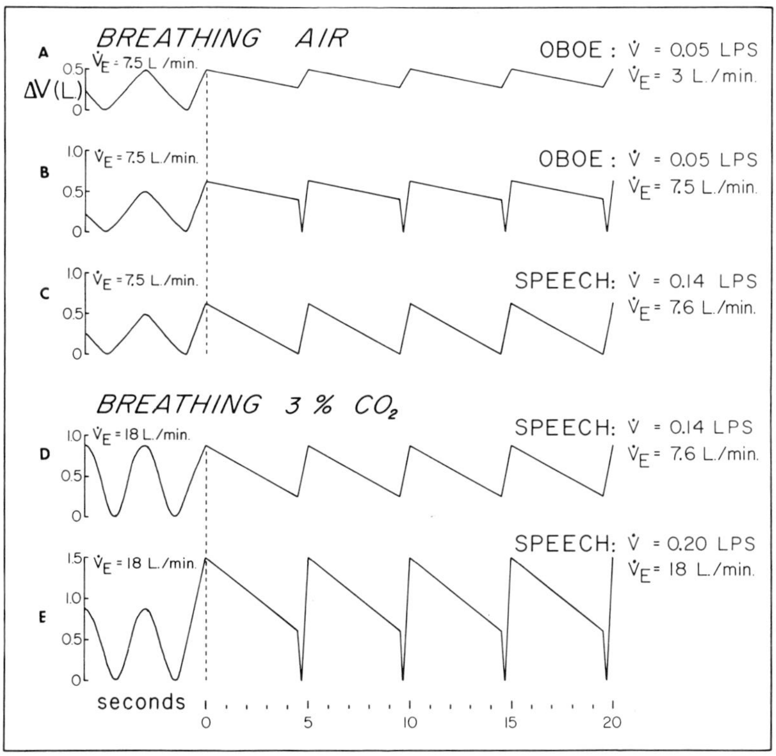

Fig. 11-12. Schematic diagram of breathing pattern during oboe playing (*A, B*), speech while breathing room air (*C*), and speech during breathing of 3% CO_2 in air (*D, E*). Resting pattern and minute ventilation ($\dot{V}_E$) at left in each graph. At right, average expiratory flow rates ($\dot{V}$) and minute ventilation ($\dot{V}_E$) during play or speech. Patterns *A* and *D* are incompatible with gas-exchange requirements ($\dot{V}_E$ too low). Hence, the player or speaker adopts pattern *B* or *E* to meet these demands. After data from references 4 and 10. Further discussion in text.

minute, tidal volume increases, and expiration is prolonged (*C*). Expiratory flow rate is assumed constant at 0.14 liters/sec. During 3 percent CO_2 breathing at rest, minute ventilation increases to 18 liters/min (*D*). If the subject maintained the same breathing pattern for speech while breathing CO_2, the minute ventilation would be only 7.6 liters/min and CO_2 would be retained. Two mechanisms that prevent this are [10] (1) the mean expiratory flow rate increases during speech, resulting in a more "breathy" but still intelligible voice, and (2) the speaker superimposes rapid expirations followed by deep inspirations upon the speech breathing pattern. The schematic curve *E* includes both mechanisms; actually, the minute ventilation decreases when speaking at rest during CO_2 breathing, so that compensation is incomplete.[10] The curves *A* and *B* show that oboe players adopt a similar breathing pattern to maintain ventilation (see p. 281).

RESPIRATION AND SPEECH IN DISEASE

There have been few quantitative studies of subglottic pressures, airflow rates, and breathing patterns in patients with speech abnormalities. Recordings of these events might help develop objective standards for diagnosing speech disorders and for assessing the effect of therapy. In re-educating patients with speech disorders, visualization of airflow rates and breathing patterns might help the patient correct malcoordination of respiratory muscle effort. For instance, a deaf-mute student might benefit from watching the normal flow pattern for various phonemes on an oscilloscope screen and trying to match this pattern. Such methods might also help stutterers and singers. Since "waste of air" seems to be common to several speech disorders and to untrained singers, visualization of airflow control might teach them how to use minimal flow rates. Monitoring muscle effort with electromyographic recordings might also be useful. Feedback from the EMG of laryngeal muscles helps to "unlearn" the habit of subvocal speech while reading.[32]

Dysarthria and aphasia. In disorders of articulation (dysarthria), muscle coordination is impaired. In patients with brain lesions, the ability to speak is often impaired while coordination of the muscles remains intact (aphasia). Recordings of subglottic pressure and flow may help to distinguish between malcoordination (dysarthria) and programming disorders (aphasia). In the latter, if there is residual speech, one would expect normal flow and pressure patterns. Such patients might be able to sing steady tones at constant loudness and pitch, while patients with dysarthria would probably have lost this ability.[18] Unfortunately, there are few reports of detailed physiological studies of speech in patients with dysarthria (parkinsonism, multiple sclerosis).[31] Hence, it is not clear how much this speech defect results from poor coordination of respiratory, laryngeal, and articulatory muscle contraction. The hypokinetic speech—reduced voice volume, monotonous voice, and dysarthria—of patients with parkinsonism relates to the delayed onset of movements and to their slowness and small amplitude. Airflow and subglottic pressure recordings might provide objective data on the effectiveness of treating this disease with drugs like L-dopa, which alter the duration of phonation and the length of pauses between utterances.[50]

Substitute vocal apparatus. Aphasia, in which speech is impossible in spite of an intact vocal apparatus, clearly demonstrates the importance of the central control system to speech. Conversely, patients who have undergone a laryngectomy for cancer learn to speak with a different effector apparatus, the entrance to the esophagus.[22] Apparently, once central speech control is fully developed, one can learn to use it to operate another peripheral apparatus. Other damage to the vocal apparatus is also compatible with good performance. For example, a patient with permanent unilateral paralysis of a vocal fold became a good choir singer after training,[1] and injecting Teflon into atrophied or paralyzed vocal folds can help restore the normal voice, even though the injected fold has no means of adjusting its tension by muscle contraction.[16]

DEVELOPMENT OF SPEECH AND LANGUAGE

Human speech is a relatively recent phylogenetic development.[44] When man assumed the upright posture, the altered position of his head led to the development of a bend in the upper airway. This increased airway resistance, as well as the dangers at the crossroads between food and air passages (Chap. 2). A more sophisticated swallowing mechanism became imperative to prevent food from entering the trachea and air from entering the stomach, even though both passed through a long pharynx. This modification required improved pharyngeal musculature and a coordinated reflex mechanism, integrated with respiratory control. The descent of the larynx to its position in modern man took place concurrently.[26] Hence, while the swallowing mechanism had obvious immediate survival value, the use of the mobile, muscular pharynx for speech may have followed almost accidentally.

The development of the articulatory capability in the supravocal tract was crucial to modern man's acquisition of speech. Monkeys can alter the shape of the supravocal tract only within narrow limits, mainly because their pharynx is short and immobile.[47] Newborn infants, too, have a short pharynx, and the configuration of their supravocal tract resembles that of nonhuman primates.[46] Analyses of the skulls of Neanderthal and Cro-Magnon man[45] indicate that the former had a short pharynx, while that of the latter resembles modern man's. Thus, Cro-Magnon man may have been able to speak, while Neanderthal man had at best very limited speech capabilities. The development of the motor apparatus for speech may be more crucial to the acquisition of speech than was formerly thought. This explains why it is impossible to teach chimpanzees to speak English. Although they have sufficient brainpower to learn language [e.g., they can learn to communicate and understand messages in other code systems (sign language) using colored plastic objects[54] or computer-controlled word symbols[56a]], they lack the vocal equipment.

The upright posture also provided another advantage for speech—it facilitated more precise regulation of subglottic pressure with the intercostal muscles and the hydraulic pull of the abdominal contents on the diaphragm.[9] Given these various structural possibilities, primitive man probably began to notice his ability to produce a larger variety of sounds that could be used to communicate with others. As he used his hands increasingly to manipulate tools, communication by gesture alone became less practical. In addition, he soon found that the voice could transmit messages to people whom he could not see. Central organization probably took place concurrently. The "improved vocalization apparatus, like the use of tools, served . . . to give the brain more to think about."[26] In turn, improved central control probably led to refined vocal output. In primates, the laryngeal output is noisy and irregular;[43] pitch control in man is much more precise.

The ontogenesis of speech in infants may represent an abbreviated form of the phylogenetic development. In newborn infants, the vocal apparatus is not suitable for speech,[46] and the central organization of speech does not function. As the vocal apparatus improves through structural changes in the supravocal tract, the infant generates some speech sounds, which in turn elicit feedback from people around him. This improves the speech "templates"[48] and stimulates the infant to make more and different sounds (see p. 284).

I speak, therefore I am? Lieberman and Crelin[45] have commented on the historical background of our concepts of speech development. Descartes' cogito ergo sum (I think, therefore I am) identified the mind as the central feature of being human. In this context, apes were nonhuman because they were not supposed to think and therefore had nothing to say. But in fact, apes can learn language,[54, 56a] although they cannot speak. Unlike Descartes, Lieberman and Crelin suggest that "Man is human because he can say so,"[45] and they stress the importance of the vocal apparatus to our ability to speak. Yet, speech, language, and thought are closely associated. The act of thinking requires some mode of expression in language. To the extent that the Premacks' chimpanzee, Sarah, interprets messages in a plastic symbol code and responds to them with an appropriate answer, she may be said to think.[54] Although man uses nonverbal modes of communication to express feelings, we cannot assess his rational thoughts unless he speaks or writes about them. Perhaps what makes us human is that we listen to others, we think, and we speak our minds.

SUMMARY

The respiratory bellows supplies power to the vocal apparatus and drives wind instruments. This power is generated by the elastic recoil of chest and lungs and by the respiratory muscles. Expiratory muscles supply driving pressure; inspiratory muscles brake the recoil forces so that low driving pressures can be maintained even at large lung volumes. Simultaneous recordings of driving (subglottal) pressure and airflow show that experienced speakers and trained singers exert precise control over their glottides and supravocal tracts. To achieve control of pitch, loudness, and quality of the voice, the muscular control of the glottis and supravocal tract is integrated with that of the respiratory muscles. Breathing patterns during speech, singing, and wind-instrument playing consist of rapid inspirations and prolonged expirations; the patterns depend on the pressure and flow requirements of the voice or instrument as well as on the need to ventilate the lungs. Volume, pressure, and flow constraints of the respiratory bellows set limits to performance, especially with wind instruments. The control of speech and similar voluntary acts requires programming of nerve impulses to the muscles in precisely quantitated and sequenced sets of motor instructions. Feedback control (auditory, proprioceptive, and tactile) helps develop these sets during learning and monitors performance afterwards. Under some conditions, special breathing patterns are used to reconcile incompatible requirements of sound production and gas exchange. The recording of respiratory events may prove helpful in diagnosing and treating speech disorders.

Human speech may have developed when man adopted the upright posture, which led to structural changes in the supravocal tract. Similar changes, including the formation of a long, mobile pharynx, occur in young children; newborn infants lack the articulatory apparatus for coordinated speech. These recent findings have a profound impact on our concepts of human language and thought and their phylogenetic and ontogenetic development.

REFERENCES

1. Aherne G: Singing with a paralysed cord. Lancet 2:1313, 1970
2. Akgün N, Özgönül H: Lung volumes in wind instrument (zurna) players. Am Rev Respir Dis 96:946–951, 1967
3. Bouhuys A: Concluding remarks, in: Sound production in man. Ann NY Acad Sci 155:379–381, 1968
4. Bouhuys A: Lung volumes and breathing patterns in wind instrument players. J Appl Physiol 19:967–975, 1964
5. Bouhuys A: Physiology and musical instruments. Nature 221:1199–1204, 1969
6. Bouhuys A: Pressure-flow events during wind instrument playing, in: Sound production in man. Ann NY Acad Sci 155:264–275, 1968
7. Bouhuys A: Sound-power production in wind instruments. J Acoust Soc Am 37:453–456, 1965
8. Bouhuys A, Mead J, Proctor DF, Stevens KN: Pressure-flow events during singing, in: Sound production in man. Ann NY Acad Sci 155:165–176, 1968
9. Bouhuys A, Proctor DF, Mead J: Kinetic aspects of singing. J Appl Physiol 21:483–496, 1966
10. Bunn JC, Mead J: Control of ventilation during speech. J Appl Physiol 31: 870–872, 1971
11. Campbell EJM, Agostoni E, Newsom Davis J: The Respiratory Muscles: Mechanics and Nerve Control, ed 2. Philadelphia, WB Saunders Co Inc, 1970
12. Cavagna GA, Margaria R: An analysis of the mechanics of phonation. J Appl Physiol 20:301–307, 1965
13. Chanaud RC: Aerodynamic whistles. Sci Am 222:40–46, 1970
14. Cherry C: On Human Communication, ed 2. Cambridge, Massachusetts Institute of Technology Press, 1966
15. Chomsky N, Halle M: The Sound Pattern of English. New York, Harper and Row, 1968
16. Cole R: Speech, in: Patterns of Orofacial Growth and Development, ASHA Reports No. 6. Washington, D.C., American Speech and Hearing Association, 1971, pp 79–95
17. Cook CD, Mead J, Orzalesi MM: Static volume-pressure characteristics of the respiratory system during maximal efforts. J Appl Physiol 19:1016–1022, 1964
18. Davis JN: Discussion remarks, in: Sound production in man. Ann NY Acad Sci 155:203, 1968
19. Dedo HH: Discussion remarks, in: Sound production in man. Ann NY Acad Sci 155:203, 1968
20. Dejours P, Wagner S, Dejager M, Vichon M-J: Ventilation et gaz alvéolaire pendant le langage parlé. J Physiol (Paris) 59:386, 1967
21. Denier van der Gon JJ, Thuring JPh: The guiding of human writing movements. Kybernetik 2:145–148, 1965
22. Diedrich WM: The mechanism of esophageal speech, in: Sound production in man. Ann NY Acad Sci 155:303–317, 1968

23. Draper MH, Ladefoged P, Whitteridge D: Expiratory pressures and air flow during speech. Br Med J 1:1837–1843, 1960
24. Dunker E: The central control of laryngeal function, in: Sound production in man. Ann NY Acad Sci 155:112–121, 1968
25. Faulkner M, Sharpey-Schafer EP: Circulatory effects of trumpet playing. Br Med J 1:685–686, 1959
26. Fenn WO: Perspectives in phonation, in: Sound production in man. Ann NY Acad Sci 155:4–8, 1968
27. Flanagan JL: Source-system interaction in the vocal tract, in: Sound production in man. Ann NY Acad Sci 155:9–17, 1968
28. Flanagan JL: Speech Analysis, Synthesis, and Perception. New York, Springer, 1965
29. Flanagan JL: The synthesis of speech. Sci Amer 226:48–58, 1972
30. Fry DB: The control of speech and voice, in Kalmus H (ed): Regulation and Control in Living Systems. London, John Wiley and Sons, 1966
31. Grewel F: Classification of dysarthrias. Acta Psych Neurol Scand 32:325–337, 1957
32. Hardyck CD, Petrinovich LF, Ellsworth DW: Feedback of speech muscle activity during silent reading: rapid extinction. Science 154:1467–1468, 1966
33. Hixon TJ: Some new techniques for measuring the biomechanical events of speech production: one laboratory's experiences. ASHA Reports No. 7. Washington, D.C., 1972, American Speech and Hearing Association, pp 68–103
34. Josephson RK, Halverson RC: High frequency muscles used in sound production by a katydid. I. Organization of the motor system. Biol Bull. 141:411–433, 1971
35. Kirchner JA, Suzuki M: Laryngeal reflexes and voice production, in: Sound production in man. Ann NY Acad Sci 155:98–109, 1968
36. Klatt DH, Stevens KN, Mead J: Studies of articulatory activity and airflow during speech, in: Sound production in man. Ann NY Acad Sci 155:42–55, 1968
37. Konno K, Mead J: Measurement of the separate volume change of ribcage and abdomen during breathing. J Appl Physiol 22:407–422, 1967
38. Ladefoged P: Linguistic aspects of respiratory phenomena, in: Sound production in man. Ann NY Acad Sci 155: 141–151, 1968
39. Ladefoged P: Three Areas of Experimental Phonetics. New York, Oxford University Press, 1967
40. Lashley KS: The problem of serial order in behavior, in Jeffress LA (ed): Cerebral Mechanisms in Behavior. New York, Wiley, 1951, pp 112–136
41. Lieberman MR, Lieberman P: Olson's "projective verse" and the use of breath control as a structural element. Language and Style 5:287–298, 1973
42. Lieberman P: Direct comparison of subglottal and esophageal pressure during speech. J Acoust Soc Am 43:1157–1164, 1968
43. Lieberman P: Primate vocalizations and human linguistic ability. J Acoust Soc Am 44:1574–1584, 1968
44. Lieberman P: The Speech of Primates. The Hague, Mouton and Co, 1972
45. Lieberman P, Crelin ES: On the speech of Neanderthal man. Linguistic Inquiry 2:203–222, 1971
46. Lieberman P, Crelin ES, Klatt DH: Phonetic ability and related anatomy of the newborn and adult human, Neanderthal man, and the chimpanzee. American Anthropologist 74:287–307, 1972
47. Lieberman P, Klatt DH, Wilson WH: Vocal tract limitations on the vowel repertoires of rhesus monkey and other non-human primates. Science 164:1185–1187, 1969
48. Marler P: A comparative approach to vocal learning: Song development in white-crowned sparrows. J. Comp Physiol Psychol (Monograph 71, No. 2, Part 2): 1–25, 1970
49. Marler P: Birdsong and speech development: could there be parallels? Am Sci 58:669–673, 1970
50. Mawdsley C, Gamsu CV: Periodicity of speech in Parkinsonism. Nature 231: 315–316, 1971
51. Mead J, Bouhuys A, Proctor DF: Mechanisms generating subglottic pressure, in: Sound production in man. Ann NY Acad Sci 155:177–181, 1968
52. Müller J: Von der Stimme und Sprache, in: Handbuch der Physiol. des Menschen, Vol II, Book 4, Part 3. Coblenz, J. Holscher, 1837

53. Negus VE: The Comparative Anatomy and Physiology of the Larynx. New York, Hafner, 1949
54. Premack AJ, Premack D: Teaching language to an ape. Sci Am 92–99, 1972
55. Pressman JJ, Kellemen G: Physiology of the Larynx, ed 2, revised by JA Kirchner, Rochester, Minn., American Academy of Ophthalmology and Otolaryngology, 1970
56. Remmers JE, Gautier H: Neural and mechanical mechanisms of feline purring. Respir Physiol 16:351–361, 1972
56a. Rumbaugh DM, Gill TV, Glasersfeld EC von: Reading and sentence completion by a chimpanzee (Pan). Science 182:731–733, 1973
57. Sears TA, Davis JN: The control of respiratory muscles during voluntary breathing, in: Sound production in man. Ann NY Acad Sci 155:183–190, 1968
58. Van den Berg J: Myoelastic-aerodynamic theory of voice production. J Speech Hearing Res 1:227–234, 1958
59. Vivona PM: Mouth pressures in trombone players, in: Sound production in man. Ann NY Acad Sci 155:290–296, 1968
60. Warren DW, Wood MT: Respiratory volumes in normal speech: a possible reason for intraoral pressure differences among voiced and voiceless consonants. J Acoust Soc Am 45:466–469, 1969
61. Woldring S: Breathing patterns during speech in deaf children, in: Sound production in man. Ann NY Acad Sci 155: 206–207, 1968
62. Young, JZ: What can we know about memory? Br Med J 14:647–652, 1970

Chapter 12

Environment and Lung Disease

This chapter reviews environmental lung diseases and introduces some practical applications of respiratory physiology. Most lung diseases result from interaction between the tissues of airways and lungs, and agents inhaled from the environment: bacteria, viruses, carcinogens, allergens, toxic chemicals, dusts, and physical stimuli. However, endogenous ("host") factors are critical in determining the type, degree, and permanence of cell injury and tissue responses induced by inhaled agents.

The first section describes how inhaled agents enter the lungs and how the tissues respond. Next, some specific environmental exposures are discussed, with emphasis on the use of lung function measurements in the detection of their effects. Lastly, prevention and control of environmental lung diseases are discussed briefly.

TRANSPORT OF INHALED AGENTS

Gas molecules, droplets, and dust particles are transported into the airways and lungs, where they elicit responses when they reach the tissues. The first concern, then, is how matter gets into the lungs and where it is deposited or absorbed.

Gases and Vapors

Gases and vapors can be absorbed from inspired air at the maximum rate $F_I \cdot \dot{V}_I$, where F_I is the fractional inspired concentration and $\dot{V}_I$ is the volume of inspired gas per unit time. The actual absorption is usually less than maximum; the ultimate effects depend on solubility, metabolic fate, excretion, and toxicity.[85] Gases may be absorbed at different sites, and their rate of uptake may be limited by different mechanisms, depending on their physical properties. Highly soluble gases (e.g., sulfur dioxide, ammonia, ozone) are absorbed by the mucus and mucosa of nose and upper airways.[34] These gases enter the bronchial tree only to the extent that the scrubbing action of the nose is saturated, or bypassed during mouth breathing. Less-soluble gases always enter the bronchial tree on inspiration. For heavy gases (e.g., sulfur hexafluoride; Chap. 4), diffusion in alveolar gas limits the rate of uptake. For lighter molecules, diffusion through the alveolocapillary membrane (e.g., many anesthetic gases; Chap. 5) may be rate limiting.

The site of the effect of gases and vapors depends largely on their solubility in mucus of upper airways and in lung tissue. Ammonia is highly soluble in mucus and also very irritating; its effect on upper airways usually leads one to withdraw from the polluted atmosphere. On the other hand, phosgene is not very soluble in watery media;[130] it is hydrolyzed in mucus to HCl and Cl_2, but this takes time. Therefore, phosgene has little effect on the upper airways. Nevertheless, phosgene or its hydrolysis products have major effects on the lung parenchyma. Chlorine occupies an intermediate position. It is not as soluble as ammonia but still exerts some effects in upper airways; parenchymal responses are frequent since much chlorine reaches lower airways as well. Oxygen is not absorbed in upper airways; its toxic effects (from prolonged administration of hyperbaric O_2 or 100 percent O_2 at 1 atm) include severe parenchymal reactions.[40]

Aerosol Particles

Droplets or solid particles in air are transported chiefly by bulk flow (Chap. 3). Most particles larger than 10 μm diameter are deposited by impaction in the nose. Smaller particles (2 to 10 μm diameter) enter the bronchial tree, where they are deposited by a combination of impaction (a function of linear air velocity, which is high in the trachea and large bronchi) and sedimentation (or settling) under the influence of gravity. Sedimentation occurs mainly in small airways, where linear air velocities are low and, hence, impaction unimportant. Particles between 0.3 and 2.0 μm in diameter are deposited largely in alveoli and terminal bronchioles. When an aerosol of round, uniform, 2 μm diameter particles is inhaled, about 50 percent of the particles are deposited in ciliated airways, and 50 percent in nonciliated ones (alveoli, alveolar ducts, and respiratory bronchioles).[109] However, most dust aerosols encountered in practice do not consist of uniform (monodisperse) particles. Commonly, they contain particles of different sizes (heterodisperse aerosols), shapes and compositions. Long and thin fibers can penetrate much deeper into the lungs than round particles of the same weight.[174] Hence, the site of deposition of heterodisperse aerosols is not easily predictable. In addition, the large particles of a heterodisperse aerosol contain most of the mass of the particles. Hence, actions that depend on the amount of matter deposited in the airways (e.g., pharmacological actions) may occur chiefly where large particles are deposited (nose, trachea, large bronchi). Dust aerosols usually contain many more small than large particles. Actions that depend on the number of particles deposited might occur principally in small airways and alveoli where most small particles are deposited.

Clearance of Dust Particles

The principal mechanisms by which dust particles are removed from the lungs are mucociliary clearance, phagocytosis, and coughing.

Mucociliary clearance (see Chap. 2). This mechanism is effective in airways down to the first generation of bronchioles. Beyond these, the ciliary beat becomes ineffective and mucus production is lacking. In that region, phagocytosis is the essential clearance mechanism.

Phagocytosis. In the healthy lung, the alveolar macrophage is the predominant phagocytic cell. During acute inflammation, polymorphonuclear cells are also mobilized. All particles deposited in alveoli are probably engulfed by phagocytic cells within a few hours. Considerable mobilization of macrophages takes place in response to subacute stimuli, such as prolonged dust exposure. Macrophages are also active in delayed hypersensitivity reactions. Within the macrophage cell, biochemical processes may lead to destruction of the particle. Some particles are taken up by lysosomes in the cells, where they are destroyed by enzymes (hydrolases). Other particles, including silica, make the lysosome membrane permeable and thus cause release of the lysosomal enzymes within the cell. This causes autodigestion, and the products of the dead macrophage cell may be an important element in initiating further tissue reactions in silicosis.[5] Thus, although macrophages provide important protection against some inhaled particles (microbes), in other instances they become active mediators in the initiation of disease: a true two-edged sword. After having ingested particles, the phagocytes may migrate via lymph vessels to regional lymph nodes, where they may die and deposit the ingested material. Other phagocytes are removed by the mucociliary clearance process.

Coughing. Coughing is an efficient bulk-transport mechanism that in a single movement can clear several milliliters of accumulated mucus, foreign matter, and infectious cellular debris from the airways. Although mainly elicited by stimuli in large airways, increased air velocities during cough extend to small airways as well. Thus, cough removes material from a large part of the bronchial tree (see also p. 179.)

Overall clearance rates. Cough clears the airways in less than a second; mucociliary clearance may take at most a few hours; clearance of phagocytosed particles takes more time. The overall rate of particle clearance from the lungs can be measured by following the clearance of radioactive particles inhaled as an aerosol. Such measurements in humans show, for example, that at the end of 24 hours about 80% of particles 3 μm in diameter have been cleared.[126] Most of the remaining particles are eventually also removed from the lungs. The lungs of South African gold miners—who may inhale more than 1000 gm dust during their years of work in the mines—contain about 20 gm dust at autopsy.[82] The time during which dust particles stay in the lungs and the time needed to elicit tissue responses are two main factors that influence the extent of lung damage induced by inhaled dust. For instance, if a response occurs within 1 hour after particle inhalation, nearly all inhaled particles may be active in eliciting a response. On the other hand, far fewer particles would have an opportunity to act if the response occurred only after, e.g., 24 hours of contact between particles and tissue.

RESPONSES OF AIRWAYS AND LUNG TISSUE

This section reviews mechanisms by which inhaled gases, vapors, fumes, and dusts may cause respiratory symptoms, disturbances in lung function, and lung tissue lesions. Excellent textbooks that provide further details on clinical and pathological aspects include those of Crofton and Douglas,[47] Morgan and Seaton,[124] and Spencer.[163]

Protective Reflexes

Protective reflexes, elicited by irritant gases from receptors in upper airways, trachea, and large bronchi,[182] cause sneezing, glottal closure, apnea (or rapid shallow breathing), and cough. These responses alert the subject to the exposure; sneezing and cough also help to clear inhaled matter. Some inhaled agents cause reflex airway constriction (see p. 311). Along with the sense of smell, these reflexes are important warning signals. The absence of such sensations and reflexes may lead to serious lung injury because the individual is not aware of being exposed (e.g., exposure to phosgene).

Increased Mucus Production

SO_2 and other irritant gases cause an acute increase in mucus production (see also Chap. 2), which may help protect the mucosa and facilitate gas absorption. The longer-term response, which includes hypertrophy of mucous glands and multiplication of goblet cells, may have some protective value as well, but it also leads to airway obstruction and cough. Chronic bronchitis is usually defined as a more or less permanent condition of increased mucus production, associated with expectoration of sputum and cough (see p. 36).

Airway Constriction

In this section, airway constriction is defined as any condition that leads to obstructive lung function loss (see p. 210 and 305). Airways may be narrowed by tumors, traumatic lesions, or foreign bodies; these are not considered here. Increased mucus production is another cause of narrowing or even closure of airway segments. This contributes to obstructive function loss in chronic bronchitis. But lung function usually does not become normal when patients with long-standing bronchitis stop smoking and are treated, even though their hypersecretion then often subsides. Their remaining function loss is probably related to changes in the walls of the airways. These changes include inflammatory swelling of the airway mucosa, which contains hypertrophic mucous glands and an increased number of goblet cells (Chap. 2), and contraction of airway smooth muscle. Atropine often improves lung function in patients with chronic bronchitis,[8] suggesting that smooth muscle contraction explains part of their obstructive function loss. But atropine also decreases mucus production (Chap. 2). It is often suspected that bronchitic patients have emphysema (see below) as well. In such cases, loss of support of the airway walls because of lung tissue destruction may contribute to obstructive function loss.

Bronchial asthma is a clinical syndrome with "widespread narrowing of the bronchial airways, which changes its severity over short periods of time either spontaneously or under treatment and is not due to cardiovascular disease."[39] The principal symptoms of asthma are wheezing and shortness of breath. The severity of these symptoms depends on the degree of airway constriction. As in bronchitis, hypersecretion of mucus (which often plugs small airways) and mucosal swelling contribute to airway narrowing. However, airway smooth muscle contraction is probably often a major factor, more important than in chronic bronchitis. Figure 12-1 shows that in asthma, severe obstructive function loss can be reversed completely with adequate treatment.

Environmental inhalants are important in the causation of asthma. However, who develops asthma in response to specific inhalants depends on host factors, in particular on immune responses and on airway hyperresponsiveness.[11, 15, 156] The immune response is a reaction between an inhaled agent (allergen; e.g., substances in house dust or pollens) and antibodies (reagins), which are bound to the surface of mast cells. The allergen-reagin reaction leads to release of chemical mediators (histamine and others). These mediators contract airway smooth muscle, stimulate mucus secretion, and promote mucosal edema. However, the immune response can be demonstrated clearly only in some patients with asthma. Other patients with asthma develop symptoms and airway constriction after inhalation of smoke or dust, after physical exercise, or without apparent exposure to risk factors. The mechanisms of airway constriction in such patients are not all clear. However, the sensitivity of airway smooth muscle to a variety of stimuli appears to be increased in most patients with asthma regardless of the etiological factors that initiate airway constriction. Perhaps asthma in response to exogenous factors develops only in persons whose airways are more sensitive to these stimuli than airways of nonasthmatic persons. The causes of airway hyperresponsiveness are not known. Increased cholinergic stimulation, changes in cell surface receptors for neurotransmitters, or alterations in intracellular biochemical events are among the factors that may contribute to airway hyperresponsiveness in asthma.

Shortness of breath in asthma is a subjective sensation that cannot be quantitated. However, this sensation is associated with lung-function changes. Although it is difficult to relate descriptions of subjective sensations to results of objective measurements, there is usually a correlation between gross changes in lung function and gross changes in dyspnea and other symptoms (Fig. 12-1). In the clinical assessment of asthma, lung function tests are of value in (1) assessing the degree of airway obstruction (Chap. 9, p. 225) and impairment of gas exchange, (2) measuring airway responses to allergens and other etiological agents, (3) quantitating airway hyperresponsiveness, (4) determining the acute effects of bronchodilator treatment, and (5) evaluating the long-term treatment and course of the disease. In these applications, functional changes reflect merely the degree of airway obstruction and do not reveal its causes.

In bronchial asthma, airway constriction can often rapidly be reversed by drugs that relax airway smooth muscle (e.g., isoproterenol and other β-adrenergic stimulants). When airway constriction is not much improved by such drugs, one may deal with chronic airway obstruction owing to chronic bronchitis, emphysema, or occupational lung diseases (see p. 317; Fig. 12-2). Some patients with chronic airway obstruction respond favorably to anticholinergic drugs[8] (see

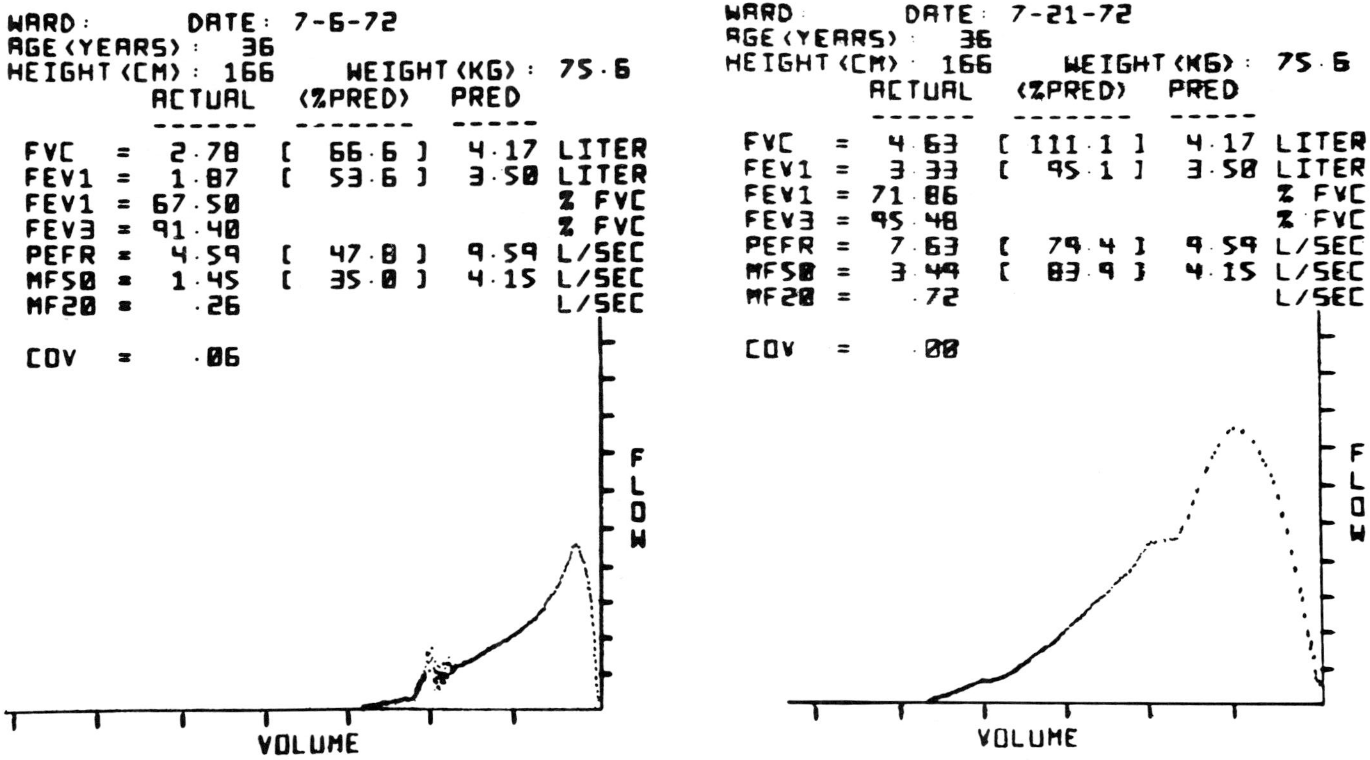

A B

Fig. 12-1. Pulmonary function test computer readout of a 36-year-old man with bronchial asthma (*A*) before and (*B*) after therapy with bronchodilator and corticosteroid drugs, which led to normalization of test results. On 7/6/72 (*A*) the patient had severe dyspnea and wheezing; on 7/21/72 (*B*) he was symptom-free. Each report contains numerical data and MEFV curve based on average expiratory flow rates during the two maximally forced expirations with the highest $FEV_{1.0}$, out of a series of 5 blows. PEFR = PEF; MF50 and MF25 = MEF50% and MEF25%; other abbreviations as in Table 9-1. See Chapter 9, p. 213 for description of test system.

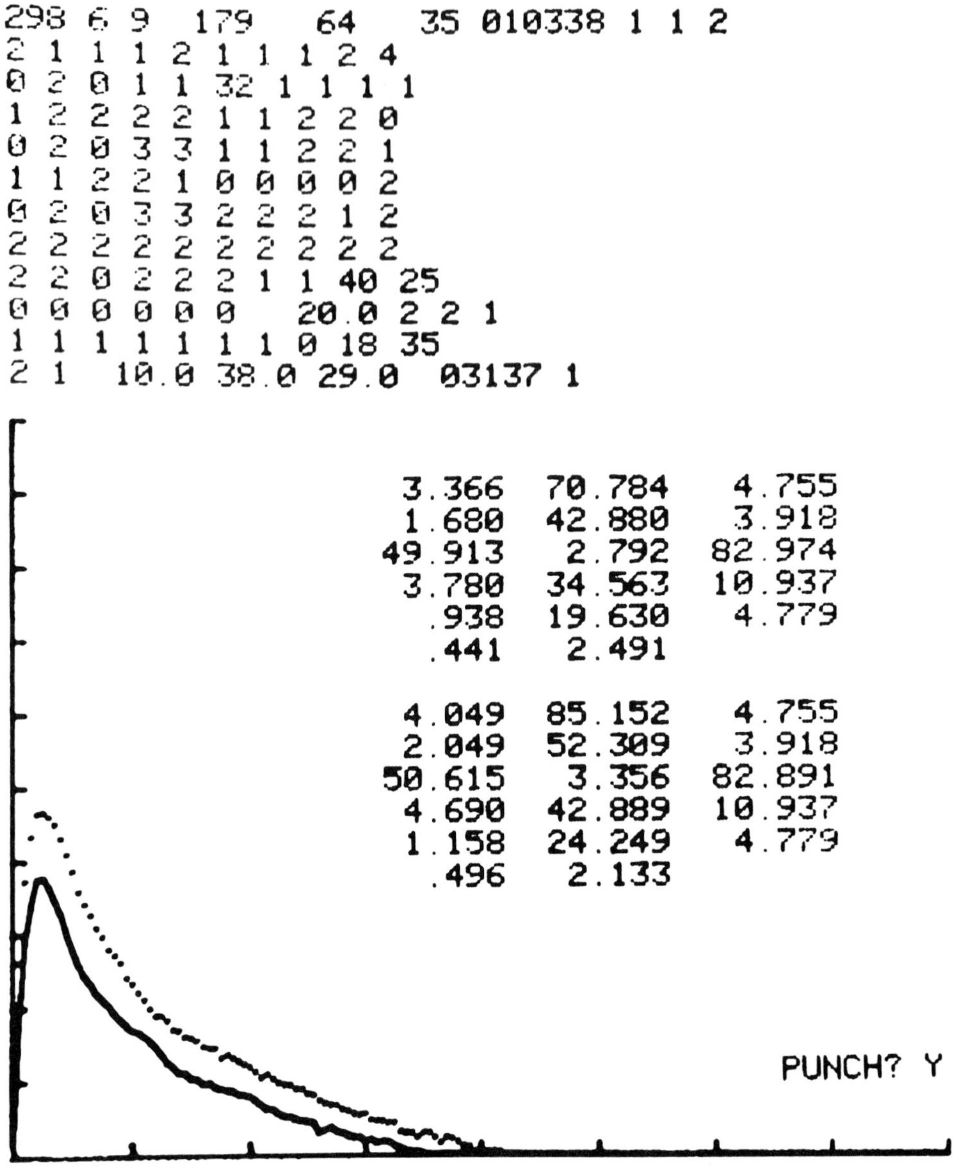

Fig. 12-2. Data output from computer test system (Chap. 9 p. 213) in a cotton cardroom worker, with MEFV curves before (*drawn line*) and after (*dashed line*) isoproterenol inhalation superimposed. Data in left upper corner are identification and questionnaire data. Data at right are numerical function values before (*top block*) and after (*lower block*) isoproterenol inhalation. Values in each block (from above down) are FVC, $FEV_{1.0}$, $FEV_{1.0}$/FVC ratio, PEF, MEF50%, and MEF25%. *Left column:* test data; *right column:* predicted values: *middle column:* test data as a percentage of predicted values. The improvement of function is considerably less than that seen in Fig. 12-1; note, however, that the result shown here occurred after only a single administration of a drug.

also Fig. 12-6). Hence, some forms of chronic airway obstruction may be amenable to drug treatment. Unfortunately, it is difficult to correlate changes in lung function during life in such patients with changes in pathological tissue responses in the airways. By analogy with their action in animals, anticholinergic drugs are believed to reduce airway constriction by reducing secretion of mucus and by relaxation of airway smooth muscle. Why one smooth muscle relaxant (isoproterenol) is sometimes inactive while others (atropine, thiazinamium, p. 318) improve function is not clear.

Other conditions. Airway constriction occurs in conditions other than those usually labeled as chronic bronchitis or asthma by clinicians. Many chemicals and dusts are able to narrow airways when inhaled in sufficient amounts by healthy persons. Cigarette smoke (p. 310) is the most common of these inhalants. Sulfur dioxide (p. 319), inert dust,[55] isocyanates,[143] enzyme detergents,[134] and hairsprays [187] are just a few others. Exposure to these substances causes obstructive function loss in healthy persons. The obstruction is reversible after short-lasting exposures. If prolonged, such exposures may contribute to chronic airway obstruction. That they do is suspected for many, likely for some, but well established only for cigarette smoke.

Immune Responses [71]

The reaginic antibody response (see p. 296) is perhaps the best understood mechanism of increased sensitivity to environmental agents. This response initiates asthma in many persons who are sensitive to pollens, house dust, or animal hair, or in those who become sensitized to occupational antigens contained in flour (baker's asthma), castor oil,[45] and other substances. The distinction between responses to these sensitizing agents, on the one hand, and responses to agents with direct toxic effects is not always clear. In general, the latter affect a larger proportion of those exposed; to determine this proportion one must study the population at risk rather than only individuals who may have been sensitized (see epidemiology, p. 306). Some occupational inhalants (platinum salts, textile dusts [p. 317]) release histamine (and perhaps other mediators as well) from nonsensitized lung tissue in vitro. For these agents, a direct toxic action on mast cells is the most likely explanation of the asthma-like symptoms they induce. If some individuals respond to exposure and others do not, this does not necessarily mean that the responders have been sensitized by an immunological process—the response to all toxic agents shows individual variability. For instance, the histamine dose needed to produce a given degree of airway constriction in guinea pigs varies about 100-fold between the most and the least sensitive animals.[53] Fortunately, immunologists have developed specific and sensitive methods to detect reagins in serum.[1] These can often provide positive evidence for a reagin-mediated response.

Immune responses different from the allergic (reaginic) response occur in a group of occupational lung diseases caused by inhalation of organic dusts, e.g., of moldy hay (farmer's lung) or of pigeon droppings (pigeon breeder's lung). These dusts contain antigenic material (e.g., from spores of fungi) that induces precipitating antibodies in the serum of exposed persons. After a period of sensitization, further exposure leads to lung disease (hypersensitivity pneumonitis) in some 10 percent of those at risk. At first there is dyspnea, fever, cough, and diffuse infiltration on the chest x-ray film (acute stage). In this stage there is an accumulation of cells (mainly leukocytes) in the alveoli and alveolar walls. Later, a chronic stage with granulomas and fibrosis (see below) develops. Lung function loss is usually restrictive (p. 305); the diffusion capacity is often decreased and there may be arterial hypoxemia. Recent studies have shown that the development of serum antibodies to the organic antigen is not sufficient to cause the disease. An additional cellular mechanism (activation of thymus-derived lymphocytes [T-cells]) may be required to produce hypersensitivity pneumonitis.[67, 123]

Lung Edema [166]

Several toxic gases (e.g., phosgene, chlorine, ozone) damage the epithelium of alveoli and terminal airways, with transudation of fluid into alveolar spaces as a consequence. Severe arterial hypoxemia results because of limited gas diffusion (Chap. 6) and a decrease of $\dot{V}_A/\dot{Q}$ ratios in large parts of the lungs (Chap. 5).

Emphysema

Emphysema is a condition marked by destruction of alveolar septae, confluence of alveoli, formation of large blebs or bullae, loss of alveolar surface area, and loss of lung elastic recoil. Two main forms are distinguished—*centrilobular* and *panacinar* emphysema. In centrilobular emphysema, the terminal airways in the center of a lobule are mainly affected and the more peripheral alveoli may be relatively intact, whereas in panacinar emphysema, alveolar units are involved. Mechanical factors influence the distribution of emphysematous lesions throughout the lungs, and there is a predilection for the lung tops (see p. 64). In recent years the ability of certain proteolytic enzymes (papain) to cause a similar pathological entity in the lungs of animals has received much attention.[76] The histological end-result of treatment of rats with papain, intratracheally or by aerosol, is very similar to human emphysema (see p. 167).

Also in recent years, a genetically determined enzyme deficiency in man has been detected, which is associated with early development of emphysema at least in homozygotic individuals.[102, 173] In this condition, there is a lack of an enzyme that inhibits the proteolytic action of trypsin (α_1-antitrypsin deficiency). How this enzyme deficiency leads to destruction of lung tissue remains a matter for speculation. It may be that shortage of factors that inhibit endogenous proteolytic enzymes can lead to breakdown of lung tissue and formation of emphysematous lesions. This hypothesis has many interesting angles—for instance, why is only lung tissue destroyed when there is a general shortage of the antitryptic enzyme?

Homozygous α_1-antitrypsin deficiency (see also Chap. 7, p. 167) is rare and accounts for at most 1 to 2 percent of all cases of emphysema. Even in these, the role of environmental factors cannot be neglected: most of these patients are also cigarette smokers. Adequate population data on the distribution of the defect are not yet available, but in any case, the majority of emphysema cases must be caused (1) by other agents or processes, or (2) by other as yet unidentified enzyme deficiencies that may also unleash proteolytic enzymes. Both hypotheses may be correct. Emphysema may well result from different disease processes, even though histological appearances at the end stage are the same.

An action of proteolytic enzymes is suspected in laundry detergent workers who have decreased elastic recoil after prolonged exposure.[119] Older textile workers with decreased ventilatory capacities have decreased elastic recoil pressures.[79] Loss of lung elastic recoil is characteristic of emphysema, but it can be recognized during life only when it is severe (Chap. 7, p. 167). Thus, emphysema in man is usually diagnosed only in its advanced stages, and the natural history of this important cause of premature death in man remains quite ill understood. In most instances, it is associated with cigarette smoking, but how smoke induces emphysema is not known.

Alveolar Cell Injury

Damage to alveolar epithelium leads to lung edema (see above) and to cellular responses that vary according to the toxic agent. High partial pressures of oxygen inactivate enzymes and can cause peroxidation of lipids; this results in cell damage. Rats exposed to 100 percent O_2 at 1 atm become cyanotic and die within 72 hours.[180] Edema, destruction of vascular endothelium, and damage to alveolar epithelium already occurred at 48 hours. Monkeys survive the same exposure longer, and a repair response can be observed in these animals. The damaged alveolar epithelium (type I cells) is replaced by type II alveolar cells, which form a cuboidal epithelial layer.[180] Apparently, type II cells with their many organelles have a much better repair capacity than type I cells, which lack these.

In paraquat poisoning, the lungs become infiltrated with macrophage cells.[68] This response also occurs with other irritant gases (phosgene, chlorine, SO_2, NO_2, O_3, croton aldehyde). The pathology of tissue proliferation in the alveoli appears qualitatively rather similar, at least in animal experiments.[77] Activation and accumulation of macrophage cells is probably a first step in many responses to foreign matter or to cell injury. In subsequent stages, granulomatous infiltrates are formed, frequently with giant cells.

Granuloma Formation and Fibrosis

In several mineral dust–induced diseases (pneumoconiosis), granulomatous and fibrous tissues are formed in the lungs. In beryllium disease, the granulomatous response predominates and fibrosis is secondary. With silica and asbestos, the initial response is an accumulation of various cells in the interstitial tissue; this is soon followed by formation of collagen and fibrous tissue. First, fine reticular fibers are formed, and later, coarse collagen fiber bundles appear. With hard metals (tungsten, cadmium) an initial inflammatory response is followed by fibrosis. Fibrosis also occurs in certain diseases—e.g., farmer's lung—caused by biological materials. Thus, fibrosis, like emphysema, is an end-stage response that may result from a variety of initial tissue responses.

In silicosis, fibrous tissue is formed in nodules; in asbestosis, fibrosis is a more diffuse process (Fig. 12-3). Perhaps long asbestos fibers elicit a more widespread response than the smaller silica particles. The original deposition pattern may also be important. Many asbestos fibers, especially curled chrysotile,

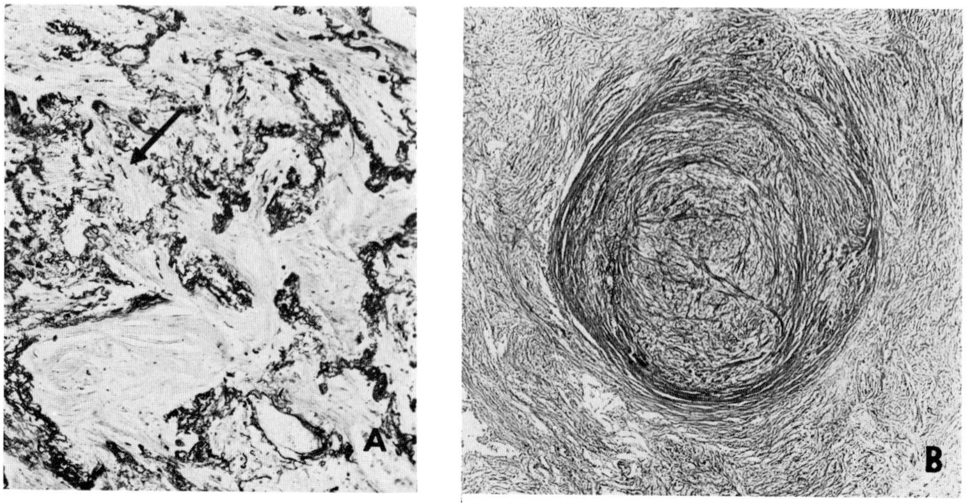

Fig. 12-3. *A*. Asbestosis (× 140). Generalized fibrosis and obliteration of alveolar spaces, with intact alveolar elastic network. Arrow indicates an asbestos particle. Modified Sheridan's stain and hematoxylin. *B*. Silicotic nodule (× 40). Note concentric arrangement of collagen fibers. Foot's reticulin stain. From reference 163, with permission from the author and Pergamon Press, Ltd (copyright 1968).

may be intercepted in small airways, whereas quartz dust particles are more likely to settle mainly in alveoli and alveolar ducts. The prevalence of siliceous rocks in many mines has made it difficult to discern fibrogenetic properties of other substances such as coal. Cases of pure carbon exposure [107] have made it clear, however, that carbon can cause fibrosis in the absence of free silica.

Silicosis and asbestosis cause restrictive lung function loss (p. 305; Fig. 9-6). However, the effects of smoking in many workers at risk may lead to airway obstruction as well. In the initial stages of pneumoconiosis, lung function loss often reflects smoking rather than industrial dust exposure. Obstructive lung function loss is particularly common among coal miners (coal workers' pneumoconiosis [CWP] [159]) who inhale not only dust containing carbon and often silica, but also gases that may promote airway obstruction.

Cancer [81]

The prevalence of lung cancer, especially bronchial carcinoma that originates in the bronchial epithelium, has greatly increased in recent decennia. To a large extent the increased prevalence is due to cigarette smoke, the most common inhaled carcinogen. Cigarette smoke contains several substances with known or suspected carcinogenic potential: aromatic hydrocarbons, phenols, radioactive isotopes, and nitrosamines. The presence of these agents in cigarette smoke convincingly supports the extensive epidemiological evidence that links smoking with lung cancer in man. However, most attempts to induce human-type bronchial carcinoma in animals by exposure to cigarette smoke have been unsuccessful. Long-term exposure (daily for more than 2 years) of beagles yielded invasive bronchial carcinomas in 2 out of 89 animals.[10] This low yield might be related to the use of a single carcinogen. There is evidence that additional exposure to other substances (co-carcinogens) may increase the likelihood of cancer. For instance, neither low-level SO_2 exposure nor intermittent exposure to low concentrations of benzo[a]pyrene was sufficient to induce lung cancer in mice; the combination of the two exposures resulted in a high incidence of lung cancer.[100] Interaction between carcinogenic substances also occurs in man: lung cancer in asbestos workers nearly always occurs in those who also smoke cigarettes.[157]

Detailed studies of occupational groups have detected several other agents that can cause lung cancer in man: coal tar (which contains 3,4-benzo[a]pyrene, a potent carcinogen),[52] uranium,[178] iron ore (hematite),[33] chloromethyl methylether (CMME, an ion-exchange resin),[66] nickel carbonyl, chrome ore and chromate, and arsenic (reviewed in ref. 50). Prevention of environmental exposures is the single most important step in reducing the incidence of lung cancer.

DETECTION AND DIAGNOSIS OF ENVIRONMENTAL LUNG DISEASE

The clinician is at a disadvantage in discerning the environmental causes of lung diseases. The patient in a hospital or clinic is often incapable of defining environmental hazards to which he may have been exposed. The only part of the environmental history that may be available to the clinician is the history of smoking habits. In the individual patient it is often impossible to weigh smoking against other exposures in terms of respective contributions to lung disease. To understand the environmental factors in lung disease, one needs to study not only the individual patient, but also others similarly exposed; in addition, one must study their environment in detail.

The main tools in detection and diagnosis are the patient's history and physical examination, chest x-ray film, and lung function tests. These methods are most effectively used in the context of epidemiological surveys. This section reviews each of these methods.

History and Physical Examination

A complete medical history—the key to diagnosing environmental lung diseases—should include details of the patient's smoking, occupation, hobbies, and residence. In population studies, standard questionnaires are essential to elicit this information and they are also of great help in clinical diagnosis. Questionnaires are designed to provide a complete record of respiratory symptoms, smoking habits, and occupational exposures as answers to carefully phrased written questions.[61] Questionnaires can be self-administered (e.g., mail surveys) or filled out by trained interviewers. In recent surveys, computer-prompted questionnaires with on-line recording of answers (stored in computer memory) proved timesaving and accurate.[25] Texts of questionnaires and instructions on their use are readily available.[15, 61, 89, 165]

Physical examination gives important clues in the diagnosis of disease in individuals. In studies of groups, however, physical examinations are usually neither practical nor necessary. More objective data on airway obstruction can be obtained from function tests, and data concerning parenchymal disease from x-ray films. Physical signs are mostly nonspecific, difficult to quantitate, and subject to errors in observation. For these reasons, physical examination is usually omitted in epidemiological studies. An exception is asbestosis, where auscultation for basal rales is important (p. 313).

Chest X-Ray Films

In mineral dust pneumoconiosis, either the dust deposit or the tissue responses it induces, or both, are radiopaque. Together with a history of exposure, the chest x-ray film is crucial for the diagnosis of these diseases.[69, 95] Unfortunately, the x-ray findings sometimes bear little relation to the patient's disability, loss of function, or the severity of symptoms. Miners with extensive lesions detected on x-ray examination may have few symptoms, whereas severely disabled miners may have no convincing roentgenographic signs. This problem arises in coal workers' pneumoconiosis as well as in silicosis. In these diseases, it is likely that disability is chiefly associated with bronchial lesions, which do not show on x-ray films. The roentgenogram remains an important tool in studies of mineral dust pneumoconiosis, but the almost exclusive reliance on this tool in the past has contributed to our present confusion concerning the functional implications of these diseases.

Chest x-ray films may detect lung cancer before symptoms appear. Unfortunately, the chances for survival of persons with asymptomatic lung cancer, detected by screening programs ("early detection"), are not clearly better than those of persons whose tumor is detected when they have developed symptoms. Whether addition of other methods (e.g., sputum cytology) to screening programs improves the results is not yet known. In any case, if screening by chest x-ray is to be done in lung cancer risk industries, it should probably be done twice rather than only once per year and should include a lateral film each time. Measures to prevent occupational carcinogen exposure should obviously be the prime means of prevention in lung cancer risk industries; in addition, workers must be urged to give up smoking.

Lung Function Tests

The physiological bases for function tests are discussed in Chapters 3 through 9. To detect disease, a sensitive test—not necessarily specific for some disease category—is needed; first, those who are normal must be distinguished from those who have some degree of disease. For diagnosis, the tests must also be specific for some functional abnormality that can be interpreted in terms of specific disease processes.

In epidemiological studies, the discriminating power of function tests is often better than in individual diagnosis. When judging function loss in a patient, one often compares the data to normal values, which can have a considerable range. In epidemiological studies, one can often compare groups at risk with control groups, and relatively small differences can then be both significant and meaningful. In longitudinal studies, each subject can serve as his own control, and this allows detection of small differences in function over a span of time.

Two main patterns of function loss occur in environmental lung disease. In silicosis and other fibrotic diseases there is *restrictive function loss.* The functional size of the lungs is decreased: total lung capacity, vital capacity, and residual volume are all reduced. The airways are not obstructed and elastic recoil may be increased because of the abundance of stiff fibrous tissue throughout the lungs. Hence, expiratory flow rates are often high, and the ratio of $FEV_{1.0}$ to VC may be close to 100 percent. The small volume combined with high flow rates results in a typical MEFV curve pattern (see Fig. 9-6, p. 210). *Obstructive function loss* occurs when small airways are partially occluded but air entry remains possible. Its effect is best seen during expiration—forced expiratory flow rates are reduced but vital capacity may be normal. Flow reduction is usually most severe at small lung volumes, since airway caliber decreases with lung volume. This results in another typical MEFV curve pattern, with a curvature opposite in direction from that in restrictive function loss (Fig. 9-6, p. 210). Obstructive function changes can be detected even in minor degrees with recordings of MEFV and PEFV curves (Chap. 9) and with methods to detect unequal degrees of gas distribution or increased airway-closing volume (Chap. 4).

Some other function tests have also been used in epidemiological studies. The single-breath diffusion capacity test (Chap. 6) is a suitable, noninvasive test of gas exchange for routine use in epidemiological studies of disease in which gas exchange may be limited in early stages (e.g., asbestosis).

Severe lung function loss limits a person's ability to do physical work and provides a basis for disability. Unfortunately, objective criteria for decreased work performance in lung disease are as yet unsatisfactory. Hyatt and associates [145] have shown that patients with obstructive lung disease have a limited exercise capacity because of their limitation in ventilatory capacity. A comparison of exercise ventilation with maximum ventilatory performance as described by the MEFV curve could be a practical test for objective disability evaluation (Fig. 12-4). Other indices of disability can be derived from measurements of diffusing capacity or arterial blood gases. For instance, if the diffusion capacity does not increase during exercise, this implies inability to increase gas exchange and thus provide for sufficient oxygen uptake to meet the requirements of the exercise. A low arterial oxygen tension implies deficient oxygenation of body tissues; this may be considered evidence of disability if it occurs during light work or at rest.

Other Methods

The identification and description of materials and organisms that damage the lungs may require help from organic chemists to identify natural products derived from plants, from mineralogists to identify mineral dusts and fibers, from botanists to identify vegetable matter, and from microbiologists to identify microbial material. For instance, identification of asbestos fibers or of silica in lung tissue proves exposure to these agents. However, when the source of exposure is known, identification of the material in the environment is easier and less traumatic to the patient than the performance of a lung biopsy. Although the biopsy may confirm exposure, it does not indicate the extent of lung disease. In fact, asbestos can be found in lungs of city dwellers who have no demonstrable lung disease.[101] For most environmental lung diseases, the epidemiological evidence that links exposure with increased risk of disease should carry far greater

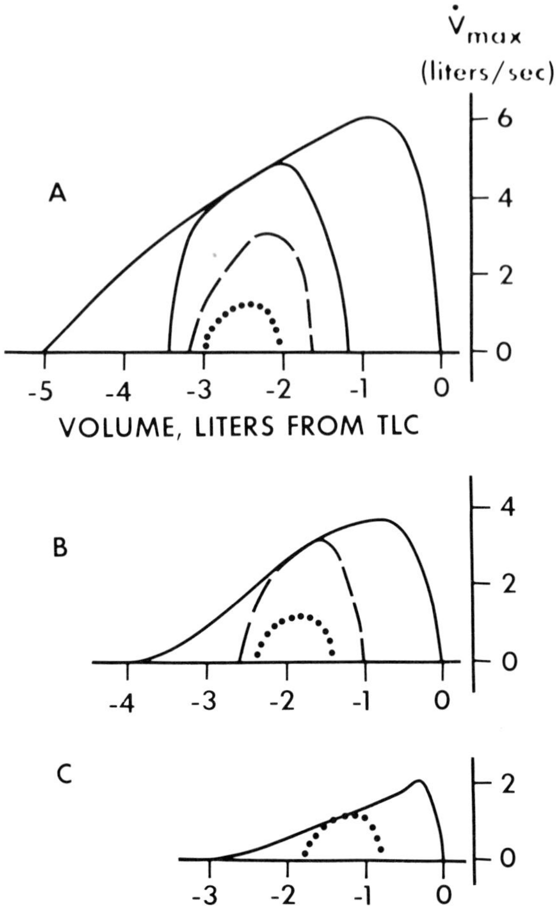

Fig. 12-4. Use of expiratory flow-volume curves to assess disabling loss of ventilatory function. *Dotted line:* tidal expiration (V_T) at rest; *dashed line:* V_T during moderate exercise; *solid line:* V_T during heavy exercise. All expiratory FV loops drawn in contour of MEFV curves in a healthy person (*A*) and in 2 patients with moderate (*B*) and severe (*C*) obstructive disease. Limits of expiratory flow are reached at rest in *C*, during moderate exercise in *B*, and during heavy work in *A*. Patient *C* is dyspneic at rest, and patient *B* during moderate exercise. From reference 18a. Used with permission of McGraw-Hill Book Co. (copyright 1974).

weight than the results of a single lung biopsy. However, in some cases, lung biopsy is essential for diagnosis.

Epidemiology [89, 112]

Potential hazards in the environment must be assessed from their effects on the health of people who live and work in that environment. When an inhaled agent is suspected of causing lung disease, one must determine who is exposed to it and if these people have lung disease. The disease may be limited to the exposed group, or it may also occur, much less frequently, in the general population. Starting from medical observations, one may ask if certain environmental exposures are common to groups of people with a specific lung disease, and, if so, how these exposures cause disease. Well-documented observations on a single case thus can provide invaluable clues, leading to the study of a group of people exposed to a common hazardous agent. The study of such population groups requires the tools of epidemiology, together with the medical and physiological methods discussed above.

The epidemiologist observes disease patterns among populations, deriving clues on etiology and natural history of diseases. By studying random groups of subjects, comparing cases with control subjects, and performing follow-up studies of defined groups of people with common characteristics (cohorts), the epidemiologist is frequently able to draw significant conclusions about a selected variable. Common epidemiological tools are discussed briefly in this section, with examples of their use in the study of environmental lung disease.

Mortality statistics often underestimate the importance of chronic diseases, since death is often ascribed to intercurrent or unrelated acute diseases.[121] Standard mortality data usually contain no information on smoking habits and occupation. Specially designed studies are usually needed to determine mortality and causes of death among people exposed to environmental risks. The increased risk of lung cancer among asbestos workers and the interaction between smoking and asbestos exposure were detected by identifying all members of a union of asbestos workers in 1942, tracing their fate into the 1960s, and determining the cause of death of those who died in the interval.[158] When members of such risk groups can be studied at the beginning of a follow-up study, factors that contribute to mortality can sometimes be determined. Thus, cigarette smoking, low $FEV_{1.0}$, the presence of chronic lung or heart disease, and occupational exposures were predictors of high mortality risks in follow-up studies of population groups over periods between 6 and 9 years.[32, 65, 86]

Morbidity data can be obtained from official sources (National Health Survey and Social Security Administration [138] in the United States), from registries of specific diseases (e.g., beryllium registry [147]), or by collection of data in population surveys. Registries can focus attention on diseases linked with specific environmental hazards. This information can help to define groups at risk, and population surveys of risk groups can then help to identify prevalence and incidence of the disease.

Cross-sectional surveys study a population at one point in time—defining the prevalence of disease (the proportion of those who are ill). *Longitudinal surveys* study a population at two or more points in time, defining prevalence as well as incidence (the number of those who become ill in a stated period of time). Cross-sectional surveys have shown the high prevalence of chronic bronchitis, chronic airway obstruction, and asthma in the general population, especially in risk groups of smokers and industrial workers. Many prevalence studies have unfortunately not been used as a base line for longitudinal surveys. Population mobility and other factors lead to high lapse rates in follow-up studies. But the initial data can help us to find out if those lost to follow-up differ from those who are seen later, e.g., in having more or less illness at the start. Laborious and time consuming as follow-up studies may be, there is little doubt that they offer the only feasible approach toward a better description of the course of chronic airway obstruction and several other lung diseases as a function of risk factors to which people may be exposed during their lifetime.

The choice of population and its size depends on the hypotheses one wishes to test. Relatively simple surveys using a standard questionnaire and a simple lung function test (usually the measurement of $FEV_{1.0}$) have given valuable information on the relative risks of smoking and occupational exposures in populations of workers in industry. A comparison of nonsmoking workers at risk and nonexposed but otherwise similar control subjects can answer the question whether those at risk have a different prevalence of respiratory symptoms or of lung function loss. Inclusion of smokers in the control and risk groups may indicate whether or not smoking and occupational exposure have additive or more than additive effects. Such studies have documented the hazards of exposure to, for example, textile dusts, coal dust, and isocyanates. However, occupational groups by definition exclude those disabled or diseased persons who retire prematurely from the work force; hence, a study group limited to active workers may reflect the occupational hazards inaccurately.[17]

Community population surveys can be used to study risk factors in the general population rather than in those in specific occupations. Selection and size of the population depend on the type and number of variables one wants to study. One can use geographical selection criteria (all inhabitants of a town or circumscribed area) or one can use groups with special age, social, or religious characteristics. Age, sex, race, and smoking habits must be taken into account in any population study. Hence, the study population must be large enough to obtain meaningful subgroups when the total population is divided according to these variables. For instance, in recent surveys of two communities in the United States about 4000 men, women, and children were studied.[120] One of the communities was in an urban, the other in a rural area. To find out whether urban or rural residence affected respiratory symptoms and lung function, we focused on those who (1) had never smoked, (2) had never worked more than 1 year in any of several occupations with known risks of lung disease (asbestos factory, mines, etc.), and (3) had always lived in either one of the two towns. There were about 400 white, nonsmoking, lifelong urban or rural resident women without significant occupational exposure, and about 160 men with the same characteristics. With smaller numbers of people in the survey, these relatively homogeneous subgroups might easily become too small for a meaningful comparison (see also p. 325).

The logistics of large-scale surveys impose many restrictions on the investigator. Physiologists tend to opt for collection of detailed data in smaller numbers of subjects; epidemiologists often favor simple methods that can be used on a larger scale. These conflicting desires can to some extent be reconciled by using computerized methods. A recently developed system [25] uses on-line data-recording methods to obtain questionnaire answers and maximum expiratory flow-volume curves; it has been used to study up to 120 people per day in community and industry surveys. Together with computer programs for data checking, tabulation, and statistical analysis, such systems may make relatively large-scale longitudinal studies on the natural history of obstructive lung disease feasible. Such studies require persistence and continued interest on the part of all concerned. There is a growing demand for medical surveillance of workers at risk in industry and for early detection of chronic bronchitis and emphysema. The benefit of such programs for better prevention and effective treatment is still a matter of dispute. However, if suitably designed, they can provide objective data on the progression of obstructive lung disease and on the risk factors involved at various stages. Perhaps such projects can eventually answer such questions as: (1) What determines which young smokers will eventually develop chronic bronchitis, loss of lung function, or both? (2) Are "early" indicators of function loss (e.g., low flow rates on MEFV curves; see p. 225) a reliable predictor of serious function loss later?

SPECIFIC EXPOSURES

Examples of common environmental exposures will be used to illustrate the material discussed in the preceding sections.

Cigarette Smoking

> Cigarette smoking is causally related to lung cancer in men; the magnitude of the effect of cigarette smoking far outweighs all other factors. The data for women, though less extensive, point in the same direction.
>
> The risk of developing lung cancer increases with duration of smoking and the number of cigarettes smoked per day, and is diminished by discontinuing smoking.
>
> For the bulk of the population of the United States, the importance of cigarette smoking as a cause of chronic bronchopulmonary disease is much greater than that of atmospheric pollution or occupational exposures.
>
> —1964 Report of the Advisory Committee to the Surgeon General of the Public Health Service, Smoking and Health [175]

Research during the past 12 years has considerably strengthened these conclusions from the 1964 Surgeon General's report. Cigarette smoking greatly increases the risk of lung cancer; it is also linked to many noncancerous respiratory and cardiovascular diseases. Even in population groups at risk of occupational exposures, the smoker may be at a disadvantage because of interactions between smoking and occupational exposures.

Mortality. One of the most impressive studies on smoking and mortality, conducted among 41,000 British physicians, showed a strong association between smoking and death from lung cancer, chronic bronchitis, and pulmonary tuberculosis.[51] Among male nonsmokers, the mortality from lung cancer was 7 deaths per 100,000 persons per year; among male smokers of 35 cigarettes per day, the comparable figure was 315 deaths per 100,000 persons. That is, if all 41,000 doctors had been nonsmokers, 34 would have died of lung cancer during the 12-year study period; if all had smoked 35 or more cigarettes per day, about 1550 would have died. Doll and Hill [51] estimated that cigarette smoking accounts for one-third of the total mortality of persons 45 to 64 years old in Great Britain of lung cancer, chronic bronchitis, and coronary thrombosis without hypertension are all attributed to smoking.

Although the excess mortality from lung cancer among smokers is now generally accepted, that from noncancerous lung and airway disease is more difficult to document. A recent study [9] has provided convincing evidence concerning the association of smoking with emphysema. These authors graded the amount of emphysema in whole-lung sections of large numbers of patients at autopsy. Few nonsmokers had anatomical lesions of emphysema, whereas smokers had a strikingly high prevalence of moderate and advanced lesions. Among continuous smokers, the degree of emphysema increased with age.

Morbidity. Studies on chronic lung disease morbidity in smokers have been reviewed elsewhere.[15] Most of these concern older men; some include women. Clear dose-response relationships (correlation between amount smoked and degree of symptoms or function loss) are not always obtained, but smokers as a group have consistently more symptoms and more airway obstruction than nonsmokers. The main factor that interferes in the dose-response relations is probably self-selection. Sensitive persons, who respond to smoking with cough and other symptoms, are not likely to become heavy smokers. In contrast, the acute response to cigarette smoking is minor in heavy smokers.[191] Industrial exposures [28] or preexisting disease (e.g., asthma) are also factors that affect smoking habits.

A clearer picture of the effects of smoking—in a population not affected by prolonged occupational exposures and other vicissitudes—can be gained from studies in young persons. Effects of smoking, in the sense of increased symptoms and decreased lung function, have been demonstrated among students in their early twenties [142] and even among high school students [155] (see Fig. 12-5 and its legend). These studies suggested that small airway obstruction often occurs after only a few years of cigarette smoking. This has recently been confirmed by histological evidence of changes in peripheral airways of young smokers.[137]

Lung function. Experimentally, smoking a cigarette causes an increase in airway resistance (Chap. 8),[129] a decrease in maximum expiratory flow rates,[191] an increase in carboxyhemoglobin content in blood,[149] and a reduction in clearance of inhaled particles from the airways in man.[141] Several of these effects also occur in long-term smokers and may be reversible during short-term abstinence (days or weeks). Delayed particle clearance in smokers is usually attributed to delayed mucociliary transport (Chap. 2).[109] However, others [37] have observed more rapid particle clearance during smoking in humans. Under suitable conditions, smoking might increase mucus production while leaving the ciliary beat unimpaired. This could increase particle transport rates. At higher dose levels, the ciliary beat may slow down or stop,[48] and transport rates would then decrease.

Smokers, even when asymptomatic, have prolonged nitrogen washout curves [38] and an increased airway closing volume.[104] Both findings suggest small-airway obstruction. Indirectly, arterial blood oxygen tensions provide added evidence. In smokers, arterial P_{O_2} may be normal in the sitting, but too low in the supine, position.[171] This decrease during the supine posture disappears after a few weeks' abstinence from smoking. Arterial P_{O_2} depends on ventilation-perfusion ratios in the lungs (Chap. 5). Arterial P_{O_2} probably decreased in smokers who were

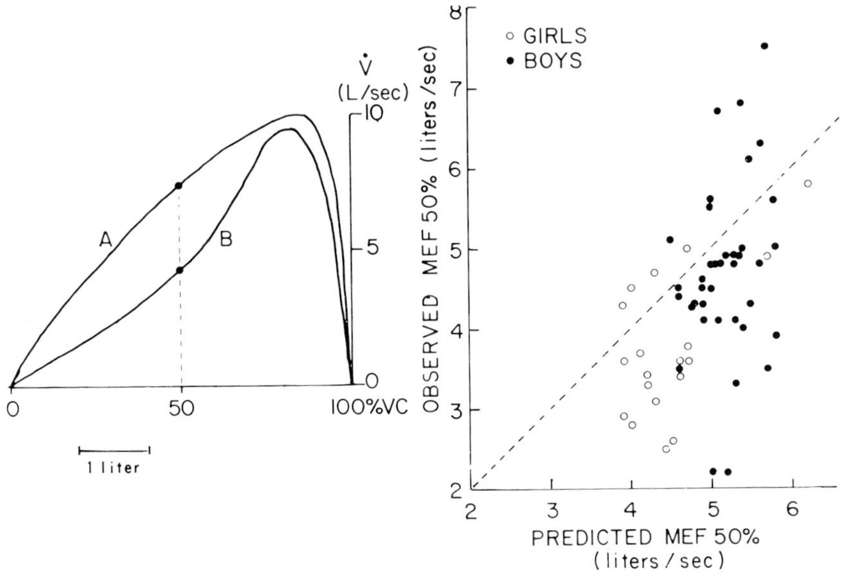

Fig. 12-5. *Left.* Maximum expiratory flow-volume curves in two 18-year-old boys. *A* is a nonsmoker who has no respiratory symptoms. *B* has smoked 16 cigarettes per day since he was 13 and has slight shortness of breath on exertion but no other respiratory symptoms. *Right.* Observed versus predicted values of MEF50% (Table 9-2) in boys smoking more than 15 cigarettes per day and in girls smoking more than 10 cigarettes per day. Line of equality (*dashed*) represents data of the average nonsmoker. Flow rates in smokers are significantly lower than predicted; the majority of points are below the line of equality. The regression equations used for the predicted values (from data in nonsmokers) are:

Boys: $\text{MEF50\%} = -5.75057 + [0.28215 \times \text{age (yrs)}] + [0.03755 \times \text{height(cm)}] - [0.00834 \times \text{weight (kg)}]$

Girls: $\text{MEF50\%} = -5.35737 + [0.20808 \times \text{age (yrs)}] + [0.02828 \times \text{height(cm)}] + [0.03036 \times \text{weight (kg)}]$

Modified from reference 155.

lying down because of increased nonuniformity of ventilation (Chap. 4), a phenomenon associated with partial obstruction of small airways. These findings, as well as the decreased flow rates on MEFV curves, all point to small-airway obstruction in smokers.

The *acute response to cigarette smoke* in man can be blocked by atropine and by isoproterenol.[110] It can be enhanced by propranolol, a β-adrenergic blocking drug.[191] Cigarette smoke contains water-soluble agents that cause airway constriction in guinea pigs.[78] The inhibitory action of atropine is consistent with the view that the acute airway constriction after smoking is due to a reflex, with its effector pathway in vagal nerve fibers.[129] But this assumption does not explain why propranolol can potentiate the acute effect of smoking. A hypothesis which explains the effects of atropine as well as those of propranolol assumes that cholinergic (vagal) stimuli sensitize airway smooth muscle to the action of constrictor agents, while opposing β-adrenergic stimuli (from adrenergic nerve endings and from circulating catecholamines) render this muscle less sensitive to constrictor stimuli (interaction theory[53, 191]). Immediate, short-lasting (minutes) effects of smoking might be of reflex origin; slowly developing and more persistent effects are better explained by an action of chemicals, perhaps involving release of chemical mediators (see p. 296). For a review of pharmacological agents in cigarette smoke, see ref. 176.

Other actions of cigarette smoke that may contribute to chronic lung disease include toxic changes in alveolar macrophage cells (p. 294), which indicate at least potential damage to lung defense mechanisms against bacterial infections. Components of cigarette smoke are able to induce activity of several enzyme systems. For instance, the microsomal enzyme that metabolizes benzo[a]pyrene, a powerful carcinogen in cigarette smoke, can be activated.[181] It is not yet clear whether enzyme induction in smokers is useful or dangerous—it might break a carcinogenic agent down to a nontoxic metabolite; it might also convert benzo[a]pyrene to the real carcinogen. It is conceivable that spontaneous or induced variations in benzo[a]pyrene-hydrolase activity levels may be related to the individual differences in sensitivity to the risk of lung cancer (see also p. 302).

Health effects of cigarette smoking have been widely publicized in recent years. Much effort has been spent, in smoking clinics and health education programs, to help people to stop smoking. In the United States, millions of adults have stopped smoking, and the social acceptability of smoking has declined. However, teen-age smoking has not decreased and may even be increasing.[176] Programs to reduce teen-age smoking should probably focus on 10- to 14-year-olds, or on even younger children; smoking habits are already more established in older children.[152] Demonstrations of acute health risks (decreased lung function, impaired athletic performance, accumulation of carboxyhemoglobin in blood) may have more impact than statistics on the likelihood of lung cancer 20 or more years later. Objective information on smoking and health should form the principal basis for programs to reduce smoking.

Occupational Exposures[140, 154]

Occupational lung diseases are caused by environmental exposures that occur during one's work. Thus, the circumstances of exposure rather than the nature of the inhalant or of its effects on the lungs determine whether a disease is included among the occupational lung diseases. For example, smokers (p. 321) and possibly city dwellers (p. 321) are exposed to potentially injurious levels of NO_2. However, only silage workers, welders, and others whose work leads to NO_2 exposures can, by definition, develop an occupational lung disease. Similarly, although many environmental inhalants, such as grass pollens, can induce asthma, only pollen exposure resulting from one's job, e.g., as a professional gardener, causes occupational asthma.

Risks of lung disease caused by dust produced during tool grinding, textile processing, coal mining, quarrying, and pottery making are as old as the activities themselves. Ramazzini[146] described these and many other occupational hazards in the early eighteenth century. But new materials and procedures discovered since then continue to increase the list of hazardous inhaled substances. Concentration of workers in factories and the faster production rates of the nineteenth and twentieth centuries have increased the amounts of inhalants as well as the number of people exposed for a substantial portion of their lives.

Two examples of occupational exposures causing lung disease are discussed in this section. One (asbestos exposure) leads to lung fibrosis and malignant tumors, the other (textile dust exposure) causes acute asthma-like disease and, later, chronic airway obstruction. For more complete reviews of occupational lung diseases, see refs. 15, 124, and 163.

Asbestos. Virtually indestructible, asbestos fibers (various forms of hydrated silicates) are widely used for their tensile strength and their thermal and electrical insulation properties. The fibers persist indefinitely when inhaled into the lungs. Three main health risks are associated with inhalation of asbestos fibers: asbestosis, lung cancer, and mesothelioma. Pleural plaques, the most frequent sign of asbestos exposure, are a benign process.

Asbestosis is a diffuse interstitial lung fibrosis (Fig. 12-3), usually a result of prolonged and heavy asbestos exposure. It is often accompanied by pleural plaques. In lung tissue, peculiar reaction products (asbestos bodies) form around asbestos fibers. These bodies, which often occur in the sputum of exposed persons, are coated asbestos fibers. Since the bodies contain iron and can also be induced by other fibers (e.g., fine glass fibers or ceramic aluminum silicate), some prefer the name ferruginous bodies rather than asbestos bodies.[49] Electron microscopic studies can distinguish asbestos fibers from these other fibers.[75, 144] Asbestos bodies in sputum indicate exposure, not necessarily disease. The diagnosis of asbestosis requires a history of exposure (usually more than 10 years in risk jobs) and certain clinical findings—bilateral rales over the lung bases; clubbing of the fingers; increased and irregular, linear, nodular markings evident on the chest x-ray film; and restrictive lung-function loss (Fig. 9-6). The diffusing capacity is usually decreased, and the patient complains of dyspnea on exertion. Obstructive lung disease is equally common among asbestos workers and control subjects;[127] the prevalence of bronchitic symptoms in asbestos workers is related to smoking and not to dust exposure, whereas dyspnea correlates with age and dust exposure and not with smoking.[114] Hence, cough is not a symptom of asbestosis, but dyspnea is.

Asbestosis, once established, progresses even after exposure is terminated. No treatment for asbestosis exists, and only supportive measures can be taken for the individual patient with asbestosis. Therefore, early detection of the disease is mainly important as a method of biological monitoring of the workroom atmosphere. The finding of asbestosis cases indicates the need for controlling workroom dust in order to protect those not yet affected. Sensitive methods are needed to detect early asbestosis in the interest of the total work force at risk. Basal rales may be among the earliest positive findings;[128] other early changes include decreases in vital capacity, single-breath diffusing capacity, or both,[128] even in persons with normal x-ray films. The arterial P_{O_2} may be low at rest or during exercise, with an increased A-a P_{O_2} difference (Chap. 5) in the presence of a normal FVC and TLC.[113] Lung compliance is usually reduced, and static recoil pressure at TLC may be increased.[97]

The functional findings in early asbestosis are consistent with the pathological finding of extensive fibrosis of the lung parenchyma, leading to increased lung stiffness and decreased gas exchange. Hence, it is important to diagnose early asbestosis even in the presence of a normal chest x-ray film, if the functional findings as well as the history support the diagnosis. In-plant surveys may detect few, if any, severe cases of asbestosis, since affected workers often retire because of disability. The prevalence of asbestosis varies with the degree and length of exposure and with the criteria used for diagnosis. In different surveys, the prevalence of chest x-ray changes varied from 26 to 90 percent in heavily exposed men working more than 30 years.[150] There is good evidence that asbestosis can be induced by long-term exposures to dust levels previously considered safe.[127]

As a cause of death among asbestos workers, *lung cancer* (see p. 302) is more important than asbestosis. Nonsmoking asbestos workers rarely get lung cancer; smoking workers are at much greater risk than other smokers.[14, 157] *Mesotheliomas,* rare and fatal tumors of the pleural and peritoneal cavities, are almost exclusively associated with asbestos exposure either in industry, in residential areas near asbestos factories, or in the neighborhood of other sources of asbestos dust. There is usually a 20- to 50-year interval between exposure and tumor development. The duration of exposure is often short or of low intensity.[115, 172] Mesothelioma is a tumor of old people; age at death in patients with mesothelioma differs little from that in the general population.[99]

In surveys of asbestos workers, the majority of lesions seen on x-ray films are pleural plaques, zones of pleural thickening, often calcified, which result from localized fibrosis. Not all plaques are caused by asbestos exposure,[148] but the association is strong enough for plaques to serve as a monitor for dust exposure. Their prevalence correlates with the extent and duration of dust exposure.[150] Their presence indicates that asbestos fibers have penetrated the pleural space.

Other effects of asbestos exposure include an excess of death from gastrointestinal cancer [148] and possibly an increased risk of cancer of the larynx.[167] The presence of asbestos fibers in drinking water of towns near sources of asbestos is of concern, as is asbestos air pollution in cities. City dwellers often have small numbers of asbestos bodies in their lungs.[160] However, there is at present no evidence that the general public in cities is exposed to increased risk of asbestos-related diseases.[148]

The mortality of heavily exposed asbestos workers over a 25-year period is about three times the expected rate, with lung cancer the major cause of death, asbestosis the second, and mesothelioma and gastrointestinal cancer accounting for additional excess mortality.[57, 58] A large proportion of such workers (about 40 percent) die of asbestos-related diseases. Early death from asbestosis may be less frequent now than in the past, since high exposure levels are less common.[73] Instead, asbestos workers die in increasing numbers from lung cancer and mesothelioma. The increased risks should be judged in relation to the lower prevalence of lung cancer and the virtual absence of mesothelioma in the general population. Thus, the overall excess mortality of asbestos workers, from all causes, is similar to the excess mortality among male smokers of 20 or more cigarettes per day.[72] "Confusion sometimes occurs between the proportion of individuals exposed who develop a disease and the excess risk of a particular disease in exposed individuals compared with the general public. The first may be relatively small and the second extremely high." [72] This statement concerning the absolute and relative risks of asbestos may be useful in counseling persons with light or moderate past asbestos exposure who are concerned about their future health.

In the United States, a Federal Standard for Asbestos [164] sets a limit to exposure levels (2 fibers/ml as of July 1, 1976) in industry and makes medical surveillance mandatory. A yearly examination, including a chest x-ray film and measurement of at least FVC and $FEV_{1.0}$, is prescribed. Whether this standard will lower future morbidity and mortality of asbestos-induced disease remains to be seen. Medical surveillance can do little to lower the risks for the individual worker: asbestosis progresses even if exposure ceases, and the risk of lung cancer depends largely on smoking habits. Nor is early detection of lung cancer or mesothelioma at present effective in improving survival. Hence the use of medical surveillance should be a biological monitor on the work environment. Detection of asbestos-induced disease should lead to improved dust control and other measures to prevent asbestos exposure. In addition, asbestos workers should be urged not to smoke.

Textile dust. Although recognized by Ramazzini and Morgagni in the eighteenth century, lung disease caused by textile (cotton, flax, soft hemp) dust exposure continues to be a risk to workers, in particular in the cotton textile industry. The clinical features of byssinosis, the most important syndrome associated with textile dust exposure, are summarized in Table 12-1.

The acute symptoms that develop on Mondays differ primarily in degree and in duration from the chronic symptoms. The former are reversible; the latter are not. Although the symptoms of byssinosis are clear-cut and not easily misinterpreted, the absence of characteristic anatomical changes visible in chest x-ray films has delayed the recognition of the disease as an occupational hazard. The clinical syndrome of byssinosis differs in many aspects from diseases caused by organic antigens, such as farmer's lung and occupational asthma. In byssinosis, chest x-ray films are not diagnostic and show, if anything, changes similar to those

Table 12-1
Main Features of Byssinosis

At risk:	Cotton, flax, and soft-hemp workers in carding, spinning, and other dusty operations.
Symptoms:	Chest tightness, shortness of breath, cough, and wheezing.
Symptoms appear:	*Initially**— on Mondays or other first workdays after absence from work;
	*Later**— also on Tuesdays and subsequent weekdays during work;
	*Eventually**—chronic shortness of breath and other respiratory symptoms, even in absence of dust exposure, and continuing after retirement from work.
Clinical grades [19, 153]:	½—occasional chest tightness or cough, or both, on first day of the working week;
	1—chest tightness on every first day of the working week;
	2—chest tightness on the first and other days of the working week;
	3—grade 2 symptoms accompanied by evidence of permanent incapacity from reduced ventilatory capacity.

* Initially = on starting employment in risk area; later = usually after more than 2–5 years' exposure to dust in a risk area; eventually = as a rule, after more than 10 years' exposure. Aggravation of symptoms on Monday continues, also in the later stages, if the worker remains at work in risk areas.

in patients with chronic bronchitis or emphysema.[153] However, objective evidence about the lung's response to dust exposure can be obtained with lung-function measurements. Byssinosis is a lung disease in which accurate function studies are essential for diagnosis.

Most data on byssinosis prevalence are based on responses to standard questions concerning chest tightness and dyspnea on Monday. These reflect the subjective experience of the workers and underestimate the prevalence of airway responses as measured with objective methods. Recent recommendations, therefore, emphasize the need to determine the worker's objective response to dust exposure.[19] Lung-function measurements should detect irreversible, long-term changes as well as acute effects of dust exposure. Airborne dust concentrations should be measured to quantitate the degree of dust exposure and to provide baseline data for control measures.

In the United States, 20 to 30 percent of cardroom workers have acute symptoms of byssinosis, even after less than 1 year employment.[31] These results agree with those in other countries and are probably representative for the industry as a whole. The risk is highest among people exposed to dust in initial processing stages and to dust of low-quality cotton; 70 percent or more of the workers in such groups may be affected. Pure cellulose fiber dust is nontoxic; hence, byssinosis is probably caused by contaminants in textile dust.

Forced expiratory volume decreases during dust exposure in cotton cardroom workers, more so on Mondays than on other weekdays.[116] Other tests, too, demonstrate that chest tightness on Monday in textile workers is associated with objective changes in lung function: nitrogen washout is prolonged,[7, 30] maximum expiratory flow rates decrease,[24, 29, 31, 177, 192] airway resistance increases,[116] and arterial P_{O_2} may decrease.[108] These changes are compatible with airway narrowing as the principal effect of acute dust exposure. The acute function changes are reversible after cessation of exposure and after inhalation of β-adrenergic stimulants (isoproterenol).[29] Although large and small airways may both be involved, small-airway narrowing correlates best with the degree of symptoms.[29]

The effects of textile dust exposure in industry can be reproduced in laboratory exposures of healthy humans to aerosols of aqueous cotton or hemp dust extracts. These exposures (of 10 minutes' duration) result in chest tightness and dyspnea,[23] prolongation of N_2-washout,[23] decreases in flow rates on flow-volume curves,[21, 188, 189] and decreases of dynamic compliance.[26] Hence, cotton and hemp dust appear to contain water-soluble agents that induce airway narrowing, probably of small airways, in healthy man. Their effect develops slowly (about 20 minutes after the end of aerosol inhalation) and may last several hours. A repeat exposure 24 hours after the first has no effect (tachyphylaxis).[23, 26] Healthy persons exposed for the first time react as severely as long-term workers.[16, 23] No special sensitization appears to be required; most people are sensitive to the dust action.

These experiments suggested that the actions of dust extract in healthy subjects, and the acute symptoms of byssinosis, might result from a nonantigenic histamine-releasing agent in the dust.[23] This could explain why most people are sensitive to the dust action, and the depletion and replenishment of histamine stores in lung tissue could explain the tachyphylaxis observed. In the worker with grade 1 byssinosis, exposure to dust on Monday would deplete the histamine stores, so that repeated exposure on Tuesday and subsequent workdays has less or no effect. Absence from exposure over a weekend would allow the histamine stores to be refilled, and dust exposure on Monday would again cause symptoms and lung-function changes. This hypothesis explains the acute effects of dust in the initial stages of byssinosis. In later stages, chronic changes in airways and lungs complicate the situation, and this may account for the more prolonged symptomatology in grade 2 byssinosis.

The histamine-release hypothesis is supported by the demonstration of histamine-releasing substances, acting on human lung tissue, in cotton-, flax-, and hemp-dust extracts.[22, 87, 135] The agent in cotton dust is derived from bracts, leaves surrounding the stem of the cotton boll. Aqueous extracts of bracts release histamine from human lungs; similar extracts of other parts of the plant do not. The release of histamine can be demonstrated in most human lung samples; sensitization procedures are not required. Thus, the histamine-releasing agent(s) in textile dusts may act directly on target cells—probably mast cells—in airway and lung tissue. The chemical nature of the agent or agents has not been established. There is no convincing evidence that antigen-antibody reactions play a role in byssinosis.

Early studies on byssinosis suggested that textile workers had more chronic lung disease than people not exposed to dust [153]—in addition to having acute distress on Mondays. Studies in communities in Spain and the United States have shown that cotton and hemp workers often retire prematurely because of disabling chronic airway obstruction.[17, 20] Hence, studies of workers active in the industry underestimate the prevalence of disabling disease. Community populations in textile industry areas include retired as well as active workers. In a Spanish town where soft-hemp (*Cannabis sativa*) fiber processing used to be the principal trade, chronic cough, dyspnea, and obstructive lung function loss were highly prevalent among older hemp workers (age 50 to 69 years), compared to control subjects in other industries nearby.[17] About one-third of the older hemp workers had disabling shortness of breath; about 20 percent of them had an $FEV_{1.0}$ less than 1 liter. Over a 7-year follow-up period, many men with disabling disease died. Among the survivors, including younger men with at least 20 years' dust exposure, $FEV_{1.0}$ decreased at a significantly faster rate than among control subjects. The incidence of chronic cough and phlegm, and of dyspnea, was also significantly higher among surviving hemp workers than among controls.[32] The survivors no longer worked with hemp during the 7-year follow-up period. Deterioration of lung function in hemp workers (in the absence of acute effects of dust exposure) begins before the age of 45 and continues even if further exposure to dust ceases.

The only community-based study of active and retired cotton textile workers, performed in the United States,[18] showed an increased prevalence of chronic respiratory symptoms and dyspnea and lower lung function among cotton workers in comparison with controls, taking into account age, sex, and smoking habits. Disabling lung function loss was less common in the U.S. population than among the Spanish hemp workers. However, the total population at risk is large, and hence the number of disabled persons is probably large in spite of a lower prevalence.

The pathological substrate for the chronic disease in textile workers is not clear, nor is its pathogenesis. The decreased maximum expiratory flow rates in older hemp workers are at least in part related to loss of lung elastic recoil.[79]

Thus, many of these workers may have parenchymal lung damage similar to that caused by emphysema (Chapter. 7, p. 167). Emphysema or chronic inflammation of the airways would be compatible with the function changes, which indicate airway obstruction not readily reversible by β-adrenergic drugs. Both emphysema and chronic bronchial lesions occur in the lungs of deceased cotton workers.[56] But since these are common lesions, a histological comparison of the lungs of nonsmoking, rural cotton workers and control subjects will be needed to define the pathological lesion induced by textile dusts per se. To some extent, the chronic disease, at least in hemp workers, may be more amenable to treatment than used to be thought. A drug with antihistaminic and anticholinergic properties (thiazinamium [Multergan®]) improved $FEV_{1.0}$ by 27 percent and FVC by 37 percent in disabled hemp workers who responded only minimally to isoproterenol.[27] Figure 12-6 shows that the drug more than offsets the gradual deterioration of $FEV_{1.0}$ over the years in these subjects.

Until adequate control of respirable dust levels becomes the rule in cotton mills, physicians will continue to see textile workers with chronic respiratory symptoms and lung function loss due at least in part to long-term exposure to respirable cotton dust. The main groups at risk are those in the opening, carding, spinning, and winding rooms in cotton mills. The diagnosis can be made from the history (Table 12-1), and confirmed by measuring the $FEV_{1.0}$, or by recording

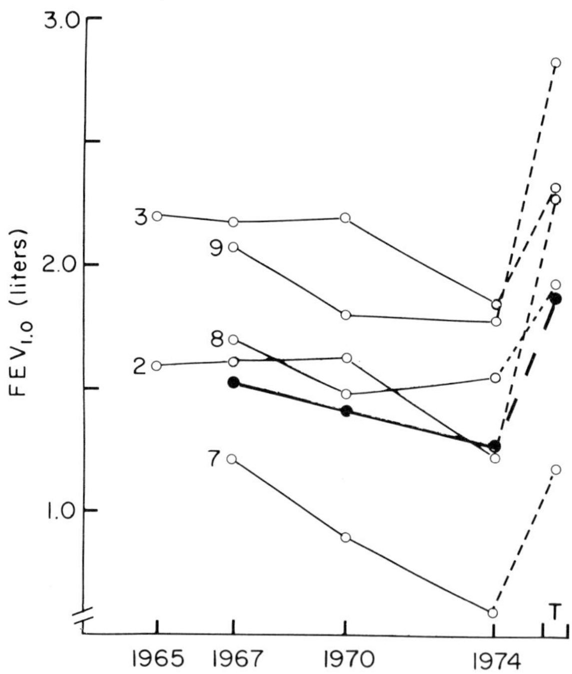

Fig. 12-6. $FEV_{1.0}$ data in retired hemp workers with chronic airway obstruction. Data on individual subjects indicated by numbers. Heavy drawn line = average values in 10 subjects seen in 1967, 1970, and 1974. Individual and average improvement of $FEV_{1.0}$ after a single dose of thiazinamium (T; 50 mg i.m.; Multergan®), from 1974 baseline levels, is shown by light and heavy dashed lines, respectively. From reference 27.

maximum expiratory flow-volume curves before and after exposure to dust during a work shift on Monday. Criteria that may assist in decisions, e.g., concerning a change to a non-dusty job, have been published.[19] Although elimination of respirable dust from the workrooms should be the prime goal of control programs, respirators and perhaps even drugs can be used to minimize acute effects of unavoidable textile dust exposure. Both disodium cromoglycate (DSCG, a drug that may act by preventing histamine release from mast cells) and ascorbic acid (vitamin C, which provides some protection against effects of histamine in man and in animals [190]) are able to prevent airway constriction induced by hemp dust extract inhalation in man.[188, 189] No trials with these drugs have been performed in the industry.

Air Pollution [169, 170, 184]

Atmospheric air often contains objectionable additives, called pollutants. Some of these can damage the airways and lungs. High death rates have occurred in the past during severe air pollution episodes (e.g., London, 1952). The health effects of more commonly occurring, lower levels of outdoor air pollution are less clear. Although these lower levels are often objectionable for many reasons, public policy in the United States bases control of air pollution largely on its health effects (primary air quality standards). Since there is no agreement on these health effects, disagreement about these standards is difficult to avoid.

Two main classes of pollution account for the majority of air-quality problems in our cities: (1) sulfur oxides and particulate pollution, and (2) photochemical smog. The former result mainly from burning coal and other types of fossil fuel containing sulfur. This type of pollution occurs in cities and industrialized areas, and it is often worst in cold and moist weather. Photochemical smog, on the other hand, results from complex chemical reactions in the atmosphere, with automobile exhaust gases as its main substrate, and requires sunlight to form its irritating components. Thus, it is worst in areas with heavy automobile traffic and a sunny climate. Carbon monoxide is an additional pollutant in areas with heavy traffic. The toxicological and epidemiological evidence concerning health effects of these forms of pollutant air masses, and of some of their constituent chemicals, will be reviewed briefly.

Sulfur oxides, mainly sulfur dioxide (SO_2) and sulfuric acid and its salts, cause chemical bronchitis when inhaled in high concentrations. In low concentrations (1 to 5 parts per million [ppm]), SO_2 decreases maximum expiratory flow rates in healthy humans.[162] Typical high levels of SO_2 in urban air are lower than that (up to 0.3 to 0.5 ppm). Although such low concentrations have no acute action on the airways in man, their long-term effects are not known. In guinea pigs, sulfuric acid and particulate sulfates cause more airway obstruction than equivalent amounts of SO_2.[6] The effect of SO_2 might thus be potentiated by formation of sulfates from SO_2 in liquid droplets in the atmosphere. However, sulfates may be relatively high in areas where atmospheric SO_2 levels are low.[91] Potential additional sources of sulfates (independent of SO_2 levels) are sea-water spray (suspected to contribute to sulfate levels in Connecticut [91]) and exhaust from automobiles equipped with catalytic converters.[161] The acute or long-term effects of sulfates on the human lung are poorly documented.

Particulates suspended in the air range from the potentially harmful to the relatively innocuous and include organic substances, pollens, viruses, metals, bacteria, and droplets. Measurements of total particulate matter in the air express in quantitative terms the dirtiness responsible for such physical effects of pollution as limitation of visibility and soiling of buildings. However, no clear relation between the air's total particulate matter and health effects is to be expected, since (1) only particles in a limited size range are inhaled and deposited in the respiratory tract (p. 293), and (2) the health effects of particles, once deposited, depend on their nature. Thus, persons with asthma develop symptoms in relatively clean air if it contains pollens to which they are sensitive, whereas dirty air may be innocuous to health if most of the suspended particles are inert.

The particle size distribution of aerosols in ambient air varies with the sources, the dispersion by air motion, and the time available for sedimentation of large particles. Thus, in relatively still air indoors, large particles settle out, and the remaining suspended matter consists chiefly of small particles (up to 91 percent ≤ 1 μm diameter [105]). Outdoors, particles ≤ 1 μm in diameter account for 50 to 75 percent of the total aerosol mass.[105] Such aerosols are deposited largely in small airways and alveoli. However, their effect depends on their nature, and the chemical composition of aerosols in ambient air is complex, including carbon compounds from auto exhaust, polymers from tire dust, and salts from sea water, soil dust, and fly ash.[70] To prevent disease, efforts to control particulate matter should focus on particles with specific damage effects (such as asbestos), rather than on the total particulate matter. Exposures near asbestos sources, for instance, may well be significant even when total particulate levels are low.

Carbon monoxide (CO)[103] is inhaled via the lungs and binds with Hb to form a blood pigment (COHb) that is inactive in oxygen transport (Chap. 6). Heavy exposures lead to rapid death because of tissue hypoxia at blood COHb levels of about 50 percent or more. Lesser exposures leading to blood COHb levels between 20 and 50 percent decrease tissue oxygenation, which affects physical and psychomotor performance. In community air pollution, even CO levels that lead to lower blood COHb levels (less than 20 percent) are of concern. Such exposures occur in heavy traffic and in tunnels. Although there is some evidence that low-level exposures interfere with performance in physiological and visual function tests, the effects of COHb levels less than 5 percent are controversial.[131]

Since the sidestream smoke of a single cigarette generates about 75 ml CO,[88] smoking is a major source of indoor CO exposure. Indoor exposure to CO also occurs during cooking on charcoal fires. CO exposure used to be common among cooks, hence the old French term *folie des cuisiniers* for the effects of CO on mental function. Outdoors, in heavy traffic areas, CO levels fluctuate during the day, with hourly averages of at most 25 mg/cu m (23 ppm) and short-lasting peaks of about 110 mg/cu m (102 ppm).[179] These levels may endanger persons who are at special risk because of lung or heart (especially coronary heart) disease.[74] For healthy persons, however, exposure to CO levels in heavy traffic is a negligible health risk. For the smoking driver, CO from cigarette smoke poses a greater risk than CO from car exhaust. Increased blood CO levels interfere with measurements of pulmonary diffusing capacity (see Chap. 6).

Ozone and other oxidants are formed when ultraviolet light acts on the mixture of hydrocarbons and nitrogen oxides emitted in automobile exhaust. Ozone, the main harmful component of oxidant smog, is a highly toxic gas. It affects the lungs when concentrations reach those prevailing, under adverse conditions, in ambient air of communities with photochemical smog. The effects of ozone [96] on the lungs are probably mediated via free oxygen radicals. Sulfur compounds (with SH or SS groups that bind free radicals) protect against O_3 toxicity in mice.[62] Free oxygen radicals may induce the formation of other compounds, e.g., lipid peroxides. Linoleic acid hydroperoxide impairs phagocytosis in rabbit alveolar macrophages;[98] ozone has a similar effect at low concentrations (0.25 ppm).[93, 94] In intact animals, ozone causes lung edema, but at concentrations higher than those that occur in photo-oxidant smog (1 to 3 ppm, 2 hours, in rats, mice, and guinea pigs [139]). In growing rats, 0.2 ppm O_3 (30 days) causes decreased lung elasticity, suggesting an effect of O_3 on lung collagen.[12] Acute toxic effects of low concentrations of ozone have also been well documented in man. They might be due to low-grade edema of lung parenchyma and airways, but the mechanisms are difficult to discern in intact humans. One to two hours' exposure to 0.6 to 0.8 ppm ozone increases airway resistance, reduces vital capacity and diffusing capacity, and decreases flow rates on MEFV curves.[13, 186] Significant decreases of $FEV_{1.0}$ and MEF50% (Chap. 9, p. 217) also occur after 2 hours at 0.37 ppm O_3.[84] These levels are in the range of O_3 levels observed in the Los Angeles area. The subjects in these experiments exercised during the exposure, increasing their ventilation rate and perhaps O_3 uptake as well. The effects seen may account for reports of respiratory distress during outdoor sports in photochemical smog episodes. Higher levels of ozone (1 to 3 ppm during 30 minutes or less) cause chest tightness, dyspnea, and cough, with a 20 percent drop in $FEV_{1.0}$ and a reduction of vital capacity and diffusing capacity.[80]

Ambient ozone exposures are not continuous; peak concentrations often occur around noon on days when climatic factors are favorable to photochemical smog formation. Thus, exposure is discontinuous, and year-round and 24-hour average values of ozone and oxidant levels are much lower than the peak values. If acute effects of peak ozone concentrations are to be avoided, they should be controlled to less than about 0.4 ppm. Research on lower-level exposures is still needed to establish a level that causes no detectable responses.

Nitrogen dioxide is an ingredient of photochemical smog and of cigarette smoke. The NO_2 concentrations inhaled by smokers may perhaps account for their increased prevalence of emphysema, which can be induced experimentally with NO_2 in rats. Most toxic effects of NO_2 in man and animals have been observed at concentrations several times higher than those observed in ambient air, which may reach up to about 0.25 ppm. A level of 15 ppm NO_2 suppresses the phagocytic activity of rabbit alveolar macrophage cells and renders the animals more sensitive to some virus infections.[2] This is related to failure of the cells to produce interferon when exposed to NO_2.[183] A concentration of 17 ppm NO_2 injures the alveolar epithelium, leads to loss of cilia in terminal bronchioles, and causes increased cell division in rat lung after 2 to 3 days' exposure. In 24 to 48 hours a repair process with cuboid cells, which are resistant to NO_2, begins. A lower concentration (2 ppm) caused similar changes, but these reversed to normal when exposure was terminated.[60, 168] In man, 5 to 8 ppm NO_2 in air increases airway resistance. This effect, which can be prevented with an antihistamine drug, may thus result from histamine release.[136] Histamine release may also explain the delayed action (maximal after 30 minutes) of NO_2 in other short-term exposures (2.5 ppm) in man.[3] For a more complete review of NO_2 toxicity see ref. 125.

Benzo[a]pyrene (p. 303) and other polycyclic hydrocarbons occur in urban air at low levels that are unlikely to contribute to the risk of lung cancer.[50] Other hydrocarbons in polluted air (e.g., aldehydes) may contribute to eye irritation in photochemical smog at levels that probably do not affect the lungs and airways. *Lead* in urban air—from car exhaust—has aroused much public concern. As a source of lead, uptake via the lungs appears to be minor compared to that from food.[44]

Toxicological studies in man and in animals show potential health risks, usually of single pollutants, but do not tell us if these risks actually occur among people living in polluted areas. Unfortunately, epidemiological studies have not yet given clear answers to that question either. Severe air pollution episodes have led to increased mortality, primarily of older people with preexisting lung or heart disease. But no clear effects of continuous lower level pollutant exposures on mortality have been established. For instance, in Los Angeles County, mortality rates among people aged 65 years and older were related to heat waves rather than to air pollution.[132] Epidemiological surveys on morbidity in relation to community air pollution have been reviewed elsewhere.[15] Repeated studies of adult men and women in Berlin, New Hampshire, showed higher ventilatory capacities and slightly lower disease prevalence in 1967 than in 1961, an improvement that might be related to a reduction in air pollution.[63, 64] Mailmen in London had a lower $FEV_{1.0}$ than rural U.K. mailmen with similar smoking habits; the difference was largest for heavy smokers and smallest in the nonsmokers.[90] Other British studies, in the 1960s, showed more lower respiratory tract infections [54] and more respiratory symptoms among children living in polluted zones than among those in clean areas.[111] However, lung function ($FEV_{1.0}$, FVC) did not differ between these groups. Four years later, air quality had improved and no differences in symptom or chest illness prevalence between the polluted and clean zones could be shown.[111] These and other studies suggest that the combination of SO_2 and particulate pollution in urban industrialized areas may contribute to respiratory disease. However, air pollution and social class are associated in Great Britain, and their separate effects on disease prevalence are not known.[43] Higher indoor pollutant levels in the homes of the poor (e.g., from kerosene heaters) might contribute to an increased prevalence of respiratory disease among those living in less affluent areas with more outdoor pollution. Indoor air pollution as a contributing cause of respiratory illness has not yet been studied carefully. Tobacco smoke,[35, 88, 151] nitrogen dioxide (e.g., from gas appliances), household and cosmetic aerosols,[187] car exhaust from attached garages, and particulates from open fires and candles are some of the sources of indoor pollution. Most of us spend the majority of our time indoors; further evaluation of indoor air pollution and its potential health effects, and of factors influencing the indoor environment (e.g., type of construction; air-conditioning and air-cleaning equipment) is clearly needed.[106, 118, 185]

In contrast to the relatively large number of epidemiological surveys on health effects of SO_2 and particulate pollution, few controlled studies on photochemical smog have been reported from areas where this type of pollution is prevalent. Thus, in spite of the demonstrated toxic properties of oxidants at levels close to those in ambient air under adverse conditions (p. 320), there is no convincing epidemiological evidence linking oxidant smog with increased prevalence or severity of respiratory disease. The lack of evidence may be largely because of the uncontrolled nature and the lack of objective methods in several surveys (reviewed in ref. 132). Nevertheless, a careful study in California of nonsmokers in an area with high oxidant levels (San Gabriel Valley) and in an area with lower oxidant levels (San Diego) showed no difference in lung function and in respiratory symptom prevalence.[42] In Los Angeles, peak flows were higher rather than lower among school children living in a high-oxidant area (up to 0.34 ppm).[117] On the other hand, studies of patients with obstructive lung disease have suggested some improvement in lung function during a stay in a controlled environment free of oxidant smog. Smoking, however, was an uncontrolled variable in most of these individuals.[132]

Interactions between pollutants have been mentioned for SO_2 and aerosols (p. 319). Recently, controlled studies [83] have shown that 2 hours' exposure to a mixture of low concentrations of SO_2 (0.37 ppm, which has no effect by itself) and of O_3 (0.37 ppm, which by itself has a slight effect on maximum expiratory flow rates [84]) caused a considerable drop in lung function ($FEV_{1.0}$: —22%; MEF50%: —46%) in healthy young nonsmokers who exercised during the experiment. This effect is of obvious practical interest since combined SO_2 and O_3 pollution occurs (although at somewhat lower levels) in industrialized areas with heavy traffic and sufficient sunlight for photochemical smog formation.

PREVENTION AND CONTROL

Environmental exposures contribute importantly to morbidity and mortality from lung diseases. Methods based on principles of respiratory physiology have provided much of the objective evidence for this statement. When it comes to prevention and control of environmental lung disease, their importance is less obvious. Cigarette smoking exceeds all other environmental exposures as a cause of premature disability and death—its prevention is largely a matter for individual decision (see p. 312). Occupational exposures need to be controlled by engineering methods: prevention of dust, gas, and fume emissions in workrooms, and removal of those that nevertheless get into workroom air. Physiological methods help to detect and quantitate respiratory health effects that may occur. However, medical surveillance of workers in risk occupations should not be used as a substitute for improvements in air quality in workrooms (see p. 315 and 319). In the study of health effects of air pollutants, sensitive lung function tests are important. Now that the widespread economic implications of outdoor air pollution control have become clear, an increasingly important question is: how much control is needed?

In comparison with smoking and occupational exposures, outdoor air pollution is probably a minor contributing cause to lung disease morbidity and mortality under most conditions. In the United States, national air quality standards have been set in order to protect the public health. These standards determine the levels of SO_2, particulates, NO_2, oxidants, carbon monoxide, and hydrocarbons that should not be exceeded in atmospheric air. Implementation of these standards [133] has led to far-reaching measures to limit pollutant emissions from mobile (automobiles) and stationary (industrial) sources. One result of these measures has been to decrease SO_2 levels by enforcing use of low-sulfur fuels for industrial use and home heating. In Connecticut and in South Carolina, SO_2 concentrations were frequently below detectable levels during the summers of 1973 and 1974.[92] Whether this degree of control of SO_2 levels is necessary to protect the public health is debatable. Control of suspended particulates in outdoor air has led to a considerable decrease of visible effects of pollution (e.g., soiling of buildings) in many cities, in particular London. It is likely that exposures to toxic components of particulates (e.g., gases adsorbed on particles) has decreased concomitantly. However, reduction in total particulates does not necessarily mean a reduction in exposure to particles with specific health effects (see p. 320).

Indirectly, reduction of particulates may, by increasing the penetration of sunlight to the lower atmosphere, increase ozone levels. Photo-oxidant smog is certainly no longer a problem peculiar to Los Angeles and its surroundings, if it ever was. Levels up to 0.12 ppm have been measured over London,[122] and up to 0.22 ppm in the New York area.[41] There are no reports of human health effects of such O_3 levels. However, 0.37 ppm O_3 caused significant lung function changes after 2 hours in healthy men (see p. 321). Ozone damage to plants has been observed in Britain (at 0.04 to 0.10 ppm peak O_3 levels)—ironically enough, to tobacco plants only.[122] Proponents of strict controls point out that the current primary air quality standard (AQS) in the United States (0.08 ppm for 1 hour) represents a safety factor of less than 5 (0.37/0.08)—a much smaller margin than adopted in other protection programs.[125] Also, concentrations less than 0.37 ppm might cause acute effects in unusually sensitive people, or in others if exposure is prolonged or repeated. On the other hand, peak concentrations of O_3 persist at most a few hours and occur only on days when conditions are favorable for photochemical smog formation. Obviously, there is a need for more data on effects of low-level O_3 exposures in humans.

Extensive monitoring of O_3 levels in the United States has recently shown that levels greater than 0.08 ppm (AQS) occur frequently in rural areas. We measured levels up to 0.09 ppm in Lebanon, Connecticut, a rural area with little traffic.[92] These levels occurred on days when the wind blew from the direction of New York. A recent report [41] documents in detail how O_3 is transported from the New York metropolitan area to points as far away as Massachusetts (about 300 km). An earlier study from England [46] suggested that O_3 might be transported over as much as 1000 km. It seems clear that local O_3 levels are to a considerable degree independent of local emissions.[36] Even upwind from New York, O_3 levels greater than 0.08 ppm occurred; [31] the same is true for a rural town (Winnsboro) in South Carolina, where 29 percent of all samples (taken in the four seasons) were higher than 0.06 ppm.[92] A decrease in primary emissions from automobiles (as during weekends) does not necessarily lower O_3 levels.[36] Clearly, enforcing the primary AQS for O_3 in the United States poses serious problems.

The ozone problem exemplifies the need for better data on health effects of air pollutants in general. A recent report for the Committee on Public Works of the U.S. Senate [4] concludes that although the data base for setting ambient air quality is unsatisfactory in several respects, recent evidence in general supports the standards that were set in 1971.[59] One may, however, wonder to what extent the prevalence of respiratory disease would decrease if these standards were fully implemented in our cities. In rural Lebanon, Connecticut, where SO_2 levels never exceeded the primary AQS and NO_2, O_3, and particulate levels rarely exceeded this standard,[92] there is nevertheless a substantial prevalence of respiratory symptoms and chest illness among nonsmoking lifetime rural residents (Table 12-2). A sensitive lung function index of airway obstruction (MEF50%; see Chap 9) showed no difference between these rural residents and nonsmoking, lifetime residents in an urban industrial area (Ansonia, Connecticut), where particulate and NO_2 levels more frequently exceeded these standards (Fig. 12-7). These results need to be interpreted with caution. Health effects obviously might occur in towns with pollutant levels higher than those in Ansonia, or short-lasting health effects not detected in our surveys might result from peak pollutant levels in Ansonia. Also, one may speculate whether the prevalence of respiratory symptoms might be lower, and lung function better, among residents of areas even less polluted than Lebanon, Connecticut, if such can be found. In any case, the results suggest that improvement of respiratory health as a result of decreased outdoor air pollution in industrialized urban areas will be difficult to document in epidemiological surveys.

The decision expressed in the Clean Air Act of 1970, i.e., to base air pollution control measures in the United States on anticipated health effects, was intended to protect the public, including persons highly sensitive to pollutants. It seems unlikely that this goal will be reached in the foreseeable future. There is no evidence that present pollutant levels in U.S. cities pose grave dangers to health. Nevertheless, risks may occur among certain at present ill-defined, high-risk groups, which

Table 12-2

Prevalence of Respiratory Symptoms and Illness Among Nonsmoking Lifetime Rural Residents (Lebanon, Connecticut)

	Age Group (yrs)							
	15–24		25–44		45–64		Total	
Symptom/Illness	M	F	M	F	M	F	M	F
n	62	88	39	86	27	63	128	237
% chronic cough (16)	5	2	3	1	7	6	5	3
% chronic phlegm (22)	3	1	5	2	4	0	4	1
% dyspnea (57–59)	2	8	0	10	4	19	2	12
% frequent chest illness (60, 3–5)	2	9	5	14	7	13	4	12
% bronchitis (71)	6	11	5	14	7	11	6	12
% pneumonia (72)	13	16	44	17	30	14	26	16
% frequent wheezing (34, 1–3)	10	6	3	0	0	8	5	4
% asthma (70)	8	2	8	2	4	0	7	2

Results from answers to standardized questions in all nonsmokers (persons who have never smoked cigarettes, pipes, or cigars, even occasionally), seen in a total community survey, who had always lived in a rural area. The percentages on each line refer to the number of positive answers to questions listed by their number in the questionnaire (see ref. 15 for text of questions and coding of answers). M = males; F = females.

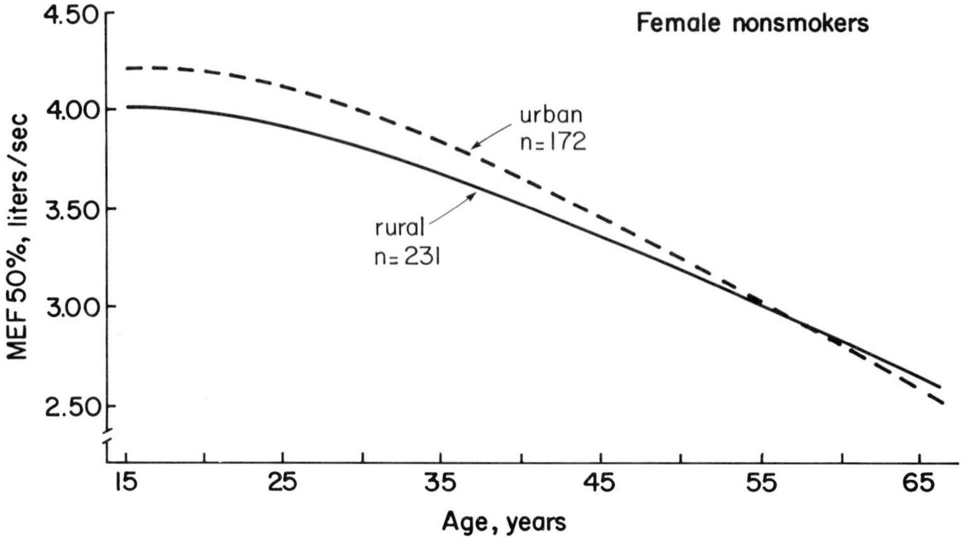

Fig. 12-7. MEF50% by age in lifelong urban or rural residents in Connecticut. The subjects are nonsmoking females with no significant occupational exposures. MEF50% was not significantly different in the two groups. The lines shown are for height equal to 160 cm and weight equal to 60 kg. The nonlinear regressions below are those that gave the best fit to the experimental data, among a series of linear and nonlinear regression equations tested.

Rural (Lebanon): $\ln \text{MEF50\%} = -3.1885 + 0.7846 \ln \text{ht} + 0.1539 \ln \text{wt} - 0.0001253\ \text{age}^2$.

Urban (Ansonia): $\ln \text{MEF50\%} = +0.8475 + 0.0177 \ln \text{ht} + 0.1341 \ln \text{wt} - 0.0001552\ \text{age}^2$.

(Unpublished material, Connecticut Lung Survey, Yale University Lung Research Center.)

may need additional protection (e.g., cessation of smoking, controlling of indoor environment). In the field of lung research, it would seem that identification of host factors that may determine individual sensitivity to environmental inhalants should be an important goal for the future. This will require intensive work on the cell biology, biochemistry, and pharmacology of the lung. Fortunately, these fields have developed rapidly in recent years. Classic respiratory physiology—the main topic of this book—provides the means to test concepts concerning responses of the airways and lungs, derived from studies at the subcellular, cellular, and tissue levels, in intact humans and animals.

REFERENCES

1. Aas K: The Biochemical and Immunological Basis of Bronchial Asthma. Springfield, Charles C Thomas, 1972
2. Acton JD, Myrvik QN: Nitrogen dioxide effects on alveolar macrophages. Arch Environ Health 24:48–52, 1972
3. Air Pollution Control Office: Air quality criteria for nitrogen oxides. Washington, D.C., Environmental Protection Agency, 1971
4. Air quality and automobile emission control. A report by the coordinating committee on air quality studies, National Academy of Sciences, National Academy of Engineering, vol 1, Summary Report; vol 2, Health Effects of

Air Pollutants. Serial No. 93-24. Washington, D.C., U.S. Govt Printing Office, 1974

5. Allison AC: Lysosomes and the toxicity of particulate pollutants. Arch Intern Med 128:131–139, 1971
6. Amdur MO: Aerosols formed by oxidation of sulfur dioxide. Arch Environ Health 23:459–468, 1971
7. Arnoldsson H, Bouhuys A, Lindell S-E: Byssinosis. Differential diagnosis from bronchial asthma and chronic bronchitis. Acta Med Scand 173:761–768, 1963
8. Astin TW: Reversibility of airways obstruction in chronic bronchitis. Clin Sci 42:725–733, 1972
9. Auerbach O, Hammond EC, Garfinkel L, Benante C: Relation of smoking and age to emphysema. Whole-lung section study. N Eng J Med 286: 853–857, 1972
10. Auerbach O, Hammond EC, Kirman D, Garfinkel L: Effects of cigarette smoking on dogs. II. Pulmonary neoplasms. Arch Environ Health 21:754–768, 1970
11. Austen KF, Lichtenstein LM (eds): Asthma: Physiology, Immunopharmacology, and Treatment. New York, Academic Press, 1973
12. Bartlett D Jr, Faulkner CS II, Cook K: Effect of chronic ozone exposure on lung elasticity in young rats. J Appl Physiol 37:92–96, 1974
13. Bates DV, Bell GM, Burnham CD, Hazucha M, Mantha J, Pengelly LD, Silverman F: Short-term effects of ozone on the lung. J Appl Physiol 32: 176–181, 1972
14. Berry G, Newhouse ML, Turok M: Combined effect of asbestos exposure and smoking on mortality from lung cancer in factory workers. Lancet 2: 476–479, 1972
15. Bouhuys A: Breathing: Physiology, Environment and Lung Disease, ed 1. New York, Grune and Stratton, 1974, pp 263–489
16. Bouhuys A, Barbero A, Lindell S-E, Roach SA, Schilling RSF: Byssinosis in hemp workers. Arch Environ Health 14:533–544, 1967
17. Bouhuys A, Barbero A, Schilling RSF, van de Woestijne KP: Chronic respiratory disease in hemp workers. Am J Med 46:526–537, 1969
18. Bouhuys A, Biris L, Mitchell CA, Ortega J, Schoenberg JB, Zuskin E: Disabling lung disease in textile workers. Am Rev Respir Dis 111:902 (abstract), 1975

18a. Bouhuys A, Gee JBL: Environmental lung disease, in Wintrobe MM, et al. (eds): Harrison's Principles of Internal Medicine, ed 7. New York, McGraw-Hill, 1974, pp 1310–1320

19. Bouhuys A, Gilson JC, Schilling RSF: Byssinosis in the textile industry; research, prevention and control. Arch Environ Health 21:475–478, 1970
20. Bouhuys A, Heaphy LJ Jr, Schilling RSF, Welborn JW: Byssinosis in the United States. N Engl J Med 277: 170–175, 1967
21. Bouhuys A, Hunt VR, Kim BM, Zapletal A: Maximum expiratory flow rates in induced bronchoconstriction in man. J Clin Invest 48:1159–1168, 1969
22. Bouhuys A, Lindell S-E: Release of histamine by cotton dust extracts from human lung tissue in vitro. Experientia 17:211–215, 1961
23. Bouhuys A, Lindell S-E, Lundin G: Experimental studies on byssinosis. Br Med J 1:324–326, 1960
24. Bouhuys A, Mitchell CA, Schilling RSF, Zuskin E: A physiological study of byssinosis in colonial America. Trans NY Acad Sci 35:537–546, 1973
25. Bouhuys A, Mitchell CA, Tuttle RW: On-line computer system for recording of respiratory questionnaires and MEFV curves. Biosci Commun 1: 219–236, 1975
26. Bouhuys A, Nicholls PJ: The effect of cotton dust on respiratory mechanics in man and in guinea pigs, in Davies CN (ed): Inhaled Particles and Vapours II. London, Pergamon, 1966, pp 75–84
27. Bouhuys A, Ortega J: Improvement of "irreversible" airway obstruction by thiazinamium (Multergan®). Pneumonologie 153:185–195, 1976
28. Bouhuys A, Schilling RSF, van de Woestijne KP: Cigarette smoking, occupational dust exposure and ventilatory capacity. Arch Environ Health 19:793–797, 1969
29. Bouhuys A, van de Woestijne KP: Respiratory mechanics and dust exposure in byssinosis. J Clin Invest 49: 106–118, 1970

30. Bouhuys A, van Duyn J, van Lennep HJ: Byssinosis in flax workers. Arch Environ Health 3:499–509, 1961
31. Bouhuys A, Wolfson RL, Horner DW, Brain JD, Zuskin E: Byssinosis in cotton textile workers. Respiratory survey of a mill with rapid labor turnover. Ann Intern Med 71:257–269, 1969
32. Bouhuys A, Zuskin E: Chronic respiratory disease in hemp workers: a follow-up study, 1967–1974. Ann Intern Med 84:398–405, 1976
33. Boyd JT, Doll R, Faulds JS, Leiper J: Cancer of the lung in iron ore (haematite) miners. Br J Ind Med 27: 97–105, 1970
34. Brain JD: The uptake of inhaled gases by the nose. Ann Otol Rhinol Laryngol 79:529–539, 1970
35. Bridge DP, Corn M: Contribution to the assessment of exposure of nonsmokers to air pollution from cigarette and cigar smoke in occupied spaces. Environ Res 5:192–209, 1972
36. Bruntz SM, Cleveland WS, Graedel TE, Kleiner B, Warner JL: Ozone concentrations in New Jersey and New York; statistical association with related variables. Science 186:257–259, 1974
37. Camner P, Philipson K, Arvidsson T: Cigarette smoking in man. Short-term effect on mucociliary transport. Arch Environ Health 23:421–426, 1971
38. Chiang ST, Wang BC: Acute effects of cigarette smoking on pulmonary function. Am Rev Respir Dis 101: 860–868, 1970
39. CIBA Guest Symposium: Terminology, definitions, and classification of chronic pulmonary emphysema and related conditions. Thorax 14:286–299, 1959
40. Clark JM, Lambertsen CJ: Pulmonary oxygen toxicity: A review. Pharmacol Rev 23:37–133, 1971
41. Cleveland WS, Kleiner B, McRae JE, Warner JL: Photochemical air pollution: transport from the New York City area into Connecticut and Massachusetts. Science 191:179–181, 1976
42. Cohen CA, Hudson AR, Clausen JL, Knelson JH: Respiratory symptoms, spirometry, and oxidant air pollution in nonsmoking adults. Am Rev Respir Dis 105:251–261, 1972
43. Colley JRT: Respiratory disease in childhood. Br Med Bull 27:9–14, 1971
44. Committee on Biologic Effects of Atmospheric Pollutants: Airborne lead in perspective. Washington, D.C., Division of Medical Sciences, National Research Council, National Academy of Sciences, 1971
45. Coombs RRA, Hunter A, Jonas WE, Bennich H, Johansson SGO, Panzani R: Detection of IgE (IgND) specific antibody (probably reagin) to castor-bean allergen by the red-cell-linked antigen-antiglobulin reaction. Lancet 1: 1115–1118, 1968
46. Cox RA, Eggleton AEJ, Derwent RG, Lovelock JE, Pack DH: Long-range transport of photochemical ozone in north-western Europe. Nature 255: 118–121, 1975
47. Crofton J, Douglas A: Respiratory Diseases. Philadelphia, FA Davis, 1969
48. Dalhamn T, Rylander R: Ciliastatic action of smoke from filter-tipped and non-tipped cigarettes. Nature 201: 401–402, 1963
49. Davis JMG, Gross P, DeTreville RTP: "Ferruginous Bodies" in guinea pigs. Arch Pathol 89:364–373, 1970
50. Doll R: Practical steps towards the prevention of bronchial carcinoma. Scott Med J 15:433–447, 1970
51. Doll R, Hill AB: Mortality in relation to smoking: Ten years' observations of British doctors. Br Med J 1:1399–1410 and 1460–1467, 1964
52. Doll R, Vessey MP, Beasley RWR, Buckley AR, Fear EC, Fisher REW, Gammon EJ, Gunn W, Hughes GO, Lee K, Norman-Smith B: Mortality of gasworkers—final report of a prospective study. Br J Ind Med 29:394–406, 1972
53. Douglas JS, Dennis MW, Ridgway P, Bouhuys A: Airway constriction in guinea pigs: interaction of histamine and autonomic drugs. J Pharmacol Exp Ther 184:169–179, 1973
54. Douglas JWB, Waller RE: Air pollution and respiratory infection in children. Br J Prev Soc Med 20:1–8, 1966
55. DuBois AB, Dautrebande L: Acute effects of breathing inert dust particles and of carbachol aerosol on the mechanical characteristics of the lungs in

man. Changes in response after inhaling sympathomimetic aerosols. J Clin Invest 37:1746–1755, 1958
56. Edwards C, Macartney J, Rooke G, Ward F: The pathology of the lung in byssinotics. Thorax 30:612–623, 1975
57. Elmes PC, Simpson MJC: Insulation workers in Belfast. 3. Mortality 1940–66. Br J Ind Med 28:226–236, 1971
58. Enterline P, de Coufle P, Henderson V: Respiratory cancer in relation to occupational exposures among retired asbestos workers. Br J Ind Med 30: 162–166, 1973
59. Environmental Protection Agency: National primary and secondary ambient air quality standards. Fed Regis 36:8186–8201, 1971
60. Evans MJ, Stephens RJ, Cabral LJ, Freeman G: Cell renewal in the lungs of rats exposed to low levels of NO_2. Arch Environ Health 24:180–188, 1972
61. Fairbairn AS, Wood CH, Fletcher CM: Variability in answers to a questionnaire on respiratory symptoms. Br J Prev Soc Med 13:175–193, 1959
62. Fairchild EJ, Murphy SD, Stokinger HE: Protection by sulfur compounds against the air pollutants ozone and nitrogen dioxide. Science 130:861–862, 1959
63. Ferris BG Jr, Higgins ITT, Higgins MW, Peters JM: Chronic nonspecific respiratory disease in Berlin, New Hampshire, 1961–1967: A follow-up study. Am Rev Respir Dis 107:110–122, 1973
64. Ferris BG Jr, Higgins ITT, Higgins MW, Peters JM, van Ganse WF, Goldman MD: Chronic nonspecific respiratory disease, Berlin, New Hampshire, 1961–1967: A cross-sectional study. Am Rev Respir Dis 104:232–244, 1971
65. Ferris BG Jr, Speizer FE, Worcester J, Chen HY: Adult mortality in Berlin, New Hampshire, from 1961–1967. Arch Environ Health 23:434–439, 1971
66. Figueroa WF, Raszkowski R, Weiss W: Lung cancer in chloromethyl methyl ether workers. N Engl J Med 288: 1096–1097, 1973
67. Fink JN, Moore UL, Barboriak JJ: Cell-mediated hypersensitivity in pigeon breeders. Int Arch Allergy Appl Immunol 49:831–836, 1975
68. Fletcher K, Wyatt I: The composition of lung lipids after poisoning with paraquat. Br J Exp Pathol 51:604–610, 1970
69. Fraser RG, Paré JAP: Diagnosis of Diseases of the Chest, vols I & II. Philadelphia, WB Saunders Co Inc, 1970
70. Friedlander SK: Chemical element balances and identification of air pollution sources. Environ Sci Tech 7:235–240, 1973
71. Gell PGH, Coombs RRA, Lachmann PJ: Clinical Aspects of Immunology, ed 3. Oxford, Blackwell Scientific Publications, 1975
72. Gilson JC: Health hazards of asbestos. Composites 3:57–59, 1972
73. Gilson JC: Problems and perspectives: The changing hazards of exposure to asbestos, in: Biological effects of asbestos. Ann NY Acad Sci 132:696–705, 1965
74. Goldsmith JR, Cohen SI: Epidemiological bases for possible air quality criteria for carbon monoxide. J Air Pollut Control Assoc 19:704–713, 1969
75. Gross P, deTreville RTP, Haller MN: Asbestos versus nonasbestos fibers. Arch Environ Health 20:571–578, 1970
76. Gross P, Pfitzer E, Tolker E, Babyak MA, Kaschak M: Experimental emphysema: its production with papain in normal and silicotic rats. Arch Environ Health 11:50–58, 1965
77. Gross P, Rinehart WE, deTreville RTP: The pulmonary reactions to toxic gases. Am Ind Hyg Assoc J 28:215–321, 1967
78. Guillerm R, Saindelle A, Faltot P, Hée J: Étude chez le Cobaye des effets bronchomoteurs de la fumée de cigarette et de quelques-uns de ses constituants. J Physiol (Paris) 57:619–620, 1965
79. Guyatt AR, Douglas JS, Zuskin E, Bouhuys A: Lung static recoil and airway obstruction in hemp workers with byssinosis. Am Rev Respir Dis 108:1111–1115, 1973
80. Hallett WY: Effect of ozone and cigarette smoke on lung function. Arch Environ Health 10:295–302, 1965
81. Hanna MG Jr, Nettesheim P, Gilbert JR (eds): Inhalation Carcinogenesis. US Atomic Energy Commission, Division of Technical Information, 1970
82. Hatch TF, Gross P: Pulmonary De-

position and Retention of Inhaled Aerosols. New York, Academic Press, 1964
83. Hazucha M, Bates DV: Combined effect of ozone and sulphur dioxide on human pulmonary function. Nature 257:50–51, 1975
84. Hazucha M, Silverman F, Parent C, Field S, Bates DV: Pulmonary function in man after short-term exposure to ozone. Arch Environ Health 27: 183–188, 1973
85. Henderson Y, Haggard HW: Noxious Gases and the Principles of Respiration Influencing Their Action. New York, Reinhold Publishing Corp, 1943
86. Higgins ITT, Gilson JC, Ferris BG Jr, Waters ME, Campbell H, Higgins MW: IV. Chronic respiratory disease in an industrial town: A nine-year follow-up study. Preliminary report. Am J Public Health 58:1667–1676, 1968
87. Hitchcock M, Piscitelli DM, Bouhuys A: Histamine release from human lung by a component of cotton bracts and by compound 48/80. Arch Environ Health 26:177–182, 1973
88. Hoegg UR: Cigarette smoke in closed spaces. Environ Health Perspect 2: 117–128, 1972
89. Holland WW (ed): Data Handling in Epidemiology. London, Oxford University Press, 1970
90. Holland WW, Reid DD: The urban factor in chronic bronchitis. Lancet 1: 445–448, 1965
91. Hosein HR, Mitchell CA, Bouhuys A: Daily variation in air quality. Arch Environ Health, in press
92. Hosein HR, Mitchell CA, Bouhuys A: Evaluation of outdoor air quality in rural and urban communities. Arch Environ Health, in press
93. Hurst DJ, Coffin DL: Ozone effect on lysosomal hydrolases of alveolar macrophages in vitro. Arch Intern Med 127: 1059–1063, 1971
94. Hurst DJ, Gardner DE, Coffin DL: Effect of ozone on acid hydrolases of the pulmonary alveolar macrophage. J Reticuloendothel Soc 8:288–301, 1970
95. Jacobson G, Bohlig H, Kiviluoto R: Essentials of chest radiography. Radiology 95:445–450, 1970
96. Jaffe LS: The biological effects of ozone on man and animals. Am Ind Hyg Assoc J 28:267–277, 1967
97. Jodoin G, Gibbs GW, Macklem PT, McDonald JC, Becklake MR: Early effects of asbestos exposure on lung function. Am Rev Respir Dis 104: 525–535, 1971
98. Khandwala A, Gee JBL: Linoleic acid hydroperoxide: Impaired bacterial uptake by alveolar macrophages, a mechanism of oxidant lung injury. Science 182:1364–1365, 1973
99. Knappmann J: Beobachtungen an 251 obduzierten Mesotheliom-Fällen in Hamburg (1958–1968). Pneumonologie 148:60–65, 1972
100. Kuschner M, Laskin S: Experimental models in environmental carcinogenesis. Am J Pathol 64:183–196, 1971
101. Langer AM, Selikoff IJ, Sastre A: Chrysotile asbestos in the lungs of persons in New York City. Arch Environ Health 22:348–361, 1971
102. Laurell CB, Eriksson S: The electrophoretic α_1-globulin pattern of serum in α_1-antitrypsin deficiency. Scand J Clin Lab Invest 15:132–140, 1963
103. Lawther PJ: Carbon monoxide. Br Med Bull 31:256–260, 1975
104. LeBlanc P, Ruff F, Milic-Emili J: Effects of age and body position on "airway closure" in man. J Appl Physiol 28:448–451, 1970
105. Lee RE Jr: The size of suspended particulate matter in air. Science 178: 567–575, 1972
106. Lefcoe NM, Inculet II: Particulates in domestic premises. II. Ambient levels and indoor-outdoor relationships. Arch Environ Health 30:565–570, 1975
107. Lister WB, Wimborne D: Carbon pneumoconiosis in a synthetic graphite worker. Br J Ind Med 29:108–110, 1972
108. Lopez-Merino V, Llopis Lombart R, Flores Marco R, Barbero Carnicero A, Gomez Guillen F, Bouhuys A: Arterial blood gas tensions and lung function during acute responses to hemp dust. Am Rev Respir Dis 107:809–815, 1973
109. Lourenço RV, Klimek MF, Borowski CJ: Deposition and clearance of 2 μ particles in the tracheobronchial tree of normal subjects—smokers and nonsmokers. J Clin Invest 50:1411–1420, 1971
110. Lovejoy FW Jr, Dautrebande L: New studies on aerosols, XX. Effects of cigarette smoke on the airway conductance in smokers and non-smokers.

Arch Int Pharmacodyn Ther 143:258–267, 1963
111. Lunn JE, Knowelden J, Roe JW: Patterns of respiratory illness in Sheffield junior school children: A follow-up study. Br J Prev Soc Med 24:223–228, 1970
112. MacMahon B, Pugh TF: Epidemiology: Principles and Methods. Boston, Little, Brown and Co., 1970
113. Mattson S-B, Ringquist T: Pleural plaques and exposure to asbestos. Scand J Respir Dis (suppl 75): 1–41, 1970
114. McDonald JC, Becklake MR, Fournier-Massey G, Rossiter CE: Respiratory symptoms in chrysotile asbestos mine and mill workers of Quebec. Arch Environ Health 24:358–363, 1972
115. McEwen J, Finlayson A, Mair A: Asbestos and mesothelioma in Scotland. An epidemiological study. Int Arch Arbeitsmed 28:301–311, 1971
116. McKerrow CB, McDermott M, Gilson JC, Schilling RSF: Respiratory function during the day in cotton workers: a study in byssinosis. Br J Ind Med 15:75–83, 1958
117. McMillan RS, Wiseman DH, Hanes B, Wehrle PF: Effects of oxidant air pollution on peak expiratory flow rates in Los Angeles school children. Arch Environ Health 18:941–949, 1969
118. McNall PE Jr: Practical methods of reducing airborne contaminants in interior spaces. Arch Environ Health 30:552–556, 1975
119. Mitchell CA: Loss of pulmonary elastic recoil in workers heavily exposed to proteolytic enzymes in the detergent industry. (Personal communication)
120. Mitchell CA, Schilling RSF, Bouhuys A: Community studies of lung disease in Connecticut: Organization and methods. Am J Epidemiol 103:212–225, 1976
121. Mitchell RS, Maisel JC, Dart GA, Silvers GW: The accuracy of the death certificate in reporting cause of death in adults. Am Rev Respir Dis 104: 844–850, 1971
122. Moore PD: Ozone over Britain. Nature 256:537, 1975
123. Moore VL, Hensley GT, Fink JN: An animal model of hypersensitivity pneumonitis in the rabbit. J Clin Invest 56:937–944, 1975
124. Morgan WKC, Seaton A: Occupational lung diseases. Philadelphia, WB Saunders Co, 1975
125. Morrow PE: An evaluation of recent NO_x toxicity data and an attempt to derive an ambient air standard for NO_x by established toxicological procedures. Environ Res 10:92–112, 1975
126. Morrow PE: Dynamics of dust removal from the lower airways; measurements and interpretations based upon radioactive aerosols, in Bouhuys A (ed): Airway Dynamics; Physiology and Pharmacology. Springfield, Charles C Thomas, 1970, pp 299–312
127. Murphy RLH, Ferris BG Jr, Burgess WA, Worcester J, Gaensler EA: Effects of low concentrations of asbestos. N Engl J Med 285:1271–1278, 1971
128. Murphy RLH Jr, Gaensler EA, Redding RA, Belleau R, Keelan PJ, Smith AA, Goff AM, Ferris BG Jr: Low exposure to asbestos: gas exchange in ship pipe coverers and controls. Arch Environ Health 25:253–264, 1972
129. Nadel JA, Comroe JH Jr: Acute effects of inhalation of cigarette smoke on airway conductance. J Appl Physiol 16:713–716, 1961
130. Nash T, Pattle RE: The absorption of phosgene by aqueous solutions and its relation to toxicity. Ann Occup Hyg 14:227–233, 1971
131. National Air Pollution Control Administration: Air quality criteria for carbon monoxide. Washington, D.C., Environmental Health Service, PHS, US Dept of Health, Education and Welfare, 1970
132. National Air Pollution Control Administration: Air quality criteria for photochemical oxidants. Washington, D.C., Environmental Health Service, PHS, US Dept of Health, Education and Welfare, 1970
133. de Nevers N: Enforcing the Clean Air Act of 1970. Sci Am 228:14–21, 1973
134. Newhouse ML, Tagg B, Pocock SJ, McEwan AC: An epidemiological study of workers producing enzyme washing powders. Lancet 1:689–693, 1970
135. Nicholls PJ, Nicholls GR, Bouhuys A: Histamine release by compound 48/80 and textile dusts from lung tissue in vitro, in Davies CN (ed): Inhaled Particles and Vapours, II. London, Pergamon, 1966, pp 69–74

136. Nieding G von, Krekeler H: Pharmakologische Beeinflussung der akuten NO_2-Wirkung auf die Lungenfunktion von Gesunden und Kranken mit einer chronischen Bronchitis. Int Arch Arbeitsmed 29:55–63, 1971
137. Niewoehner DE, Kleinerman J, Rice DB: Pathologic changes in the peripheral airways of young cigarette smokers. N Engl J Med 291:755–758, 1974
138. Occupational Characteristics of Disabled Workers, by Disabling Condition: Disability Insurance Benefit Awards Made in 1959 to 1962 to Men under Age 65. Publication No. 1531, US Dept of Health, Education and Welfare, 1967
139. Okulicz WC: Lung biogenic amines and pulmonary edema in ozone exposed rats, mice, and guinea pigs. MPH thesis, New Haven, Yale University, 1971
140. Patty FA (ed): Industrial hygiene and toxicology, in Fassett DW, Irish DD (eds): Toxicology, ed 2, vol II. New York, Interscience Publishers, 1963
141. Pavia D, Thomson ML, Pocock SJ: Evidence for temporary slowing of mucociliary clearance in the lung caused by tobacco smoking. Nature 231:325–326, 1971
142. Peters JM, Ferris BG Jr: Smoking, pulmonary function, and respiratory symptoms in a college age group. Am Rev Respir Dis 95:774–782, 1967
143. Peters JM, Murphy RLH, Pagnotto LD, van Ganse WF: Acute respiratory effects in workers exposed to low levels of toluene diisocyanate (TDI). Arch Environ Health 16:642–647, 1968
144. Pooley FD: Electron microscope characteristics of inhaled chrysotile asbestos fibre. Br J Ind Med 29:146–153, 1972
145. Potter WA, Olafsson S, Hyatt RE: Ventilatory mechanics and expiratory flow limitation during exercise in patients with obstructive lung disease. J Clin Invest 50:910–919, 1971
146. Ramazzini B: De Morbis Artificum Diatriba. Wright WC (ed). Chicago, University of Chicago Press, 1940
147. Redding RA, Hardy HL, Gaensler EA: Beryllium disease: a 16-year follow-up case study. Respiration 25:263–278, 1968
148. Report of the Advisory Committee on Asbestos Cancers to the Director of the International Agency for Research on Cancer. Br J Ind Med 30:180–186, 1973
149. Rode A, Shephard RJ: The influence of cigarette smoking upon the oxygen cost of breathing in near-maximal exercise. Med Sci Sports 3:51–55, 1971
150. Rossiter CE, Bristol LJ, Cartier PH, Gilson JC, Grainger TR, Sluis-Cremer GK, McDonald JC: Radiographic changes in chrysotile asbestos mine and millworkers of Quebec. Arch Environ Health 24:388–400, 1972
151. Russell MAH, Cole PV, Brown E: Absorption by non-smokers of carbon monoxide from room air polluted by tobacco smoke. Lancet 1:576–579, 1973
152. Salber EJ: Smoking among teen-agers. Bull NY Acad Med 44:1521–1525, 1968
153. Schilling RSF: Byssinosis in cotton and other textile workers. Lancet 2: 261–265, 319–325, 1956
154. Schilling RSF (ed): Occupational Health Practice. London, Butterworths, 1973
155. Seely JE, Zuskin E, Bouhuys A: Cigarette smoking: Objective evidence for lung damage in teen-agers. Science 172:741–743, 1971
156. Segal MS, Weiss EB (eds): Bronchial Asthma; Chap 29, Experimental asthma in man and in animals, by A Bouhuys. Boston, Little, Brown and Co, 1976
157. Selikoff IJ, Churg J, Hammond EC: Asbestos exposure and neoplasia. JAMA 188:22–26, 1964
158. Selikoff IJ, Churg J, Hammond EC: The occurrence of asbestosis among insulation workers in the United States. Ann NY Acad Sci 132:139–155, 1965
159. Selikoff IJ, Key MM, Lee DHK (eds): Coal workers' pneumoconiosis. Ann NY Acad Sci 200:1–861, 1972
160. Selikoff IJ, Nicholson WJ, Langer AM: Asbestos air pollution. Arch Environ Health 25:1–13, 1972
161. Shapley D: Auto pollution: EPA worrying that the catalyst may backfire. Science 182:368–371, 1973
162. Snell RE, Luchsinger PC: Effects of sulfur dioxide on expiratory flow rates and total respiratory resistance in normal human subjects. Arch Environ Health 18:693–698, 1969
163. Spencer H: Pathology of the Lung, ed 2. Oxford, Pergamon Press, 1968
164. Standard for exposure to asbestos dust.

Title 29: Labor, Part 1910, Occupational Safety and Health Standards. Fed Regis 37:11318–11322, 1972
165. Standards for epidemiologic surveys in chronic respiratory disease. National Tuberculosis & Respiratory Disease Association, 1969
166. Staub NC: Pulmonary edema. Physiol Rev 54:678–809, 1974
167. Stell PM, McGill T: Asbestos and laryngeal carcinoma. Lancet 2:416–417, 1973
168. Stephens RJ, Freeman G, Evans MJ: Early response of lungs to low levels of nitrogen dioxide. Arch Environ Health 24:160–179, 1972
169. Stern A (ed): Air Pollution, vol I (2 ed): Air Pollution and Its Effects. New York, Academic Press, 1968
170. Stokinger HE: Toxicity of airborne chemicals: Air quality standards—A national and international view. Annu Rev Pharmacol 12:407–422, 1972
171. Strieder DJ, Kazemi H: Hypoxemia in young asymptomatic cigarette smokers. Ann Thorac Surg 4:523–531, 1967
172. Stumphius J: Epidemiology of mesothelioma on Walcheren Island. Br J Ind Med 28:59–66, 1971
173. Talamo RC, Allen JD, Kahan MG, Austen KF: Hereditary $alpha_1$-antitrypsin deficiency. N Engl J Med 278: 345–351, 1968
174. Timbrell V: Inhalation and biological effects of asbestos, in Mercer TT, Morrow PE, Stöber W (eds): Assessment of Airborne Particles. Springfield, Charles C Thomas, 1972, pp 429–445
175. US Public Health Service: Smoking and Health. Report of the Advisory Committee to the Surgeon General of the Public Health Service. Washington, D.C., US Dept of Health, Education and Welfare, PHS publication no 1103, 1964
176. US Public Health Service: The Health Consequences of Smoking, A Report of the Surgeon General: 1972. Washington, D.C., US Dept of Health, Education and Welfare, DHEW no (HSM) 72–7516, 1972
177. Valić F, Zuskin E: Effects of different vegetable dust exposures. Br J Ind Med 29:293–297, 1972
178. Wagoner JK, Archer VE, Lundin FE Jr, Holaday DA, Lloyd JW: Radiation as the cause of lung cancer among uranium miners. N Engl J Med 273: 181–188, 1965
179. Waller RE, Commins BT, Lawther PJ: Air pollution in a city street. Br J Ind Med 22:128–138, 1965
180. Weibel ER: Oxygen effect on lung cells. Arch Intern Med 128:54–56, 1971
181. Welch RM, Loh A, Conney AH: Cigarette smoke: Stimulatory effect on metabolism of 3,4-benzpyrene by enzymes in rat lung. Life Sci [I] 10:215–221, 1971
182. Widdicombe JG: Respiratory reflexes, in Fenn WO, Rahn H (eds): Handbook of Physiology, Section 3: Respiration, vol. I. Washington, D.C., American Physiological Society, 1964, pp 585–630
183. Williams RD, Acton JD, Myrvik QN: Influence of nitrogen dioxide on the uptake of parainfluenza-3 virus by alveolar macrophages. J Reticuloendothel Soc 11:627–636, 1972
184. World Health Organization: Health hazards of the human environment. Geneva, 1972
185. Yocom JE, Clink WL, Cote WA: Indoor-outdoor air quality relationships. J Air Pollut Control Assoc 21:251–259, 1971
186. Young WA, Shaw DB, Bates DV: Effect of low concentrations of ozone on pulmonary function in man. J Appl Physiol 19:765–768, 1964
187. Zuskin E, Bouhuys A: Acute airway responses to hairspray preparations. N Engl J Med 290:660–663, 1974
188. Zuskin E, Bouhuys A: Byssinosis: airway responses in textile dust exposure. J Occup Med 17:357–359, 1975
189. Zuskin E, Bouhuys A: Protective effect of disodium cromoglycate against airway constriction induced by hemp dust extract. J Allergy Clin Immunol 57:925–940, 1976
190. Zuskin E, Lewis AJ, Bouhuys A: Inhibition of histamine-induced airway constriction by ascorbic acid. J Allergy Clin Immunol 51:218–226, 1973
191. Zuskin E, Mitchell CA, Bouhuys A: Interaction between effects of beta blockade and cigarette smoke on airways. J Appl Physiol 36:449–452, 1974
192. Zuskin E, Wolfson RL, Harpel G, Welborn JW, Bouhuys A: Byssinosis in carding and spinning workers. Arch Environ Health 19:666–673, 1969

Index

a
b
c
d
7 e
8 f
9 g
0 h
1 i
8 2 j